Clinical Massage Therapy
A Structural Approach to Pain Management

Clinical Massage Therapy

A Structural Approach
to Pain Management

JAMES WASLASKI, AA, LMT, CPT

PEARSON

Boston   Columbus   Indianapolis   New York   San Francisco   Upper Saddle River

Amsterdam   Cape Town   Dubai   London   Madrid   Milan   Munich   Paris   Montreal   Toronto

Delhi   Mexico City   Sao Paulo   Sydney   Hong Kong   Seoul   Singapore   Taipei   Tokyo

Publisher: Julie Levin Alexander
Editor-in-Chief: Mark Cohen
Executive Editor: John Goucher
Assistant Editor: Nicole Ragonese
Editorial Assistant: Rosalie Hawley
Director of Marketing: David Gesell
Executive Marketing Manager: Katrin Beacom
Marketing Specialist: Michael Sirinides
Managing Production Editor: Patrick Walsh
Production Project Manager: Christina Zingone
Operations Specialist: Alan Fischer

Design Director: Jayne Conte
Art Director: Karen Salzbach
Media Editor: Amy Peltier
Media Project Manager: Lorena Cerisano
Media Coordinator: Ellen Martino
Full-Service Project Management: Rebecca Lazure
Illustrator: Body Scientific International
Photographer: Kristen Oliver
Composition: Laserwords Maine
Printer/Binder: Courier/Kendallville
Cover Printer: Lehigh-Phoenix Color/Hagerstown

Notice: The authors and the publisher of this volume have taken care that the information and technical recommendations contained herein are based on research and expert consultation, and are accurate and compatible with the standards generally accepted at the time of publication. Nevertheless, as new information becomes available, changes in clinical and technical practices become necessary. The reader is advised to carefully consult manufacturers' instructions and information material for all supplies and equipment before use, and to consult with a health care professional as necessary. This advice is especially important when using new supplies or equipment for clinical purposes. The authors and publisher disclaim all responsibility for any liability, loss, injury, or damage incurred as a consequence, directly or indirectly, of the use and application of any of the contents of this volume.

Credits: Chapter Outline: oleg66/iStockphoto.com; Case Study: crystalfoto/shutterstock; Precautionary Note: Oleksii Natykach/shutterstock; Learning Objectives: crolique/shutterstock; Expert Opinion: LoopAll/shutterstock.

Library of Congress Cataloging-in-Publication Data
Waslaski, James.
    Clinical massage therapy : a structural approach to pain management / James Waslaski.
        p. ; cm.
    ISBN-13: 978-0-13-706362-8
    ISBN-10: 0-13-706362-8
    1. Massage therapy.   2. Sports injuries—Treatment.   3. Pain--Treatment.
I. Title.
    [DNLM: 1. Massage—methods.   2. Athletic injuries—therapy.   3. Musculoskeletal Diseases—therapy.   4. Pain—therapy. WB 537]
        RM721.W297 2012
        615.8'22—dc23   2011019557

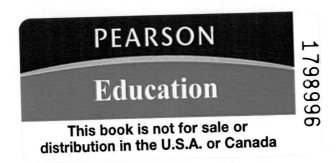

This book is not for sale or distribution in the U.S.A. or Canada

1798996

10 9 8 7 6 5 4 3 2 1

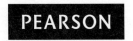

www.pearsonhighered.com

ISBN-13: 978-0-13-706362-8
ISBN-10:   0-13-706362-8

Dedication

I would like to dedicate this book to my mother, June Waslaski. On November 20, 2010, she lost her battle to cancer. About two months before her death, she was able to attend the AMTA National Massage Convention to meet the many loving people in this great profession. All I have become, and all that I will continue to achieve in this life, is due to the unselfish and unconditional love of my beautiful mother, June. Throughout her life she taught me the importance of honesty, integrity, unconditional love, and putting God and people first. Her last words to me when we said goodbye were "I will be with you in the sky, as you continue your travels to fulfill God's plan by helping others facilitate healing throughout the world." I love you, Mom. Your beautiful spirit will live on through this incredible work. Thanks for shaping my destiny.

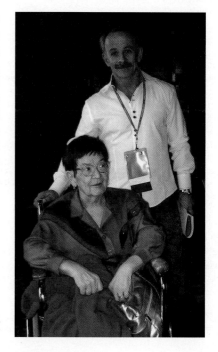

June Waslaski
June 13, 1935–November 20, 2010

Brief Contents

Foreword   ix

Preface   xi

Acknowledgments   xv

About the Author   xvii

About the Illustrators   xix

Reviewers   xxi

Chapter 1   The Twelve-Step Approach: Assessment, Treatment, and Client Self-Care   2

Chapter 2   Pelvic Stabilization—The Key to Structural Integration   38

Chapter 3   Knee and Thigh Conditions   84

Chapter 4   Lower Leg, Ankle, and Foot Conditions   116

Chapter 5   Shoulder Conditions   146

Chapter 6   Cervical Spine Conditions   202

Chapter 7   Elbow, Forearm, Wrist, and Hand Conditions   234

Appendix A   End-of-Chapter Questions—Answer Key   263

Appendix B   Notes   265

Appendix C   Suggested Readings   269

Glossary   271

Index   275

Foreword

It was at the 1998 Boston New England Conference where I first had the pleasure of meeting James Waslaski. We literally "bumped" into one another as I wandered around the hotel lobby searching for a familiar face. Although I'd been involved in bodywork (Rolfing) for many years, I'd not attended a massage conference and James, sensing my insecurity, immediately put me at ease with his kind, playful, and teasing spirit. Although much water has passed under the bridge since those early convention days, many special remembrances live on. By far, my fondest memories were of our weeklong co-teaching events in Costa Rica (Pain Management in Paradise) and James's very popular "Seminars at Sea" cruises.

There's nothing quite like the physical, emotional, and intellectual bonds that form when you have the opportunity to eat, live, and learn together for a week. From the first day of our initial co-teaching gig, we knew—and the class knew—this would not be your typical workshop. A stimulating, fun-filled, and unpredictable magic filled the air. As I observed James during his presentations, it was like watching an accomplished athlete perform his sport. With almost effortless motion, the athlete, like the master practitioner, is so good at what he does, has practiced it so many times, that it seems almost effortless. But we all know better.

Passion for the work drives some, like James Waslaski, to generously share their lifelong collection of touch therapy experiences and I'm delighted he has accomplished this in his meticulously written and handsomely illustrated textbook *Clinical Massage Therapy: A Structural Approach to Pain Management.* Although *Clinical Massage Therapy* requires extensive study in therapeutic assessment, manipulation, and restoration of movement, the book's goal is to teach practicing somatic therapists a straightforward, pain-free treatment protocol for reducing pain and correcting dysfunction. Thousands of manual therapists have learned this popular multidisciplinary method over the years and the results speak for themselves. It has been said that pain management may be recession-proof. If so, this text is a "must have" for every practitioner's collection.

As you delve into *Clinical Massage Therapy,* James will lead you on a step-by-step journey that ends by establishing structural and functional balance for a wide variety of musculoskeletal disorders, chronic pain conditions, and sports injuries. You will learn practical ways to filter the results of a client's history, palpatory findings, and functional tests through a philosophic lens based on basic science and clinical reasoning. Throughout the book, James emphasizes how impaired or altered functioning of the neuromuscular system leads to stress and pain that impedes optimal athletic performance and enjoyment of daily activities.

Many of us know James as a very generous, hardworking, and giving educator who's dedicated his life to helping therapists elevate their somatic skills while encouraging them to have fun, be vulnerable, and to appreciate the knowledge this great profession has to offer. This is accomplished through attitude—the way we treat people who come to us for pain management. Therapeutic touch establishes and maintains the confidence, trust, and healing relationship required to make technique effective. *Clinical Massage Therapy* is human contact at its best and James delivers human contact and all it offers for a better healing relationship and a better world.

Erik Dalton, PhD
Author of *Advanced Myoskeletal Techniques*
and Dynamic Body and Founder of the Freedom From Pain Institute

Preface

Clinical Massage Therapy: A Structural Approach to Pain Management was written to help take today's clinical massage therapist to the next level by eliminating most forms of complicated musculoskeletal pain patterns due to repetitive stress and sports injuries.

Based on current scientific research and clinical studies, this text is designed to provide manual therapy students and practitioners with a set of therapeutic techniques that can prevent or eliminate multifaceted pain conditions. From this foundation, readers will learn and be able to apply an effective range of therapeutic approaches for evaluating and treating clients with chronic pain, sports injuries, and structural imbalances. The book's multimodal and multidisciplinary approach enhances skills and training practices for a variety of health care professionals including physical and occupational therapists, athletic trainers, personal trainers, strength and conditioning coaches, chiropractors, osteopaths, nurses, manipulative therapists, and physicians.

This text seeks to bridge all manual therapy disciplines through a unique twelve-step approach based on soft-tissue and structural balancing, and can be integrated as a new model for most manual therapy training programs. The ultimate goal is to inform, inspire, and guide current and upcoming manual therapy practitioners toward the astounding potential available in today's pain management and performance enhancement therapies.

APPROACH: STRUCTURAL BALANCE AND CORE STABILIZATION

This book involves a different concept of treatment for chronic pain than is currently used by most clinical massage therapists. The use of a physical therapy approach allows today's practitioner to consistently monitor and evaluate treatment progress, via client movement evaluation and special orthopedic tests. In this context, clients feel most comfortable wearing shorts and a sports top or swimsuit. However, proper draping techniques are always demonstrated for the benefit of those therapists working in a spa setting.

Please be advised that the twelve-step approach presented in this book does not follow a formula and should not be considered a "cookbook" approach to manual therapy. Rather, it is a unique system that helps you quickly identify the "key" areas of pain and dysfunction so that appropriate treatment

techniques can be matched to the underlying pathology. The work must always be performed pain-free. Consistent attention is given to restoring musculoskeletal balance by correcting structural asymmetries prior to treating each individual clinical symptom.

Overall, the recommended treatment sequence in this book is to restore balance to opposing muscle groups throughout the body. This is accomplished by first lengthening short, tight muscle groups and then tonifying the opposing weak, inhibited tissues. The most effective treatment protocol begins by addressing myofascial tension, tight muscle bands, muscle belly trigger points, scar tissue, joint capsule adhesions, and finally the resulting joint pain. Tight muscle bands can be teased apart with gentle cross-fiber gliding strokes, while trigger points are addressed by direct, moderate pressure, with all work performed pain-free. Please note that it is in the client's best interest to avoid using the word *pain* in the therapeutic setting because it may trigger a negative nervous system response.

This book's approach to scar tissue also sets it apart from more conventional treatment methods, which typically recommend deep cross-fiber friction, in one direction only, to realign the scar tissue's injured or disorganized muscle fibers. However, an examination of collagen formed after an injury reveals the potential problem with this approach. Scar tissue at the injury site consists of a fiberglass-like matrix of collagen fibers oriented in multiple directions and multiple layers, causing pain and limiting the client's range of motion. A much more effective technique is to use multidirectional friction to mobilize the scar tissue, followed by pain-free movement, pain-free eccentric muscle contractions, and pain-free stretching or pain-free strengthening to restore normal muscle resting lengths throughout the body. Unlike simple cross-fiber friction, the multidirectional forces focus on softening the thickest fibers in the collagen matrix, superficial to deep, so the pain-free movement and eccentric muscle contractions can facilitate functional and more aligned scar tissue. This unique strategy makes it possible for the area of scar tissue to remain smooth to palpation after treatment and enables the client to remain pain-free.

It is believed that no single modality is the answer for treating all conditions. Rather, it is the synergy of many modalities and disciplines integrated together that allows the therapist to treat each client in a truly individualized manner. This book offers such an approach.

ORGANIZATION AND STRUCTURE

This text introduces a variety of rehabilitation disciplines and massage modalities to treat specific clinical pathologies. *The goal is to organize complex therapeutic pain management concepts into user-friendly and understandable modalities to quickly evaluate, test, and treat commonly seen pain syndromes.*

The treatment principles outlined in the first chapter establish the foundation for treating specific clinical conditions according to body region:

Chapter 1 explains the twelve-step assessment, treatment, and self-care approach and each step's application. It includes a full body map illustrating structural balance and alignment of the body. As you reference the body map and apply the twelve steps throughout the book, a consistent pattern will emerge: assessment, treatment, and client self-care which, when combined, can be used to treat a wide range of conditions.

Chapters 2 through 7 are organized by body region:

- Chapter 2 provides in-depth coverage of pelvic stabilization, a unique core structural balancing approach to pain management. You will learn how to balance the major muscle groups to facilitate myoskeletal alignment of the pelvis, sacrum, and lumbar spine.
- Chapter 3 addresses knee and thigh problems such as iliotibial band friction syndrome, chondromalacia, hamstring strains, patellar tendinosis, medial and lateral collateral ligament sprains, and meniscus injuries.
- Chapter 4 focuses on lower leg, ankle, and foot dysfunctions. Conditions such as Achilles tendinosis, shin pain, anterior compartment syndrome, ankle sprains, and plantar fascial pain are covered.
- Chapter 5 is dedicated to commonly seen thoracic and shoulder problems. Rotator cuff injuries, thoracic outlet, shoulder impingement, and frozen shoulder are among the many conditions discussed.
- Chapter 6 focuses on cervical spine conditions such as whiplash, atlas–axis mobilization, lateral shearing forces, facet joint dysfunction, nerve entrapment, cervical sprains and strains, limited range of motion, and migraine headaches.
- Chapter 7 addresses elbow, forearm, wrist, and hand problems, including elbow tendinosis, carpal tunnel syndrome, joint arthritis, and much more.

FEATURES

The following features appear throughout the text to enhance the understanding of the basic principles and how to apply them.

- **Anatomical Artwork:** The most exciting feature of this text is the detailed anatomical artwork using photographic overlays. Designed to precisely illustrate the true underlying pathology of each and every condition, special state-of-the-art effects are used liberally. This groundbreaking artwork allows you to see exactly

what muscles or structures should be worked on, and in precisely what order.
- **Twelve-Step Flow Chart:** A distinguishing feature of the *Clinical Massage Therapy* textbook is the inclusion in Chapter 1 of a twelve-step flow chart. This helpful tool clearly explains the goals not only of each step but also for each client condition.

As an additional learning tool, the chapters explain the structures involved in common clinical conditions such as adhesive capsulitis, thoracic outlet, whiplash, carpal tunnel syndrome, among others. Although massage therapists are not allowed to diagnose, it is important to understand diagnostic terms in order to better apply assessment and treatment skills. That way, specific massage modalities, or manual therapy disciplines, can better address the cause of each diagnosis identified by the client's primary health care provider. Commonly diagnosed conditions are explained, along with a corresponding "path" for identifying the necessary steps to best address each clinical condition.

- **Learning Objectives:** Performance-driven objectives that serve as a checklist of skills you will learn as you work through the chapter.
- **Body Map:** Illustrates the relationships among the different body parts and highlights the core muscles involved, the names of those muscles, and the conditions to be discussed. A full body map appears in Chapter 1, and each body region chapter includes a map that focuses on that specific region.
- **Directional Arrows:** Color coded arrows illustrate client and therapist movements. Arrows are blue to indicate movement by the therapist, and yellow to indicate movement by the client, to aid in understanding certain techniques.
- **Expert Opinion:** A boxed feature inserted throughout the text consisting of input and suggestions, in narrative format, of various approaches and techniques from leading pain management experts.
- **Precautionary Note:** Boxed alerts telling the therapist what *not* to do if a client has a certain condition.
- **Body Mechanics:** Instructions on proper body mechanics are demonstrated and discussed in Chapter 1 to minimize energy required, optimize technique outcomes, and prevent injuries to the clinical massage therapist.
- **Video Clips:** Professionally edited video clips are included at www.myhealthprofessionskit.com, with precise demonstrations of some of the key techniques. Within a window of various video clips, there are real dissections inserted to clearly highlight what is happening inside the body during each technique.
- **Case Studies:** Actual client stories that illustrate conditions resulting from everyday activities and how the twelve-step approach is used to create pain-free movement and optimal performance.
- **Review Questions:** Appear at the end of each chapter. The questions will help reinforce key points in the chapter, and will serve as preparation for a certification exam.

- **Glossary:** Appears at the end of the book and defines all of the key terms.

It is vital to understand why the book is titled *Clinical Massage Therapy* rather than *Medical Massage Therapy*. The field of medical massage should include all massage-related disciplines that have a positive effect on pain or disease in the body. There are many such complementary massage-related disciplines: posturology, functional assessment, neuromuscular therapy, lymphatic drainage, craniosacral therapy, myoskeletal alignment, visceral manipulation, orthopedic massage, myofascial release, structural integration, Trager energy work, active isolated stretching, and many other disciplines.

The name *Clinical Massage Therapy* was chosen to reflect the author's interest in all components of the neuromuscular system. The intent of this manual therapy method is to assess and correct systemwide structural and functional imbalances, and to enhance athletic performance. The causes and contributing factors involved in myoskeletal pain are always addressed prior to treating and eliminating the client's symptoms. This systems approach has evolved from many years of experience in health-related fields such as emergency medicine, sports massage, personal training, and orthopedic massage. Thus, *clinical massage therapy,* much like *medical massage,* can be considered an umbrella term that includes a variety of restorative and enhancement-based manual therapy techniques to correct a wide range of client complaints.

In his worldwide travels teaching this work, the author has been blessed to facilitate in healing hundreds of people who were previously given no hope for pain-free living. In many cases, their recovery has created a domino effect, enhancing not only the quality of their own life but also that of their family and friends. It is sincerely hoped the information shared in this book serves to expand that domino effect of facilitating healing in individuals suffering from complicated pain conditions worldwide.

Acknowledgments

This book would never have been possible without the many years of hard work by Sheri Wells. Sheri started taking notes in many of my seminars about ten years ago. After years of assisting my seminars, and hundreds of revisions in what became our *Orthopedic Massage Manual,* along with countless hours of editing text and photographs, the hard work of Sheri Wells became the manuscript of this book. Sheri has also spent many years guiding me through the difficult challenges of the entire book. Words cannot express my eternal gratitude for her role in this textbook. I would also like to thank my teaching assistant Michelle Mokracek from New Jersey for making a phone call to George Werner, Executive Vice President Operations at Pearson Education. That call was certainly a defining moment in the publication of this book. My heartfelt thanks also goes out to the over 200 teaching assistants, throughout the world, that assist me at each seminar in sharing this work. Their invaluable input has certainly been pivotal in refining the work in this book, and their friendships will last forever.

I would also like to give special thanks to John Goucher for believing in my ability as an author while he was still with Lippincott, Williams, and Wilkins, prior to getting involved with this book at Pearson. A special thanks also goes out to Mark Cohen for working with me to get this book accepted by Pearson.

The magic of this textbook happens with the staff at Pearson. The hard work and guidance by Nicole Ragonese and John Goucher kept me accountable, better organized, educated, and on track. The difficult task in the critical editing and review process would not have been possible without all the help from Rebecca Lazure, our awesome project manager. The incredible photography and artwork were the magic of Marcelo Oliver and Body Scientific International, and his lovely wife Kristen and Kristen Oliver Photography.

I wish to thank ATI Enterprises, and in particular the ATI North Richland Hills, TX, for hosting the photo shoot. The following ATI individuals were particularly helpful in ensuring the shoot went smoothly: Deidra Bennett, Shelli Davis-Redford, Brandon Dowdy, and Carol Rogers.

My seven-year journey in writing this textbook would never have been completed without the constant encouragement and valuable contributions from my wife, Fran, and great friend, Erik Dalton. Their organization and encouragement, during the many times I began to doubt myself, were pivotal in seeing this project to completion. In addition to being a wife and mother, my beautiful wife Fran was the model throughout the book. She encouraged me to pray more each time I felt overwhelmed. Erik Dalton consulted with me on a great portion of this book, but most importantly he called me almost weekly to check in and encourage me. He is indeed a true and unconditional eternal friend. Special thanks also goes to my office manager Allison Treta, for running our company, which places me at about 42 seminars per year around the world, so I could focus on this book, product development, and teaching seminars. Thanks also to my beautiful daughter Alex for constantly reminding me to slow down and enjoy life's journey.

I would also like to thank my minister, Pastor Paul Cole, for being my counselor when the heat was turned up by my reviewers and other industry leaders to make me accountable for the protocols and techniques presented in this book.

Finally, I would like to thank all of the industry leaders and colleagues who taught me this work, and the thousands of students throughout the world who helped me refine my work through their challenging questions and honest feedback.

Most importantly, I want to thank God for giving me a passion and spiritual purpose to share this work throughout the world. I now know that my purpose on this earth is to share the work of my great teachers and mentors, to facilitate healing in patients who may have lost hope for living without pain. Through this book, my vision is that thousands of manual therapists will be better prepared to improve the quality of life of their clients.

About the Author

James Waslaski teaches approximately 40 seminars per year around the globe. He has served as the American Massage Therapy Association (AMTA) sports massage chair and the Florida State Massage Therapy Association (FSMTA) professional relations chair. He developed a series of orthopedic massage and sports injuries DVDs and has authored manuals on advanced orthopedic massage, advancements in event and clinical sports massage, and client self-care. James worked at the 1996 Olympic Games and taught sports massage at the Olympic training center in Melbourne Australia, just prior to the 2000 Olympic Games in Sydney. James has worked with the New York Yankees and frequently consults with athletic trainers and massage therapists working for top professional sport teams throughout the world.

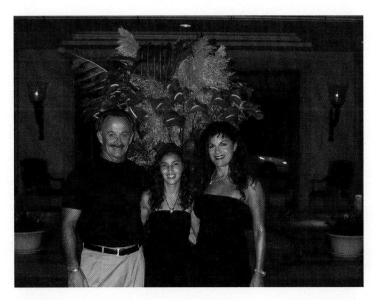

Waslaski presents at state, national, and international massage, chiropractic, and osteopathic conventions including key note addresses at the FSMTA, World of Wellness, New England Regional Conference, Irish National Massage Convention, Scottish National Massage Convention, and the Australian National Massage Convention. His audience includes massage and physical therapists as well as athletic trainers, chiropractors, osteopaths, nurses, physicians, occupational therapists, physiotherapists, and high-end sports and athletic trainers.

James is the President of The Center for Pain Management, and lives in Colleyville, Texas with his wife Fran and stepdaughter Alex. Waslaski is a certified personal trainer with the National Academy of Sports Medicine (NASM). He received the 1999 FSMTA International Achievement Award and was inducted in 2009 into the Massage Therapy Hall of Fame. Visit www.orthomassage.net for additional information.

About the Illustrators

Marcelo Oliver is President and founder of Body Scientific International, LLC. He holds a masters degree in Medical and Biological Illustration from the University of Michigan. For the past 20 years, his passion has been to condense complex anatomical information into visual education tools for students, patients and medical professionals. Body Scientific's contributing artists in this publication were Marcelo Oliver (art director), Carol Hrejsa (medical illustrator) and Kristen Oliver (professional photographer). Their contribution in the publication was key in the creation and editing of the artwork. Body Scientific invites you to visit their websites at www.bodyscientific.com and kristenoliverphotography.com.

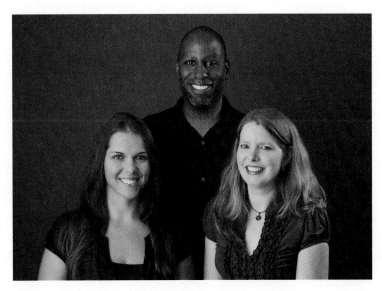

Reviewers

Elizabeth Aerts, BS, MBA, NCTMB
Formerly of The School of Integrative Therapies
Holmdel, New Jersey

Adrienne F. Asta, NCTMB, BA
Cortiva Institute—Somerset School of Massage Therapy
Wall, New Jersey

Patty Berak, NCBTMB, BHSA, CHt, MBA
Baker College of Clinton Township
Clinton Township, Michigan

Gabrielle J. Ham-Jones, BS, CMT
Massage Institute of Maryland
Catonsville, Maryland

Steven D. Koehler, ND, BS, AAS, LMBT
Carteret Community College
Morehead City, North Carolina

Lisa Melendez, LMT, NCTMB
South Carolina Massage and Esthetics Institute
Myrtle Beach, South Carolina

Jennifer O'Connell, LMT
Abaton Center of Healing Arts
Albuquerque, New Mexico

Roger Olbrot
Myotherapy College of Utah
Salt Lake City, Utah

Suzanne Shonbrun, BA
California Institute of Massage & Spa Services
Sonoma, California

Victoria J. Stone, MA, NCMT
Blue Ridge School of Massage & Yoga
Blacksburg, Virginia

Contents

Foreword   ix

Preface   xi

Acknowledgments   xv

About the Author   xvii

About the Illustrators   xix

Reviewers   xxi

Chapter 1   The Twelve-Step Approach: Assessment, Treatment, and Client Self-Care   2

Twelve Steps to Pain Management   5
Definitions   7
Step 1: Client History   7
Step 2: Assess Active Range of Motion (AROM)   7
Step 3: Assess Passive Range of Motion (PROM)   14
Step 4: Assess Resisted Range of Motion (RROM)   15
Steps 5–12: Path to Pain-Free Movement   15
Step 5: Area Preparation   18
Step 6: Myofascial Release   19
Step 7: Cross-Fiber Gliding Strokes/Trigger Point Therapy   20
Step 8: Multidirectional Friction   23
Step 9: Pain-Free Movement   25
Step 10: Eccentric Scar Tissue Alignment   25
Step 11: Stretching (During Therapy/Client Self-Care)   26
Step 12: Strengthening (Client Self-Care)   28
Origins of the Twelve-Step Approach   29
Tendinosis Techniques and Scar Tissue Mobilization   29
Tendinosis Techniques   29
Scar Tissue Mobilization   30
A New Hypothesis   31
Case Study   32
Draping   35
Chapter Summary   37
Review Questions   37

Chapter 2   Pelvic Stabilization—The Key to Structural Integration   38

Twelve-Step Approach to Pelvic Stabilization   40
Degenerative Disc Disease   40
Bulging Discs and Herniated Discs   40
Osteophytes   40
Step 1: Client History   41
Step 2: Assess Active Range of Motion (AROM)   41

Step 3: Assess Passive Range of Motion (PROM)   43
Step 4: Assess Resisted Range of Motion (RROM)   43
Psoas Major, Iliacus (Iliopsoas), and Joint Capsule   43
Step 2: Assess Active Range of Motion (AROM)   44
Step 3: Assess Passive Range of Motion (PROM)   44
Step 11: Stretching (During Therapy)   48
Step 2: Assess Active Range of Motion (AROM)   50
Quadratus Lumborum (QL) and Erector Spinae   50
Step 3: Assess Passive Range of Motion (PROM)   50
Step 6: Myofascial Release   52
Step 7: Trigger Point Therapy   52
Step 6: Myofascial Release   52
Step 11: Stretching (During Therapy)   53
Step 8: Multidirectional Friction   53
Step 9: Pain-Free Movement   54
Step 10: Eccentric Scar Tissue Alignment   54
Step 4: Assess Resisted Range of Motion (RROM)   55
Step 6: Myofascial Release   55
Step 3: Assess Passive Range of Motion (PROM)   56
Lateral Hip Rotators or Medial Hip Rotators and Adductors   56
Step 3: Assess Passive Range of Motion (PROM) for Lateral Hip Rotation   56
Step 3: Assess Passive Range of Motion (PROM) for Medial Hip Rotation   58
Lateral Hip Rotator Protocol   59
Step 4: Assess Resisted Range of Motion (RROM)   59
Step 6: Myofascial Release   59
Step 7: Cross-Fiber Gliding Strokes/Trigger Point Therapy   60
Step 6: Myofascial Release   60
Step 11: Stretching (During Therapy)   60
Step 8: Multidirectional Friction   62
Step 9: Pain-Free Movement   62
Step 10: Eccentric Scar Tissue Alignment   62
Step 4: Assess Resisted Range of Motion (RROM)   62
Step 3: Assess Passive Range of Motion (PROM)   63
Medial Hip Rotators and Adductors   63
Step 4: Assess Medial Hip Rotation Resisted Range of Motion (RROM)   63
Step 3: Assess Adductor Passive Range of Motion (PROM)   63
Step 4: Assess Adductor Resisted Range of Motion (RROM)   63
Step 6: Myofascial Release   63
Step 7: Trigger Point Therapy   65

Step 11: Stretching Adductors (During Therapy) 65

Step 11: Stretching Medial Hip Rotators (During Therapy) 65

Step 8: Multidirectional Friction 66

Step 9: Pain-Free Movement 66

Step 10: Eccentric Scar Tissue Alignment 66

Step 4: Assess Resisted Range of Motion (RROM) 66

Step 3: Assess Passive Range of Motion (PROM) 66

Quadriceps and Iliotibial Band (ITB) 66

Quadriceps 67

Step 3: Assess Passive Range of Motion (PROM) 67

Step 4: Assess Resisted Range of Motion (RROM) 67

Step 6: Myofascial Release 68

Step 7: Cross-Fiber Gliding Strokes/Trigger Point Therapy 68

Iliotibial Band (ITB) 69

Step 6: Myofascial Release 69

Step 7: Cross-Fiber Gliding Strokes/Trigger Point Therapy 69

Step 11: Stretching (During Therapy) 70

Step 8: Multidirectional Friction 70

Step 9: Pain-Free Movement 71

Step 10: Eccentric Scar Tissue Alignment 71

Quadriceps 71

Step 11: Stretching (During Therapy) 71

Step 8: Multidirectional Friction 72

Step 9: Pain-Free Movement 72

Step 10: Eccentric Scar Tissue Alignment 72

Step 4: Assess Resisted Range of Motion (RROM) 72

Step 3: Assess Passive Range of Motion (PROM) 72

Hamstrings 72

Step 2: Assess Active Range of Motion (AROM) 72

Step 3: Assess Passive Range of Motion (PROM) 72

Step 4: Assess Resisted Range of Motion (RROM) 72

Step 6: Myofascial Release 73

Step 7: Cross-Fiber Gliding Strokes/Trigger Point Therapy 75

Step 11: Stretching (During Therapy) 75

Step 8: Multidirectional Friction 77

Step 9: Pain-Free Movement 77

Step 10: Eccentric Scar Tissue Alignment 77

Step 4: Assess Resisted Range of Motion (RROM) 77

Step 2: Assess Active Range of Motion (AROM) 77

Step 11: Stretching (Client Self-Care) 77

Step 12: Strengthening (Client Self-Care) 81

Case Study 81

Chapter Summary 82

Review Questions 82

Chapter 3   Knee and Thigh Conditions 84

Twelve-Step Approach to Knee and Thigh Conditions 86

Anterior Cruciate Ligament (ACL) and Posterior Cruciate Ligament (PCL) Instability 86

Step 1: Client History 86

Step 2: Assess Active Range of Motion (AROM) 88

Step 3: Assess Passive Range of Motion (PROM) 89

Step 4: Assess Resisted Range of Motion (RROM) 90

Patellar Tendinosis and Chondromalacia 91

Quadriceps Protocol 91

Step 4: Assess Resisted Range of Motion (RROM) 91

Step 5: Area Preparation 92

Step 6: Myofascial Release 92

Step 7: Cross-Fiber Gliding Strokes/Trigger Point Therapy 93

Step 8: Multidirectional Friction 93

Step 9: Pain-Free Movement 94

Step 10: Eccentric Scar Tissue Alignment 94

Step 4: Assess Resisted Range of Motion (RROM) 94

Step 11: Stretching (During Therapy) 95

Plantaris Strain 96

Step 4: Assess Resisted Range of Motion (RROM) 96

Step 5: Area Preparation 96

Step 6: Myofascial Release 96

Step 7: Cross-Fiber Gliding Strokes/Trigger Point Therapy 97

Step 11: Stretching (During Therapy) 97

Step 8: Multidirectional Friction 97

Step 9: Pain-Free Movement 98

Step 10: Eccentric Scar Tissue Alignment 98

Step 4: Assess Resisted Range of Motion (RROM) 98

Popliteus Strain 98

Step 4: Assess Resisted Range of Motion (RROM) 99

Step 5: Area Preparation 99

Step 6: Myofascial Release 100

Step 7: Cross-Fiber Gliding Strokes/Trigger Point Therapy 100

Step 8: Multidirectional Friction 100

Step 9: Pain-Free Movement 100

Step 10: Eccentric Scar Tissue Alignment 100

Step 4: Assess Resisted Range of Motion (RROM) 101

Medial Meniscus Injury and Medial Collateral Ligament (MCL) Sprain 101

Step 4: Assess Resisted Range of Motion (RROM) 101

Step 5: Area Preparation 102

Step 8: Multidirectional Friction 102

Step 9: Pain-Free Movement 103

Step 10: Eccentric Scar Tissue Alignment 103

Step 4: Assess Resisted Range of Motion (RROM) 104

Iliotibial Band Friction Syndrome 104

Step 4: Assess Resisted Range of Motion (RROM) 105

Step 5: Area Preparation 105

Step 6: Myofascial Release 105

Step 7: Cross-Fiber Gliding Strokes/Trigger Point Therapy 106

Step 11: Stretching (During Therapy) 107

Step 8: Multidirectional Friction 107

Step 9: Pain-Free Movement 107
Step 10: Eccentric Scar Tissue Alignment 107
Step 4: Assess Resisted Range of Motion (RROM) 107
Lateral Meniscus Injury and Lateral Collateral Ligament (LCL) Sprain 107
Step 4: Assess Resisted Range of Motion (RROM) 107
Step 5: Area Preparation 108
Step 8: Multidirectional Friction 108
Step 9: Pain-Free Movement 108
Step 10: Eccentric Scar Tissue Alignment 109
Step 4: Assess Resisted Range of Motion (RROM) 109
Step 11: Stretching (Client Self-Care) 109
Step 12: Strengthening (Client Self-Care) 112
Case Study 113
Chapter Summary 114
Review Questions 114

Chapter 4 Lower Leg, Ankle, and Foot Conditions 116
Twelve-Step Approach to Lower Leg, Ankle, and Foot Conditions 118
Step 1: Client History 118
Step 2: Assess Active Range of Motion (AROM) 118
Step 3: Assess Passive Range of Motion (PROM) 120
Step 4: Assess Resisted Range of Motion (RROM) 120
Achilles Tendinosis 120
Gastrocnemius Protocol to Address Achilles Tendon Pain 120
Step 4: Assess Resisted Range of Motion (RROM) 120
Step 5: Area Preparation 120
Step 6: Myofascial Release 120
Step 7: Cross-Fiber Gliding Strokes/Trigger Point Therapy 121
Step 11: Stretching (During Therapy) 122
Step 8: Multidirectional Friction 122
Step 9: Pain-Free Movement 122
Step 10: Eccentric Scar Tissue Alignment 123
Step 4: Assess Resisted Range of Motion (RROM) 123
Soleus Protocol 123
Step 4: Assess Resisted Range of Motion (RROM) 123
Step 6: Myofascial Release 123
Step 7: Cross-Fiber Gliding Strokes/Trigger Point Therapy 123
Step 11: Stretching (During Therapy) 124
Step 8: Multidirectional Friction 124
Step 9: Pain-Free Movement 125
Step 10: Eccentric Scar Tissue Alignment 125

Step 4: Assess Resisted Range of Motion (RROM) 125
Step 6: Myofascial Release 125
Posteromedial Shin Splints 126
Tibialis Posterior Protocol 126
Step 5: Area Preparation 127
Step 4: Assess Resisted Range of Motion (RROM) 127
Step 6: Myofascial Release 127
Step 11: Stretching (During Therapy) 128
Step 8: Multidirectional Friction 128
Step 9: Pain-Free Movement 128
Step 10: Eccentric Scar Tissue Alignment 128
Step 4: Assess Resisted Range of Motion (RROM) 128
Flat Feet and Fallen Arches or Pronation 128
Plantar Fasciitis 129
Step 4: Assess Resisted Range of Motion (RROM) 129
Step 5: Area Preparation 129
Step 6: Myofascial Release 130
Step 7: Cross-Fiber Gliding Strokes 130
Step 11: Stretching (During Therapy) 131
Step 8: Multidirectional Friction 132
Step 9: Pain-Free Movement 132
Step 10: Eccentric Scar Tissue Alignment 132
Step 4: Assess Resisted Range of Motion (RROM) 133
Anterior Compartment Syndrome (ACS) 133
Step 4: Assess Resisted Range of Motion (RROM) 133
Step 5: Area Preparation 134
Step 6: Myofascial Release 134
Step 7: Cross-Fiber Gliding Strokes/Trigger Point Therapy 135
Step 4: Assess Resisted Range of Motion (RROM) 136
Anterolateral Shin Splints 136
Step 5: Area Preparation 136
Step 4: Assess Resisted Range of Motion (RROM) 136
Step 8: Multidirectional Friction 136
Step 9: Pain-Free Movement 136
Step 10: Eccentric Scar Tissue Alignment 137
Step 4: Assess Resisted Range of Motion (RROM) 137
Inversion Ankle Sprain and Strain 137
Step 4: Assess Resisted Range of Motion (RROM) 138
Step 6: Myofascial Release 138
Step 11: Stretching (During Therapy) 138
Step 8: Multidirectional Friction 139
Step 9: Pain-Free Movement 139
Step 10: Eccentric Scar Tissue Alignment 139
Step 4: Assess Resisted Range of Motion (RROM) 139

Stress Fracture   140
   Step 11: Stretching (Client Self-Care)   140
   Step 12: Strengthening (Client Self-Care)   142
Case Study   144
Chapter Summary   144
Review Questions   145

Chapter 5   Shoulder Conditions   146
Twelve-Step Approach to Shoulder Conditions   148
   Step 1: Client History   149
   *Step 2: Assess Active Range of Motion
     (AROM)*   149
   *Step 3: Assess Passive Range of Motion
     (PROM)*   152
   *Step 4: Assess Resisted Range of Motion
     (RROM)*   152
Specific Muscle Resistance Tests   152
   Biceps (Long Head) and Coracobrachialis   153
   Subscapularis   153
   Pectoralis Minor   153
   Pectoralis Major   154
   Supraspinatus   154
   Infraspinatus   155
   Teres Minor   155
   Middle Deltoid   155
   Rhomboid Major and Minor   155
General Shoulder Protocol   156
   Joint Capsule Work   156
   "Velvet Glove" Technique   158
Pectoralis Major   159
   Step 5: Area Preparation   159
   Step 6: Myofascial Release   160
   *Step 7: Cross-Fiber Gliding Strokes/Trigger Point
     Therapy*   160
Pectoralis Minor   161
   Step 5: Area Preparation   161
   *Step 7: Cross-Fiber Gliding Strokes/Trigger Point
     Therapy*   161
   Step 11: Stretching (During Therapy)   162
   Step 8: Multidirectional Friction   163
   Step 9: Pain-Free Movement   164
   Step 10: Eccentric Scar Tissue Alignment   164
   *Step 4: Assess Resisted Range of Motion
     (RROM)*   164
Subclavius   165
   *Step 7: Cross-Fiber Gliding Strokes/Trigger Point
     Therapy*   165
   Step 11: Stretching (During Therapy)   165
Biceps and Coracobrachialis   166
   Step 5: Area Preparation   166
   Step 6: Myofascial Release   166
   *Step 7: Cross-Fiber Gliding Strokes/Trigger Point
     Therapy*   166
   Step 11: Stretching (During Therapy)   167
   Step 11: Stretching (During Therapy)   168

   Step 8: Multidirectional Friction   168
   Step 9: Pain-Free Movement   169
   Step 10: Eccentric Scar Tissue Alignment   169
   *Step 4: Assess Resisted Range of Motion
     (RROM)*   170
Upper Trapezius and Middle Deltoid   170
   Step 5: Area Preparation   170
   Step 6: Myofascial Release   171
   *Step 7: Cross-Fiber Gliding Strokes/Trigger Point
     Therapy*   171
   *Step 4: Assess Resisted Range of Motion
     (RROM)*   172
   Step 8: Multidirectional Friction   172
   Step 9: Pain-Free Movement   173
   Step 10: Eccentric Scar Tissue Alignment   173
   *Step 4: Assess Resisted Range of Motion
     (RROM)*   174
Subscapularis   174
   Step 5: Area Preparation   174
   Step 6: Myofascial Release   174
   *Step 7: Cross-Fiber Gliding Strokes/Trigger Point
     Therapy*   175
   Step 11: Stretching (During Therapy)   175
Rhomboids   176
   Step 5: Area Preparation   176
   Step 6: Myofascial Release   176
Triceps and Posterior Deltoid   177
   Step 5: Area Preparation   178
   Step 6: Myofascial Release   178
   *Step 4: Assess Resisted Range of Motion
     (RROM)*   179
   Step 8: Multidirectional Friction   179
   Step 9: Pain-Free Movement   179
   Step 10: Eccentric Scar Tissue Alignment   179
   *Step 4: Assess Resisted Range of Motion
     (RROM)*   180
   *Step 4: Assess Resisted Range of Motion
     (RROM)*   180
   Step 8: Multidirectional Friction   180
   Step 9: Pain-Free Movement   180
   Step 10: Eccentric Scar Tissue Alignment   181
   *Step 4: Assess Resisted Range of Motion
     (RROM)*   181
Scapula Reposition   181
   Step 5: Area Preparation   181
   Step 6: Myofascial Release   182
Supraspinatus and Upper Trapezius   182
   Step 5: Area Preparation   183
   *Step 7: Cross-Fiber Gliding Strokes/Trigger Point
     Therapy*   183
   Step 11: Stretching (During Therapy)   184
   Step 8: Multidirectional Friction   184
   Step 9: Pain-Free Movement   185
   Step 10: Eccentric Scar Tissue Alignment   185
   *Step 4: Assess Resisted Range of Motion
     (RROM)*   186

Infraspinatus and Teres Minor 186
    Step 5: Area Preparation 186
    Step 6: Myofascial Release 186
    Step 7: Cross-Fiber Gliding Strokes/Trigger Point
       Therapy 187
    Step 4: Assess Resisted Range of Motion
       (RROM) 187
    Step 8: Multidirectional Friction 188
    Step 9: Pain-Free Movement 188
    Step 10: Eccentric Scar Tissue Alignment 188
    Step 4: Assess Resisted Range of Motion
       (RROM) 189
Common Conditions 190
    Thoracic Outlet Syndrome 190
    Step 11: Stretching (During Therapy) 191
    Step 11: Stretching (During Therapy) 191
    Frozen Shoulder (Adhesive Capsulitis) 192
    Rotator Cuff Injuries 193
    Supraspinatus Tendinosis 193
    Infraspinatus Tendinosis and Teres Minor
       Tendinosis 194
    Subscapularis Tendinosis versus Bicipital and
       Coracobrachialis Tendinosis 194
    Subacromial Bursitis 194
    Upper Crossed Syndrome 195
    Step 11: Stretching (Client Self-Care) 195
    Step 12: Strengthening (Client Self-Care) 197
Case Study 199
Chapter Summary 200
Review Questions 201

Chapter 6 Cervical Spine Conditions 202
Twelve-Step Approach to Cervical Spine Conditions 204
    Precautionary Tests 204
    Step 1: Client History 206
    Step 2: Assess Active Range of Motion (AROM) 206
    Step 3: Assess Passive Range of Motion
       (PROM) 208
    Step 4: Assess Resisted Range of Motion
       (RROM) 208
Cervical Spine Protocol 210
    Cervical Mobilization 210
    Dura Mater and Dural Sheath Mobilization 210
    Dura Mater and Dural Sheath Mobilization
       Protocol 210
    Atlanto-Occipital/Atlanto-Axial Lateral Mobilization
       Protocol 211
    Atlanto-Occipital/Atlanto-Axial Anterior-Posterior
       Mobilization Protocol 212
    Velvet Glove Myofascial Release Technique 214
Sternocleidomastoid (SCM) and Scalenes 217
    Step 6: Myofascial Release 217
    Step 7: Cross-Fiber Gliding Strokes/Trigger Point
       Therapy 218
    Step 11: Stretching (During Therapy) 219
    Step 11: Stretching (During Therapy) 220
    Step 11: Stretching (During Therapy) 220

Interspinales, Rotatores, and Intertransversarii 222
    Interspinales ("Yes") 223
    Step 6: Myofascial Release 223
    Rotatores ("No") 223
    Step 6: Myofascial Release 223
    Intertransversarii ("I Don't Know") 223
    Step 6: Myofascial Release 223
Suboccipital Muscles 224
    Step 6: Myofascial Release 224
    Cervical Joint Capsule Work and C1–C2
       Mobilization 225
    Step 11: Stretching (During Therapy) 226
    Step 8: Multidirectional Friction 227
    Step 9: Pain-Free Movement 227
    Step 10: Eccentric Scar Tissue Alignment 227
    Step 4: Assess Resisted Range of Motion
       (RROM) 227
    Step 11: Stretching (During Therapy) 227
    Step 8: Multidirectional Friction 227
    Step 9: Pain-Free Movement 227
    Step 10: Eccentric Scar Tissue Alignment 227
    Step 4: Assess Resisted Range of Motion
       (RROM) 227
Levator Scapula 227
    Step 11: Stretching (During Therapy) 228
    Step 8: Multidirectional Friction 228
    Step 9: Pain-Free Movement 228
    Step 10: Eccentric Scar Tissue Alignment 228
    Step 4: Assess Resisted Range of Motion
       (RROM) 228
    Step 11: Stretching (Client Self-Care) 230
    Techniques for Client Self-Care 230
    Step 12: Strengthening (Client Self-Care) 231
    Neck Extensors 231
Case Study 232
Chapter Summary 232
Review Questions 233

**Chapter 7 Elbow, Forearm, Wrist, and Hand
Conditions** 234
Twelve-Step Approach to Elbow, Forearm, Wrist,
    and Hand Conditions 236
    Step 1: Client History 236
    Step 2: Assess Active Range of Motion (AROM) 236
    Step 3: Assess Passive Range of Motion
       (PROM) 238
    Step 4: Assess Resisted Range of Motion
       (RROM) 239
Medial Epicondylosis (Golfer's Elbow) 239
    Step 2: Assess Active Range of Motion (AROM) 240
    Step 3: Assess Passive Range of Motion
       (PROM) 240
    Step 4: Assess Resisted Range of Motion
       (RROM) 240
    Step 6: Myofascial Release 240
    Step 7: Cross-Fiber Gliding Strokes/Trigger Point
       Therapy 241

Step 6: Myofascial Release Flexor Tendons   242
Step 11: Stretching (During Therapy)   244
Step 8: Multidirectional Friction   244
Step 9: Pain-Free Movement   244
Step 10: Eccentric Scar Tissue Alignment   244
Step 4: Assess Resisted Range of Motion (RROM)   244
Step 6: Myofascial Release   244
Step 6: Myofascial Release   245
Step 11: Stretching (During Therapy)   245
Step 8: Multidirectional Friction   246
Step 9: Pain-Free Movement   246
Step 10: Eccentric Scar Tissue Alignment   246
Step 4: Assess Resisted Range of Motion (RROM)   246
Lateral Epicondylosis (Tennis Elbow)   246
Step 2: Assess Active Range of Motion (AROM)   247
Step 3: Assess Passive Range of Motion (PROM)   247
Step 4: Assess Resisted Range of Motion (RROM)   247
Step 6: Myofascial Release   248
Step 7: Cross-Fiber Gliding Strokes/Trigger Point Therapy   248
Step 8: Multidirectional Friction   249
Step 9: Pain-Free Movement   249
Step 10: Eccentric Scar Tissue Alignment   249
Step 4: Assess Resisted Range of Motion (RROM)   250
Step 6: Myofascial Release   250
Step 4: Assess Resisted Range of Motion   250
Step 8: Multidirectional Friction   250
Step 9: Pain-Free Movement   251
Step 10: Eccentric Scar Tissue Alignment   251

Step 4: Assess Resisted Range of Motion (RROM)   251
Carpal Tunnel Syndrome   251
Step 6: Myofascial Release   252
Step 11: Stretching (During Therapy)   253
Thumb Strain or Sprain   255
Step 6: Myofascial Release   255
Step 4: Assess Resisted Range of Motion (RROM)   255
Step 8: Multidirectional Friction   256
Step 9: Pain-Free Movement   256
Step 10: Eccentric Scar Tissue Alignment   256
Step 4: Assess Resisted Range of Motion (RROM)   256
Step 11: Stretching (During Therapy)   256
Degenerative Arthritis   256
Treatment   256
Trigger Finger   257
Step 11: Stretching (Client Self-Care)   258
Step 12: Strengthening (Client Self-Care)   258
Case Study   260
Chapter Summary   260
Review Questions   261

Appendix A   **End-of-Chapter Questions—Answer Key**   263

Appendix B   **Notes**   265

Appendix C   **Suggested Readings**   269

Glossary   271
Index   275

1

The Twelve-Step Approach: Assessment, Treatment, and Client Self-Care

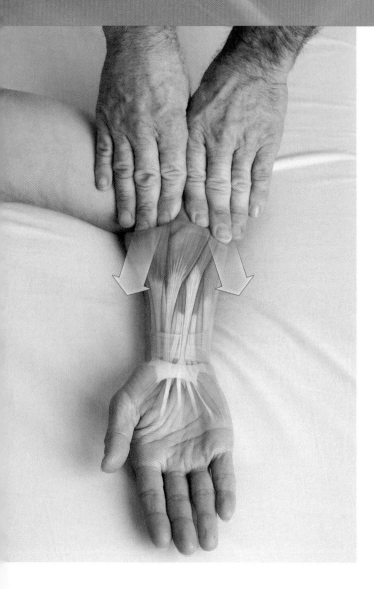

 CHAPTER OUTLINE

Twelve Steps to Pain Management

Origins of the Twelve-Step Approach

Tendinosis Techniques and Scar Tissue Mobilization

A New Hypothesis

LEARNING OBJECTIVES

Upon completing this chapter the reader will be able to:

- Understand and implement the twelve-step assessment, treatment, and self-care approach
- Steps 1–4: History and Assessment
  - Step 1: Client History
  - Step 2: Assess Active Range of Motion (AROM)
  - Step 3: Assess Passive Range of Motion (PROM)
  - Step 4: Assess Resisted Range of Motion (RROM)
- Steps 5–12: Path to Pain-Free Movement
  - Step 5: Area Preparation

- Step 6: Myofascial Release/Compression
- Step 7: Cross-Fiber Gliding Strokes/Trigger Point Therapy
- Step 8: Multidirectional Friction
- Step 9: Pain-Free Movement
- Step 10: Eccentric Scar Tissue Alignment
- Step 11: Stretching (During Therapy/Client Self-Care)
- Step 12: Strengthening (Client Self-Care)

KEY TERMS

Active assisted stretching 26

Active range of motion (AROM) 7

Collagen 23

Cross-fiber gliding strokes 20

Eccentric contraction 25

Hypothesis 31

Ischemia 27

Muscle–tendon junction 15

Myofascial release 19

Passive range of motion (PROM) 14

Pathology 15

Periosteal junction 15

Post isometric relaxation 27

Proprioceptive neuromuscular facilitation (PNF) 26

Proprioceptors 27

Reciprocal inhibition 27

Resisted range of motion (RROM) 15

Scar tissue 23

Sprain 23

Strain 23

Structural integration 4

Tendinitis 7

Tendinosis 7

Tendon tension 29

Tenosynovitis 7

Trigger point 20

When a clinical massage therapist sees a client whose physician has diagnosed him or her with a clinical condition such as thoracic outlet or carpal tunnel syndrome, the therapist has several immediate needs: a quick reference to understanding the client's underlying musculoskeletal anatomy, the ability to perform a thorough assessment, and the skill to formulate the most effective treatment and client self-care regimen for that specific condition. Advanced clinical massage therapy is a structural approach to pain management in which a twelve-step sequence will allow you to eliminate the underlying cause of each clinical condition before addressing the symptom(s). For the purposes of this book, advanced clinical massage therapy may be defined as therapeutic assessment, manipulation, and movement of locomotor soft tissues (muscles, tendons, ligaments, fascia, and joint capsules) to prevent, reduce, or eliminate chronic pain or injuries throughout the body.[1] A multidisciplinary and multimodality approach is utilized to restore structural balance throughout the body, which allows focus on the prevention and rehabilitation of musculoskeletal dysfunctions, trauma, sports injuries, and chronic pain. **Structural integration** helps the body return to structural and functional postural alignment by removing tensions and restrictions in areas that have been held tight and by further balancing myofascial relationships throughout the entire body (Figures 1-1 ■, 1-2 ■, and 1-3 ■).[2]

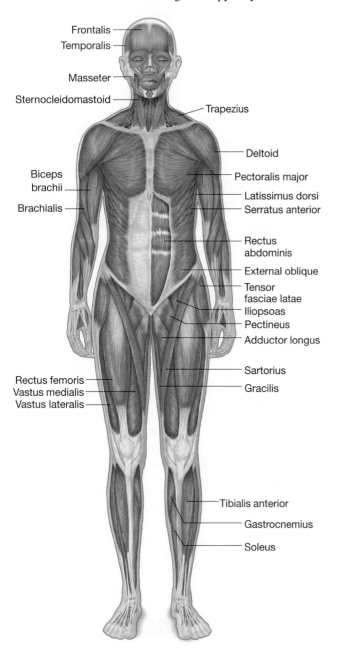

FIGURE 1-1

Anterior View of Ideal Posture.

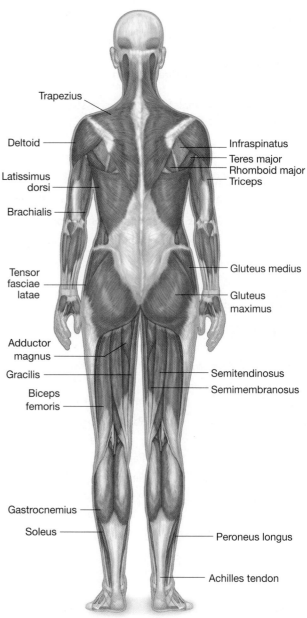

FIGURE 1-2

Posterior View of Ideal Posture.

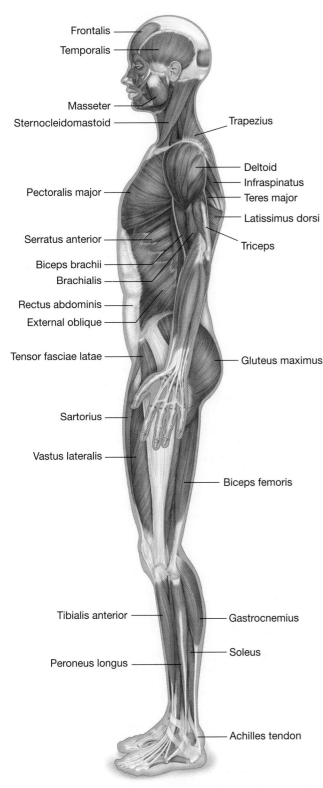

FIGURE 1-3
Lateral View of Ideal Posture.

Improper alignment of the myoskeletal system compromises nerves, blood vessels, organs, and most other body structures, leading to osseous, neural, myofascial, and vascular degeneration. Complicated pain conditions,

underlying forms of disease, and structural pathology often result. Instability in the body's core musculature results in compensations and complications throughout the entire neuromyoskeletal system. Therefore, many painful conditions are rooted in structures located far away from the site of the pain. A classic example occurs when large muscle groups such as the iliopsoas and quadriceps co-contract to produce anterior pelvic tilting, the result of which is a compensatory low shoulder. This common misalignment often affects cervical, thoracic, and upper extremity structures.[3]

Therapists must learn safe and pain-free techniques to manipulate muscle groups in an organized fashion to facilitate or enhance alignment of the myoskeletal system, working superficial to deep, but starting with the core muscles. This chapter will teach you how to employ a systematic twelve-step approach that will help your clients achieve structural balance, eliminate pain and dysfunction, and allow you to provide an individualized approach to client wellness.

TWELVE STEPS TO PAIN MANAGEMENT

The twelve-step approach to pain management consists of a set of detailed functional assessment skills for specific pain conditions that will help you formulate an individualized treatment plan based on the client's history. Although some clients may present similar or identical pain conditions, each requires a unique treatment plan. Using the twelve-step approach, you will learn to choose the appropriate massage modality or treatment protocol for a specific clinical condition, while encouraging the client to participate in his or her own treatment. This concept is something that most health care professionals (such as doctors, chiropractors, physical therapists, athletic trainers, etc.) currently follow.

The twelve-step flow chart identifies the steps, and shows the general order the therapist should follow to allow the client history and functional assessments to define the most appropriate treatment and self-care plans. (Figure 1-4 ■). As the treatment protocols in later chapters reveal, steps 5 through 12 may not all be needed, but those steps required should always occur in numerical order. You will always follow steps 1 through 4, but the utilization of the remaining eight steps can vary depending on both the client's condition—whether or not an injury is present—and his or her response to the preceding step. You will work through each step thoroughly, proceeding from one step to the next only after each area of tension is appropriately released or the step can be completed pain-free. It is vital that the twelve-step approach is not used as a "cookbook" approach to therapy, since it will vary with each client.

To apply the twelve-step approach successfully, you must be able to accomplish two tasks:

1. Identify the appropriate therapeutic techniques needed to address specific structures

Twelve-Step Flow Chart

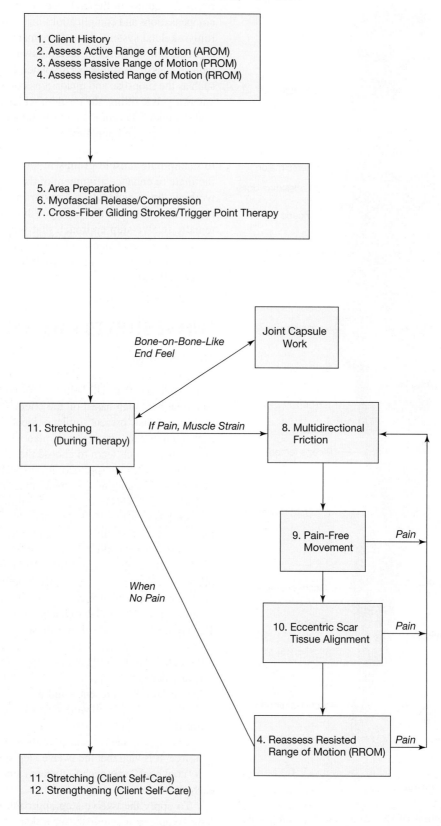

FIGURE 1-4

Twelve-Step Flow Chart.

2. Differentiate among soft-tissue problems caused by

- Myofascial restrictions
- Musculoskeletal problems
- Skeletal alignment problems
- Trigger point tension
- Joint capsule adhesions
- Strained muscle fibers
- Scar tissue
- Nerve compression

Your goals in applying the twelve steps are

- To restore structural balance and postural alignment
- To create pain-free movement by balancing opposing muscle groups throughout the body
- To increase joint space throughout the body
- To create aligned or functional scar tissue
- To restore normal muscle resting lengths throughout the body

Definitions

Tendinitis is inflammation of tendons or of muscle–tendon attachments.

Tendinosis is tearing of tendon fibers in the absence of an inflammatory process.

Tenosynovitis is the inflammation of a tendon sheath or adhesions within the tendon sheath.

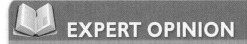

EXPERT OPINION

The clinical massage therapist should constantly interact with the client, working pain-free, between soft-tissue imbalances and damage, joint capsule adhesions, and emotional guarding. To enhance each technique, combine intention, compassion, presence in therapy, a positive healing dialogue, client education, and client visualization throughout the entire session. This allows the therapist to become a facilitator of the healing process.

Step 1: Client History

Your first step in defining the client's specific treatment plan is to obtain a thorough client history (Figure 1-5 ■). This history is important for several reasons. First, it will give you a comprehensive view of the client's soft-tissue conditions. This information will help you identify which specific muscle groups or structures are involved, thus helping you determine what modality or treatment plan to use. This

information is crucial, since treatment plans can vary widely depending on which tissues or structures are injured. Finally, the history also provides valuable insight into your client's physical and emotional states.

TECHNIQUE FOR ASSESSING CLIENT HISTORY

Goal: to obtain a thorough medical history including precautions and contraindications for treatment of the client's condition.

The client history includes but is not limited to the following:

- Current condition: symptoms acute or chronic
- Previous conditions
- Daily activities limited by condition
- Self-care routines
- Previous successful treatments
- Current stress level
- Sleep, diet, exercise habits
- Occupation
- Repetitive motions performed at work, while playing sports, or while engaged in a hobby
- Contract for care

You should also request basic information such as current medications the client is taking, any current medical condition and symptoms of that condition, precautions or contraindications, and whether a doctor's approval is needed for you to perform massage. In addition, ask the client a few focused questions about when, where, and how his or her problem began. Encourage the client to describe the area of pain and anything that alleviates or worsens it. This feedback should help you determine what type of problem the client is experiencing. For example, if the client experiences discomfort during movement, this suggests that the problem most likely lies in the contractile structures such as the muscles and tendons. If the client describes the pain as electric, radiating, sharp, or shooting, then the problem may involve compression of the nerves.

It is essential to reevaluate the client each time he or she returns for therapy. A previous history or even another therapist's assessment or diagnosis is not reliable because the client's current condition may have improved, worsened, or been misdiagnosed. The point of therapy is to alter the client's condition, so if he or she has sought therapy previously, it is likely that on the next visit the pain may be different. Pay attention to the client's clinical diagnosis, but set it aside and reevaluate your client starting with the next step in the twelve-step approach.

Step 2: Assess Active Range of Motion (AROM)

Assessing a client's **active range of motion (AROM)** will help you determine which muscles are restricted and what is preventing them from performing a normal range of motion without pain. *(Text continues on page 14.)*

Health History for Massage Therapy Treatment

Name _____ Date of initial visit _____

Address _____ Phone _____

Occupation _____ Date of birth _____

Name of physician _____ Phone _____

Other health care provider _____

Referred by _____

1. Have you had massage therapy before?   Yes   No

2. For women: Are you pregnant?   Yes   No
   If yes, how many months? _____

3. Do you have any difficulty lying on your front, back, or side?   Yes   No
   If yes, please explain _____

4. Do you have allergic reactions to oils, lotions, ointments, liniments, or other
   substances put on your skin?   Yes   No
   If yes, please explain _____

5. Do you wear contact lenses ☐ dentures ☐ a hearing aid ☐?

6. Do you sit for long hours at a workstation, computer, or driving?   Yes   No
   If yes, please describe _____

7. Do you perform any repetitive movement in your work, sports, or hobby?   Yes   No
   If yes, please describe _____

8. Do you experience stress in your work, family, or other aspect of your life?   Yes   No
   How would you describe your stress level?
   Low Medium High Very high
   If high, how do you think stress has effected your health?
   muscle tension ☐ anxiety ☐ insomnia ☐ irritability ☐ other_____

9. Is there a particular area of the body where you are experiencing tension,
   stiffness, or other discomfort? (see body map)   Yes   No
   If yes, please identify _____

In order to plan a massage session that is safe and effective, we need some general information about your medical history.

10. Are you currently under medical supervision?   Yes   No
    If yes, please explain _____

11. Are you currently taking any medication?   Yes   No
    If yes, please list _____

12. Insurance company _____ Policy # _____
    ID # _____ Group # _____ Claim # _____
    Phone number _____

(1 of 2)

FIGURE 1-5
Client Intake Form.

13. Please check any condition listed below that applies to you:

    _____ Skin condition (e.g., acne, rash, skin cancer, allergy, easy bruising, contagious condition)

    _____ Allergies

    _____ Past accident, injury, or surgery (e.g., whiplash, sprain, broken bone, deep bruise)

    _____ Muscular problems (e.g., tension, cramping, chronic soreness)

    _____ Joint problems (e.g., osteoarthritis, rheumatoid arthritis, gout, hypermobile joints, recent dislocation)

    _____ Lymphatic condition (e.g., swollen glands, nodes removed, lymphoma, lymphedema)

    _____ Circulatory or blood conditions (e.g., atherosclerosis, varicose veins, phlebitis, arrhythmias, high or low blood pressure, heart disease, recent heart attack or stroke, blood clots, anemia)

    _____ Neurologic condition (e.g., numbness or tingling in any area of the body, sciatica, damage from stroke, epilepsy, multiple sclerosis, cerebral palsy)

    _____ Digestive conditions (e.g., ulcers)

    _____ Immune system conditions (e.g., chronic fatigue, HIV/AIDS)

    _____ Skeletal conditions (e.g., osteoporosis, bone cancer, spinal injury)

    _____ Headaches (e.g., tension, PMS, migraines)

    _____ Cancer

    _____ Emotional difficulties (e.g., depression, anxiety, panic attacks, eating disorder, psychotic episodes). Are you currently seeing a psychotherapist for this condition? Yes No

    _____ Previous surgery, disease, or other medical condition that may be affecting you now (e.g., polio, previous heart attack or stroke, previously broken bones, abdominal aortic aneurysm)

    _____ Elective surgery or procedures

    Comments:

    _____

    _____

    _____

14. Is there anything else about your health history that you think would be useful for your massage practitioner to know to plan a safe and effective massage session for you?

    _____

    _____

    _____

15. Has your physician or other health care provider recommended massage for any of the conditions listed above?   Yes   No

    If yes, please explain _____

16. Do you have any particular goals in mind for this massage session related to any of the conditions mentioned above?   Yes   No

    If yes, please explain _____

I understand that I should see a doctor or other appropriate health care provider for diagnosis and treatment of any suspected medical problem. It may be beneficial for my massage practitioner to speak to my doctor about my medical condition to determine how massage may help the healing process, and to avoid worsening the condition. I will be asked for permission to contact my doctor, if the massage practitioner thinks that it might be useful. I also understand that it is my responsibility to keep my massage practitioner informed of any changes in my health, and any medications that I may begin to take in the future.

Signature _____ Date _____

(2 of 2)

FIGURE 1-5 *(Continued)*

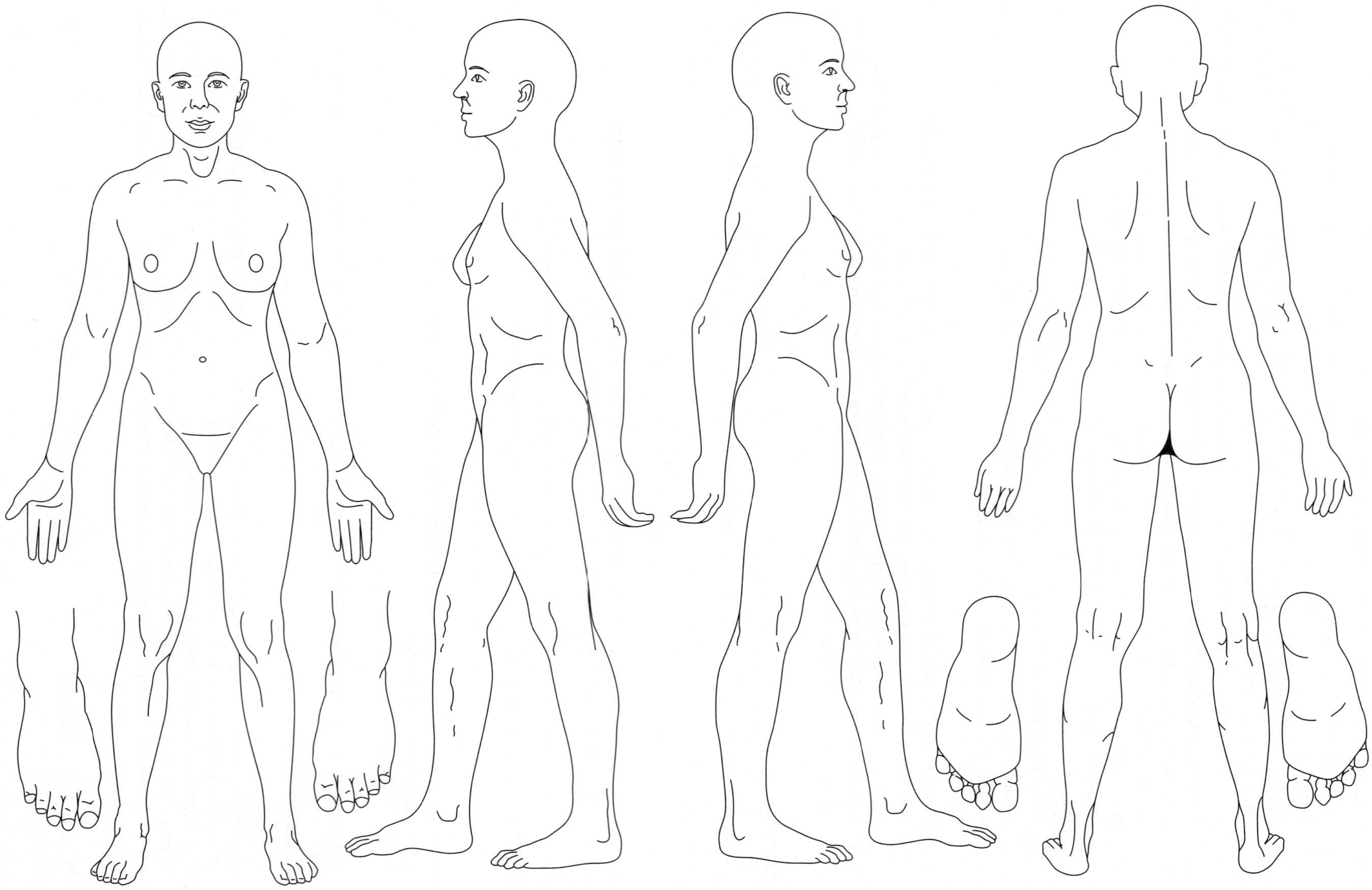

Body map to show areas of pain

FIGURE 1-5 (*Continued*)

General Agreement and Consent

I, _____ understand that the massage therapy given to me by _____ is for the purpose of general health and wellness, relaxation, improved circulation, pain management, and other effects supported by experience and research. Massage therapy is performed here within the scope of practice of massage therapists in this state.

I understand that massage therapists do not diagnosis medical conditions, nor do they prescribe medical treatments or medications, nor do they perform spinal manipulation or chiropractic adjustments.

I understand that massage therapy is not a substitute for examination by a medical provider, and that it is recommended that I seek medical attention first for any illness, injury, or disorder that I might have.

I understand that massage therapy can be a valuable complement to health care provided by medical doctors, chiropractic physicians, naturopathic physicians, practitioners of traditional Chinese medicine, and psychiatrists and psychologists. I agree to keep my massage therapist informed of any medical treatment I am receiving with the understanding that it may impact the massage therapy I receive.

I have stated all my known medical conditions, treatments, and medications, and I agree to keep the massage therapist updated on any changes.

My signature below confirms my agreement to the general policies, privacy policy, and consent statements above.

Name _____ Date _____

Witness _____ Date _____

FIGURE 1-5 *(Continued)*

SOAP NOTE CHART
CONTINUING MASSAGE SESSION

Practitioner's Name _____   Date _____

Client's Name _____

S: Reason for massage, complaints, reports

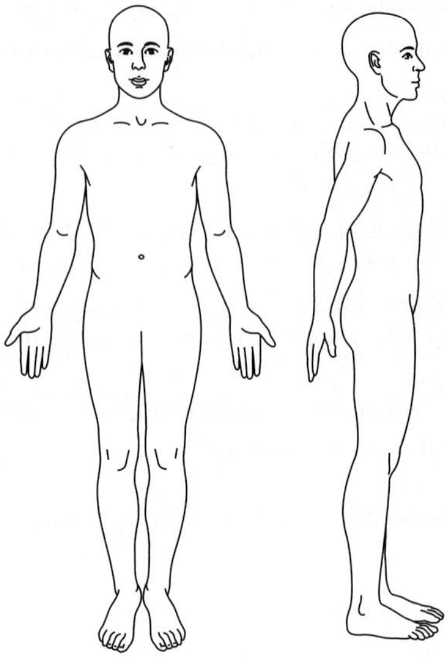

O: Observations, qualitative/quantitative measurements

A: Primary and secondary goals for the session; contraindications

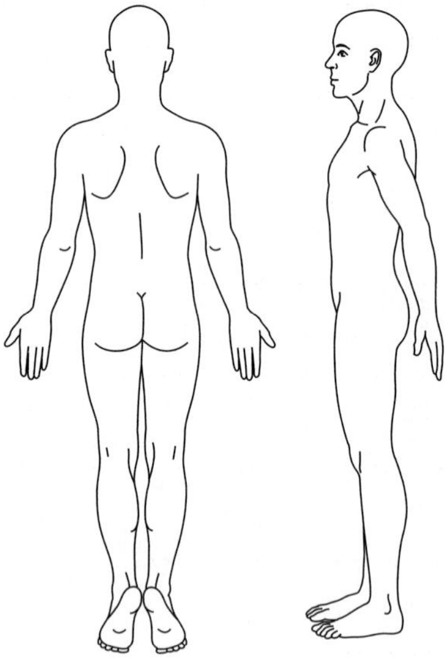

P: Duration of massage; areas addressed; techniques used; results; suggested home care

Practitioner Signature _____   Date _____

Symbols:

Primary **1°**	Secondary **2°**	Change **Δ**	Increase **↑**	Decrease **↓**	Tension **≡**
Adhesion **X**	Pain **P**	Numbness **〰**	Inflammation **✳**	TrP **⊗**	

FIGURE 1-5 *(Continued)*

Intake Form for Outreach Events

Massage Therapist _____ Date _____

WELCOME! To ensure a safe and healthy experience of massage therapy, please tell your massage therapist the following:

- If you have a medical condition that may be adversely affected by massage
- If you are taking medication that affects circulation or ability to sense pain
- If you have high or low blood pressure
- If you have had a serious illness or injury recently
- If you are pregnant
- Any areas the massage therapist should avoid

Your signature below indicates that you have given the massage therapist the information requested and give your consent to receive massage. The massage therapist and the sponsoring organization are not responsible for unforeseeable adverse reactions to the massage received.

Name   Time

1. _____
   print   signature

2. _____
   print   signature

3. _____
   print   signature

4. _____
   print   signature

5. _____
   print   signature

6. _____
   print   signature

7. _____
   print   signature

8. _____
   print   signature

9. _____
   print   signature

10. _____
   print   signature

Form # _____ MT Initials _____

FIGURE 1-5 *(Continued)*

TECHNIQUE FOR ASSESSING AROM

Goal: to assess range of motion of single-plane movements performed solely by the client to identify tight or restricted muscle groups.

- Demonstrate for the client the movement to be performed, emphasizing that the movement must be performed with zero discomfort.
- These movements are performed solely by the client.
- Evaluate the uninjured, unrestricted, normal side first.

As the client performs the movement, note the following:

- Degree of range of motion achieved.
- Abnormal movement patterns, or restricted areas.
- Location and movement performed at the onset of pain.
- Abnormalities in the client's posture. Is he or she compensating or splinting the area due to discomfort or protection from anticipated pain?

You want to discover what is restricting the muscles from performing the normal range of motion, pain-free. Become a healing detective by looking for the cause of the problem.

Step 3: Assess Passive Range of Motion (PROM)

To assess **passive range of motion (PROM),** you perform the movements on the clients, rather than the client performing the movements as in AROM. The purpose of assessing PROM is to differentiate between inert tissues (bones, ligaments, joint capsules, and cartilage) and contractile tissues (muscles and tendons). Knowing what is abnormal can help you determine whether the restriction in the joint is muscle–tendon related (soft-tissue pathology) or caused from abnormal joint pathologies like joint arthritis, adhesive capsulitis, torn ligaments, damaged cartilage, or hypermobile joints.

When you assess PROM you need to determine the "end feel" of the physiological barrier at the end of each joint's range of motion.[4] Some common end feel descriptions include:

- **Tissue stretch or soft and leathery:** The stretch of soft tissues around the joint. (i.e., ankle dorsiflexion)
- **Bone-on-bone:** Occurs when two bones contact each other and stop the range of motion (i.e., elbow extension).
- **Bone-on-bone-like:** Feels like bone-on-bone but is actually adhesions within the hip or shoulder joint capsules (i.e., adhesive capsulitis of the shoulder). Joints like the hips and shoulders should not present with a bone-on-bone-like end feel. This is referred to as adhesive capsulitis.
- **Tissue compression:** Occurs when the range of motion is stopped by muscle contacting muscle (i.e., elbow flexion).
- **Ligamentous:** Occurs when ligaments stop the movement of a joint (i.e., ankle plantar flexion).

- **Springy block:** A pathological end-feel that is associated with a loose body in the joint (i.e., motions of the knee where a torn meniscus is present and there is a loose body of cartilage in the joint). Springy block can also be felt in the knee if there is a fixated fibular head dysfunction from excess lateral rotation of the tibia/fibula.

TECHNIQUE FOR ASSESSING PROM

Goal: to assess the range of motion end feel of single-plane movements performed on the client. Passive motions focus on the inert tissues. In passive movements the contractile tissues are moved, but not engaged.

- The therapist brings the client's joint through each full pain-free range of motion, by moving the muscles into a lengthened position.
- Gently stretch that tissue.
- If the client experiences muscle–tendon discomfort or neuromuscular tension during the stretch, ask him or her to isolate the specific spot with one finger and point to it.

When performing PROM, you should always be sensitive to the client's breathing and patterns of guarding. Your overall confidence, combined with a calming voice, can help the client relax.

As in AROM, observe the following and then compare notes between AROM and PROM.

- Degree of range of motion achieved.
- End feel when the movement stops.
- Abnormal or restricted movement patterns.
- Site and movement performed at the onset of pain.
- Abnormalities in the client's posture. Is he or she compensating or splinting the area due to discomfort or protection from anticipated pain?
- Joint play.

According to Dr. John Mennell there are movements within a joint: active, passive, and joint play. His research states that joint play occurs within the paraphysiological space within a joint. Without 1/8 inch of normal joint play nutrients cannot be exchanged, thus degeneration occurs. "Voluntary movements cannot be achieved unless certain well-defined movements of joint play are present."[5] The following are four basic truths about joint play from Dr. Mennell's work:

1. When a joint is not free to move, the muscles that move it are not free to move.
2. Muscles cannot be restored to normal if the joint that they move is not free to move.
3. Normal muscle function is dependent on normal joint movement.
4. Impaired muscle function perpetuates and may cause deterioration in normal joints.

Step 4: Assess Resisted Range of Motion (RROM)

Assessing **resisted range of motion (RROM)**, also know as manual resistance testing, is critical to determine if the client's pain is the result of a *muscle–tendon strain* and will identify the exact location of the strained fibers. It will also help you differentiate between myofascial pain, neuromuscular pain, and muscle–tendon strain pain. Problems usually occur at the **periosteal junction,** where the tendon attaches to the bone, or at the **muscle–tendon junction,** where the muscle fibers become tendons (Figure 1-6 ■).

The weakest transition is the muscle–tendon junction and therefore the most common area of strain. However, both of these junctions are weak areas of transition and easily injured. Your assessment skills will allow you to isolate the client's condition and determine the **pathology** present so that it can be treated effectively and appropriately with the exact modality or technique.

TECHNIQUE FOR ASSESSING RROM

Goal: to assess if there is a muscle–tendon strain present, which muscle–tendon unit or structure is involved, and exactly where it is located.

- Find a comfortable position to test the muscle.
- Start with the muscle in a neutral position.
- Test the normal side first. Give kinesthetic cues or show the client the movement to be performed.
- Ask the client to contract the tested muscle using only 20 percent force, and if there is no pain you can apply reverse resistance (in the opposite direction).

- Start with light reverse resistance to avoid pain, and increase the intensity of the reverse resistance only until the client can identify the specific area of muscle–tendon strain. Sometimes the pain of a small, deep muscle strain will not surface until the muscle is fully stretched and contracted with more intensity, as it is tested.
- You, not the client, control the amount of force being applied to avoid pain or the possibility of creating a secondary injury by being too aggressive.
- If the client experiences discomfort during this movement, ask the client to isolate the specific area by pointing to it with one finger. The site the client points to is the location of the muscle–tendon injury.
- Listen to the client. The client helps direct the treatment by indicating where the pain or discomfort is located.

Steps 5–12: Path to Pain-Free Movement

BODY MECHANICS

Prior to getting into the treatment part of this twelve-step series, it is important to talk about body mechanics and the most effective application of specific techniques. To prevent injuries in your own body, and optimize the effectiveness of each technique, learning proper body mechanics is critical. When using your body weight, rather than muscle force, clinical massage can require a lot less effort than other forms of massage therapy. Keep in mind that part of your session is spent doing assessment and special orthopedic testing, part of your time doing treatment, and part of your time teaching self-care techniques. With proper body mechanics in the treatment portion, you will have a long career as a clinical massage therapist because you will not get fatigued or injured. Sometimes something as simple as lowering the height of your table and adjusting the height of your stool can have a profound effect on your body mechanics and the energy required to do effective manual therapy. Many therapists have a short career due to exhaustion, injury, or burnout. Adopting the following practices may help prevent you from falling into that category (Figures 1-7 ■ to 1-23 ■).

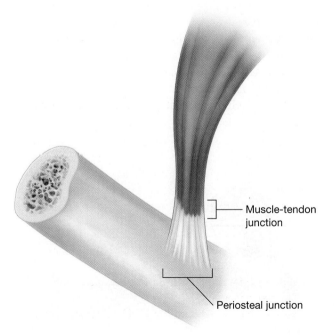

FIGURE 1-6
Muscle–Tendon Strain.

Muscle-tendon junction

Periosteal junction

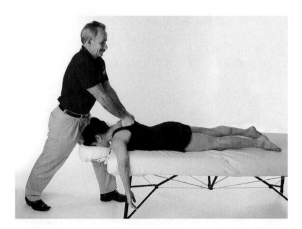

FIGURE 1-7
Align Body, Neck and Spine Straight, and Arms Straight.

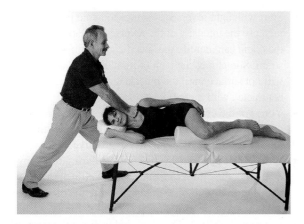

FIGURE 1-8

Pressure and Depth Comes from Good Body Alignment.

- Keep the joints through which your weight passes relatively straight, and avoid hyperextension of your joints.
- Use your body weight rather than muscle to apply pressure.
- Let movement come from your center of gravity— hips and legs—rather than from your arms and shoulders.
- Use your fists or knuckles to mobilize the deep investing fascia.

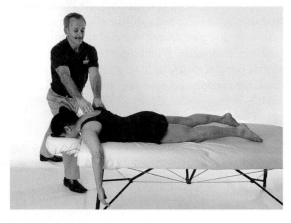

FIGURE 1-9

Arms, Wrists, and Fingers Straight.

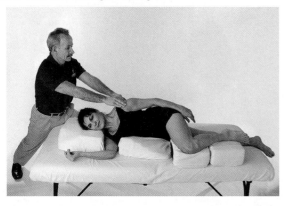

FIGURE 1-10

Body Support Systems Aid Good Body Mechanics.

- Keep your arms and wrists relatively straight, as pressure is generated from the hips.
- Keep your neck from being in prolonged flexion.
- Keep your fingers straight to avoid excessive joint pressure while mobilizing fascia.

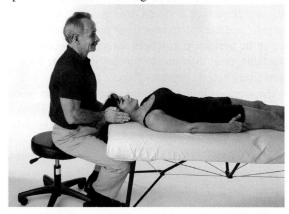

FIGURE 1-11

Straight Upper Body, Hips, and Knees close to 90 Degrees.

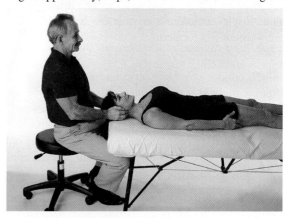

FIGURE 1-12

Traction Comes from Upper Body.

- When doing cervical compression or decompression, lean forward and backward with your entire body, keeping back and neck straight.
- Keep your elbows bent at about 90 degrees and relax your shoulders.

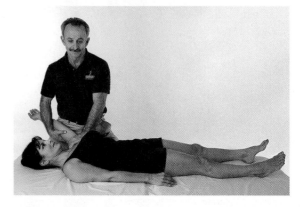

FIGURE 1-13

Joint Capsule Work Comes from Hips and Legs.

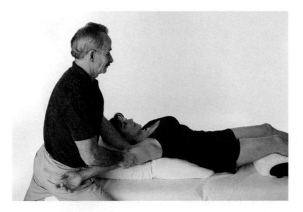

FIGURE 1-14
Stabilize Scapula During Joint Capsule Work.

- When doing shoulder joint capsule work, rest the client's forearm on your hip. This allows you to compress and decompress the client's shoulder capsule using hip movement.
- Keep your back and neck straight and apply gentle, even pressure around the client's elbow while your other hand keeps the scapula from moving.

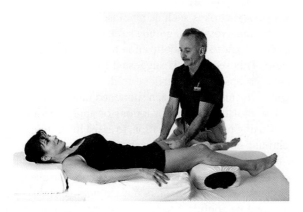

FIGURE 1-15
Myofascial Pressure and Depth Come from Therapist's Entire Body.

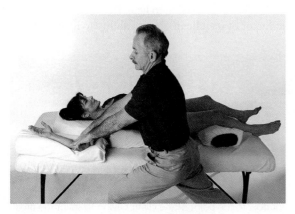

FIGURE 1-16
Ideal Body Mechanics Minimizes Energy and Maximizes Results.

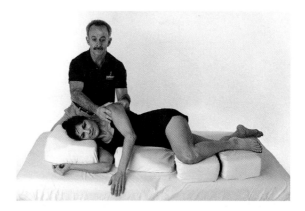

FIGURE 1-17
Body Support Systems Enhance Side Lying Subscapularis Work.

- Use cushions, such as body support systems, to allow for better body mechanics for you and to position the client's body for more effective therapy.

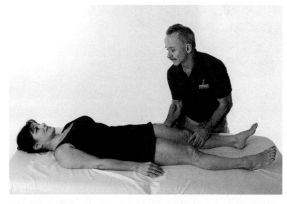

FIGURE 1-18
Support Elbow into Hip to Minimize Energy and Maximize Results.

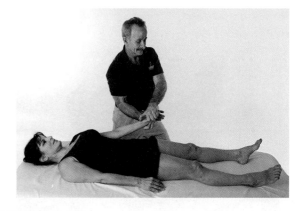

FIGURE 1-19
Support Elbow and Rotate from Hips.

- Transfer weight from your pelvis to your arm.

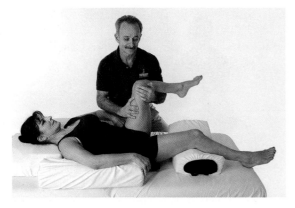

FIGURE 1-20
Compression and Traction Comes from Therapist's Hips and Legs.

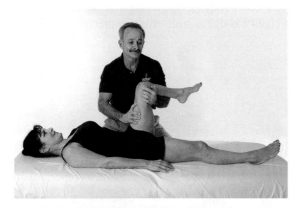

FIGURE 1-21
Maintain Straight Upper Body.

- When doing hip capsule work, keep your back and neck straight. Bend at your knees and rotate from your hips.
- Compress and decompress using your hips and knees.
- Make sure to protect the client's knee, and apply even pressure on the muscles with your hands. Squeezing the muscle with your fingertips can cause pain.

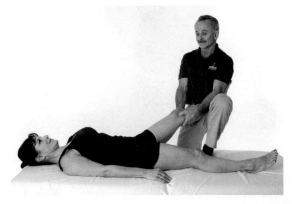

FIGURE 1-22
Hip Decompression Using Therapist's Entire Body.

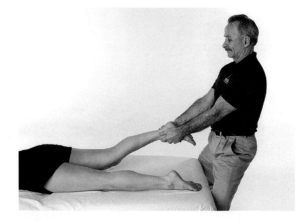

FIGURE 1-23
Traction Comes from Entire Body Leaning Back.

- When you traction or decompress the hip, knee, or ankle joints, lean back with your entire body, keeping your hips, back, and neck straight.

Step 5: Area Preparation

The goal is to prepare the area by applying moist heat or heating ointments to facilitate myofascial release.

Preparing the area for clinical massage involves general massage strokes such as myofascial spreading, gentle compression, cross-fiber gliding strokes, trigger point work, and gentle scar tissue mobilization to encourage soft-tissue release. This sequence is suggested to release short, tight muscle groups from superficial to deep, moving from the origin to the insertion of each shortened muscle group.

Use moist heat, oils, or lotions or apply heating ointments, using minimal lubrication, to assist in warming areas of chronic, nonacute pain. You should observe and evaluate the results of the technique, the depth of pressure, and the speed of movement used to release the tissue. The client may experience discomfort, pain, or muscle spasms. Use positive words and be confident to help repattern and interrupt the pain response to the client's brain. You can help the client visualize letting go of the pain by using words such as "feel the release" or "feel the tissue softening" during therapy. Give the client permission to heal. Remember, you are only a facilitator of the client's innate ability to heal.

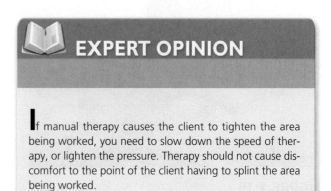

EXPERT OPINION

If manual therapy causes the client to tighten the area being worked, you need to slow down the speed of therapy, or lighten the pressure. Therapy should not cause discomfort to the point of the client having to splint the area being worked.

Always treat the cause of pain before treating the symptoms or specific area of pain. The use of ice on the muscle belly is not recommended unless there is inflammation (heat, redness, or swelling). Ice causes the fascia to become less mobile and can restrict soft-tissue mobilization. This is counterproductive to the mobilization and healing process that the therapy work is promoting. Ice is more commonly used to treat joint pain, due to resultant inflammation, tendinitis, and calcification during the acute and subacute phase of an injury. However, the application of products like Bio-freeze can calm the pain receptors in nonacute tender areas to allow for deeper and more effective treatments (Figure 1-24 ■).

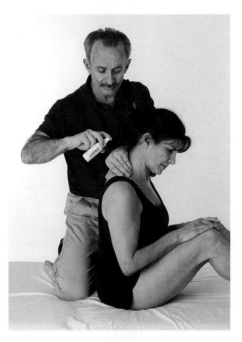

FIGURE 1-24
Application of Biofreeze Prior to or After Treatment to Calm the Pain Receptors.

Step 6: Myofascial Release

Fascia surrounds every muscle, muscle fiber, and component in the body. It is the connective tissue that holds the body together. As such, any injury, accident, muscle imbalance, or immobility can create tight or restricted fascia. You should perform **myofascial release** techniques that will expand the connective tissue, thus maximizing blood flow to the ischemic tissues and promoting healing. Investigators at Ball State University found that soft-tissue mobilization increases fibroblast recruitment and promotes healing.[6] To maximize space and to restore the client's connective tissue to a functional, neutral, and anatomical position you need to direct the fascia back to its normal position in the body.

Myofascial release is one of the most important of the twelve steps. It always precedes and enhances deeper, more specific work. It creates space around muscle tissue and is a preparatory step to further access structures within and around the muscles. Myofascia responds to heat, pressure,

movement, and gentle stretch. Myofascial work is the primary modality to be used on pain described by the client as general, covering a broad area, or diffuse and the client is unable to pinpoint the exact area of pain.

TECHNIQUE FOR MYOFASCIAL RELEASE

Goal: to warm, soften, and mobilize the fascia, and to move the fascial layers back to normal resting positions. This facilitates musculoskeletal balance throughout the body. You want to restore all opposing muscle groups throughout the body to their normal resting lengths.

- Apply light lubricant with palmar friction to create warmth (Figure 1-25 ■). A product with ideal viscosity is suggested, such as Prossage Heat, to hook the deep investing fascia without too much glide.
- Release fascia at a 45-degree angle into the tissue using the palms of your hands, or back of your fists, and then progress to using your knuckles or finger pads. Always move the fascia back to its normal resting position. This usually means starting with the client face up to release the strong flexors before working the usually weak antagonistic extensors (Figure 1-26 ■).
- Apply compression to the muscle belly, between each myofascial sequence, to increase blood flow. The increased blood flow can bring more warmth and oxygen at the capillary level and enhance deeper, pain-free myofascial responses (Figure 1-27 ■).
- Work superficial layers to progressively deeper layers.
- Work slowly and with very little lubrication to hook and mobilize the fascial layers.

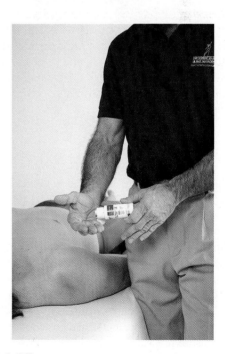

FIGURE 1-25
Prossage Heat Enhances Myofascial Release.

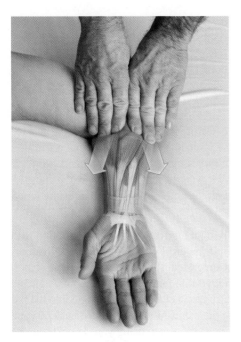

FIGURE 1-26
Myofascial Spreading to Forearm.

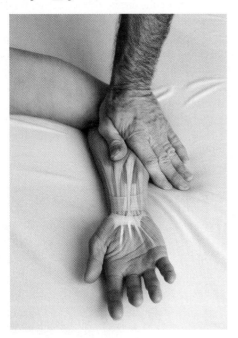

FIGURE 1-27
Compression Broadening to Forearm Muscles.

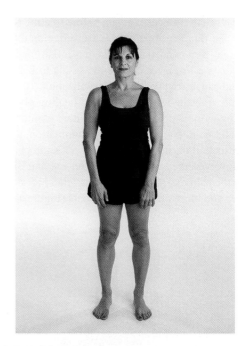

FIGURE 1-28
Medially Rotated Shoulders.

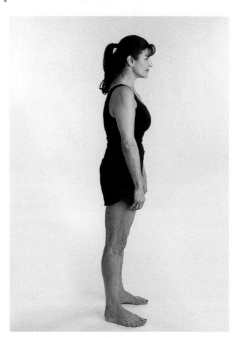

FIGURE 1-29
Forward Head Posture.

Start on the shortened or contracted, tight muscles to bring the joint to a neutral position. For example, most clients' shoulders are medially rotated, with a forward head posture, due to tight pectorals, subscapularis, SCMs, and scalene muscles. (Figures 1-28 ■ and 1-29 ■). This misalignment creates weak, inhibited and sometimes overstretched rhomboids, infraspinatus, teres minor, and posterior cervical muscles. Focus on releasing the muscle groups in front of the neck and shoulders, rather treating the pain in the back, as is the tendency of many therapists. As a result, less neuromuscular treatment or trigger point therapy will be needed.

Step 7: Cross-Fiber Gliding Strokes/Trigger Point Therapy

Cross-fiber gliding strokes and **trigger point** therapy are two different techniques of releasing tissues. Which one is appropriate to use depends on the client's condition. While working through tender areas, you will need to learn to differentiate among the following:

- **Active muscle belly trigger points.** Actively refers pain locally or to another location. (Most trigger points refer pain elsewhere in the body along nerve

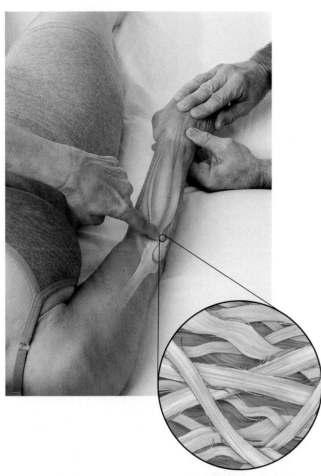

Disorganized scar tissue

FIGURE 1-30
Muscle Resistance Test for Strain.

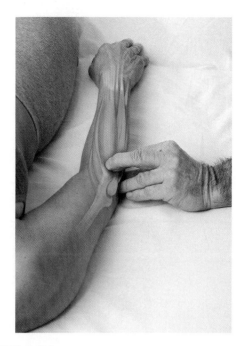

FIGURE 1-31
Multidirectional Friction.

origin to insertion on tight or contracted muscle groups to create length, and usually from insertion to origin on weak and inhibited muscle groups to create relaxation. Keep in mind that your ultimate goal is to restore normal muscle resting lengths to opposing muscle groups throughout the body. This is much more effective and gentler than stripping through muscle fibers, and enhances the release of that muscle group beyond what doing only trigger point work would accomplish.

pathways.) These tender sites need trigger point therapy, based on the Travell trigger point theories.[7]

- **Tight muscle fiber pain.** Located directly under your pressure, this requires cross-fiber gliding strokes to loosen up tight muscle fibers that often feed and contribute to active, latent, and satellite trigger points.
- **Scar tissue.** Pain is located by doing a muscle resistance test and is referred to as a muscle–tendon strain (Figure 1-30 ■). This requires multidirectional friction (step 8) to soften the matrix of dysfunctional scar that limits movement and creates pain with movement (Figure 1-31 ■).

CROSS-FIBER GLIDING STROKES

Cross-fiber gliding techniques are used when a client has tight muscles creating restrictions in the tissue. The gliding strokes are beneficial because they help spread apart tight muscle bands, affecting the fibers by releasing restrictions, so the muscle fibers can move freely and more independently. Cross-fiber gliding strokes should be performed prior to trigger point work to loosen tight muscle fibers that feed active and latent muscle belly trigger points. Tease the tight muscle fibers apart as you evaluate for trigger points. Work from

TECHNIQUE FOR APPLYING CROSS-FIBER GLIDING STROKES

Goal: to tease apart tight muscle bands in contracted, shortened muscle groups and to relax the tight bands in weak, inhibited, or overstretched muscle groups (Figure 1-32 ■).

- Use your thumbs, knuckles, or supported fingers.
- Move back and forth across the longitudinal muscle fibers or area of restricted tissue.
- Perform strokes called cross-fiber gliding strokes, working across and along the entire length of the muscle.
- Repeat using slower, deeper strokes performed pain-free, until the tissue softens.
- Add additional compression strokes to the muscle belly to enhance pain-free cross-fiber work.
- Add additional deeper myofascial spreading techniques to enhance softening and release of muscle fibers. Work from superficial to deep.
- Sequence cross-fiber strokes, compression, and myofascial spreading as needed to keep the work pain-free. There is synergy among these three techniques to increase hyperemia.

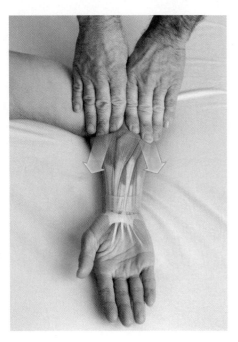

FIGURE 1-32
Myofascial Spreading, Forearm Muscles.

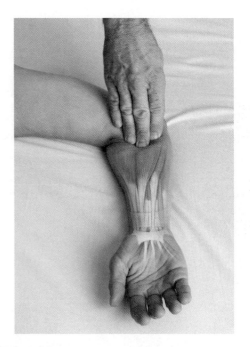

FIGURE 1-33
Cross-Fiber Gliding Strokes/Trigger Point Work.

TRIGGER POINT THERAPY

Trigger points are small, painful nodules located in tight muscles. Active muscle belly trigger points actively refer pain elsewhere in the body, along nerve pathways in a predictable pattern. When direct pressure is applied to active muscle belly trigger points, they refer or radiate pain away from the site of pressure along nerve pathways in a predictable pattern. A latent trigger point is one that exists but does not yet refer pain actively, but may do so when direct pressure is applied (Figure 1-33 ■).[8] By applying trigger point therapy, with moderate and sustained direct pressure for 10 to 12 seconds to the tender site, the therapist can diminish or eliminate the pain created by active and latent muscle belly trigger points.

Dr. A. Cathie points out that many trigger points (he calls them trigger "spots") correspond to points where nerves pierce fascial investments.[9] Hence sustained tension or traction on the fascia may lead to varying degrees of fascial entrapment of neural structures and consequently a wide range of symptoms and dysfunctions. Any appropriate manual treatment, movement, or exercise is likely to modulate these negative effects and reduce trigger point activity. A degree of normal function may return when the soft-tissue circulatory environment is improved and the stress-producing elements, whether of biomechanical, biochemical, or psychological origin, are reduced or removed. Trigger points may occur in numerous body structures; however, only those occurring in myofascial structures are named myofascial trigger points.

A clinical massage therapist's focus is primarily on treating active and latent muscle belly trigger points, to help restore normal muscle resting lengths. That is why the release of a trigger point is followed with digital compression and fascial stretch. Trigger points may also occur in skin, ligaments, joint capsules, and periosteal and scar tissue. Stretching a muscle before releasing its active muscle belly trigger points might further inflame or stress the attachments. Clinical experience and research suggest that "key" predictable trigger points exist, which if deactivated relieve activity in satellite trigger points that are located in other muscle areas rather than the original source of pain (Figure 1-34 ■).[10]

TECHNIQUE FOR APPLYING TRIGGER POINT THERAPY

Goal: to release active and latent trigger points in the muscle belly if they are found.

Ask the client the following question when you locate a tender area of congested tissue:

- "Does the pain radiate or refer to another location other than where I apply direct pressure?" Evaluate for a predictable pattern based on the Travell trigger point theories for active and latent muscle belly trigger points.[11]
  - If yes, this is a trigger point. Apply direct, moderate pressure for 10 to 12 seconds until a proprioceptive change occurs and the tissue releases or softens.
  - Follow this with gentle compressions over the area to pump blood to the ischemic tissue and further soften the area.
  - Gently stretch the fascia feeding the ischemic, tender area since you are addressing active and latent myofascial trigger points with this technique.

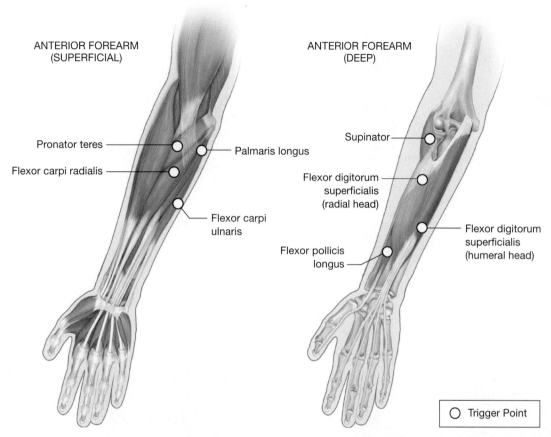

ANTERIOR FOREARM
(SUPERFICIAL)

ANTERIOR FOREARM
(DEEP)

Pronator teres

Flexor carpi radialis

Palmaris longus

Flexor carpi
ulnaris

Supinator

Flexor digitorum
superficialis
(radial head)

Flexor pollicis
longus

Flexor digitorum
superficialis
(humeral head)

○ Trigger Point

FIGURE 1-34
Trigger Points.

It is important to work pain-free. If you sense that the client is guarding or apprehensive during therapy, then that should be your cue to ease up on your pressure.

Focus on performing trigger point work on the contracted, tight muscles. Creating structural balance around the joint often eliminates painful trigger points, tender points, and myofascial pain patterns in the weak, inhibited, and sometimes overstretched muscle groups. Then they can be more effectively strengthened as part of client self-care.

Step 8: Multidirectional Friction

Multidirectional friction is performed if the client experiences increased pain to a specific area during your assessment of resisted range of motion or during a deep stretch (step 4). During RROM, if the client experiences pain in a specific area—which indicates a muscle–tendon **strain** or ligament **sprain**—multidirectional friction techniques are most appropriate. A strain involves injury to the muscle, muscle–tendon junction, or periosteal junction, whereas a sprain is an injury to the ligamentous tissue. Typically, injuries occur either at the muscle–tendon junction or at the periosteal junction. After an injury, damaged tissue heals with **collagen** fiber formation or scar tissue creating adhesions, resulting in pain and limited movement. The collagen

fibers form a fiberglass-like matrix in multiple directions and multiple layers (Figure 1-35 ■).

Multidirectional friction can free up the collagen (**scar tissue**) that is causing pain, thickening, and limitations in the client's range of motion especially since the original dysfunctional scar has certain thicker fibers that run in multiple directions due to immobilization following pain or injury.

TECHNIQUE FOR APPLYING MULTIDIRECTIONAL FRICTION

Goal: to soften the collagen matrix by working in multiple directions to prepare for a more functional alignment of scar tissue fibers.

● Perform the resisted range of motion (RROM) test to locate the scar tissue (Figure 1-36 ■).
● Use a supported finger to massage the tissue in different directions for a total of only 20 to 30 seconds. Performing this technique begins to soften the collagen fibers. The skin must move with the stroke to affect the underlying strained or sprained fibers (Figure 1-37 ■). Close your eyes to enhance palpation, and tune in to the direction of each multidirectional

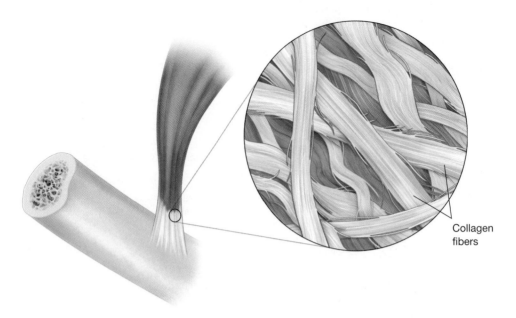

Collagen
fibers

FIGURE 1-35
Multidirectional Scar.

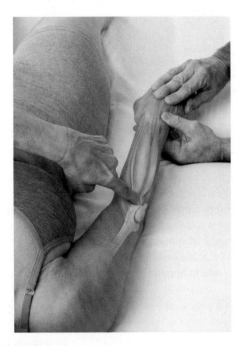

FIGURE 1-36
Muscle Resistance Test for Strain.

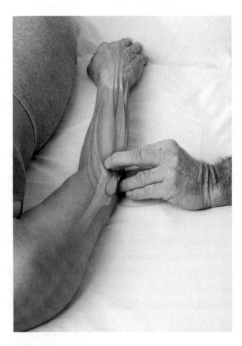

FIGURE 1-37
Multidirectional Friction.

stroke. Find the fiber direction or directions that are thicker and more restricted and work on softening or releasing them. Do not overwork the area. Use only enough pressure to soften the fiber matrix.

- Perform this technique several times, working from superficial to deep.
- Follow it each time with pain-free movement and pain-free eccentric alignment (explained in steps 9 and 10 and in a later section of this chapter titled "Scar Tissue Mobilization").

The reason for 20 to 30 seconds of multidirectional friction, performed several times, is to avoid the secondary inflammation that is often associated with therapy that consists of 6 to 12 minutes of deep cross-fiber friction. The original scar is multilayered and multidirectional and thus you can help avoid inflammation and additional fibroblast formation by working for shorter time periods and into progressively deeper layers, followed by pain-free movement and pain-free eccentric muscle contractions. This breaks down the scar in layers without the side effect of inflammation. It is not the friction technique that realigns the scar, rather the pain-free movement and pain-free eccentric muscle contraction that follow the friction technique.

Step 9: Pain-Free Movement

Pain-free movement following multidirectional friction begins the process of realigning scar tissue fibers to create functional scar tissue. The softened scar matrix migrates in the direction of muscle–tendon movement. Once pain-free movement is achieved, along with balanced muscles around the joints of the body, structural integration can occur. An aligned and balanced body with correct posture allows for greater ease of movement with little or no pain.

TECHNIQUE FOR ASSESSING PAIN-FREE MOVEMENT

Goal: to determine if the client can actively perform specific movement without pain. If so, this gives permission to proceed with pain-free eccentric scar tissue alignment techniques.

- Reassess the client's active range of motion (AROM—step 2).
- Ask the client if he or she was able to perform the movement pain-free. Have the client *actively* perform the specific single-plane movement several times for neuromuscular reeducation. In the example of extensor tendinosis, ask for full wrist flexion and extension.
- Range of motion should be increased and pain-free.
- Proceed to step 10, eccentric scar tissue alignment.

If the client performed the movement and it was not pain-free, return to multidirectional friction (step 8), working a little slower and deeper. Continue to mobilize the tissue and reassess until the client achieves pain-free movement. The client's movement must be pain-free before you proceed to step 10.

Step 10: Eccentric Scar Tissue Alignment

There are three kinds of muscle contraction: eccentric, concentric, and isometric. **Eccentric contraction** is when the muscle–tendon unit lengthens against mild resistance. Concentric contraction is when the muscle–tendon unit shortens against resistance. Isometric contraction is when no movement occurs in the muscle–tendon unit as resistance is applied. Performed pain-free on a client with a muscle–tendon strain, an eccentric muscle contraction creates improved collagen fiber regeneration and organization so that the muscle–tendon achieves the necessary tensile strength for normal function. The multidirectional collagen organizes into fibers that are oriented parallel to each other in the direction of the opposite forces, produced during the muscle–tendon lengthening of the eccentric contraction. This affects even deeper layers of scar tissue resulting in functional, pain-free scar tissue alignment (Figures 1-38 ■ and 1-39 ■).[12] Eccentric contraction is performed after

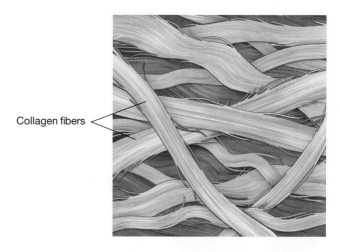

Collagen fibers

Disorganized Scar Tissue

FIGURE 1-38
Disorganized Collagen.

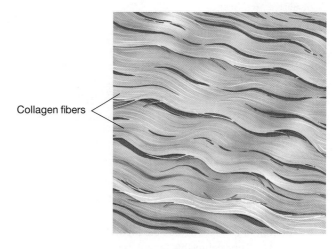

Collagen fibers

Organized Scar Tissue

FIGURE 1-39
Organized Collagen.

multidirectional friction (step 8) and pain-free movement (step 9) are achieved.

TECHNIQUE FOR APPLYING ECCENTRIC SCAR TISSUE ALIGNMENT

Goal: to apply pain-free eccentric contraction by lengthening an injured muscle–tendon unit against mild resistance to realign or redirect the scar tissue (Figure 1-40 ■).

- Activate and begin to restructure the myofibrils by having the client actively lengthen the specific muscle involved to its full (pain-free) range of motion.

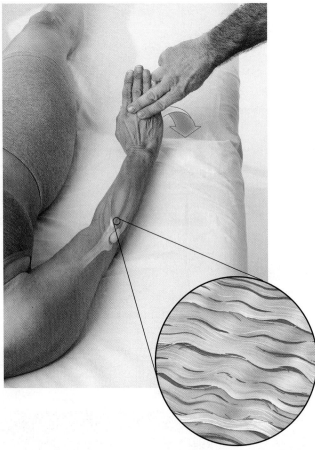

Functional scar tissue

FIGURE 1-40

Eccentric Muscle Contraction.

- Ask the client to very gently contract and shorten the specific involved muscle.
- Attempt to gently lengthen the involved muscle–tendon unit, to its normal resting length, by providing a pain-free pressure that is barely greater than the force of the client's contraction, asking the client to "barely resist, but let me win (Figure 1-40)."
- Start with the pressure of only two fingers. The pressure should minimally overcome the client's contraction and allow the muscle to lengthen, pain-free.
- Ask the client to increase resistance if he or she has zero discomfort. This progressively increased *pain-free* force of movement is performed to help realign the deeper layers of scar tissue. The greatest error when performing the eccentric alignment procedure is being too aggressive and not keeping the technique pain-free each time.
- Perform a resisted test on the involved muscle. If the client is still experiencing pain at the specific spot, repeat step 8 (multidirectional friction), working pain-free and progressing deeper, followed by steps 9 and 10 (pain-free movement and eccentric scar tissue alignment). Continue to reassess and repeat up to three times per treatment if needed until the pain is gone.

Step 11: Stretching (During Therapy/Client Self-Care)

During therapy, stretches will be utilized to create normal range of motion and normal resting length in the client's shortened or contracted muscle groups. Explain these stretches to the client, as client self-care involves clients performing many of these same stretches at home to maintain structural balance and pain-free movement following their therapies.

STRETCHING (DURING THERAPY)

When you view the twelve-step flow chart you will notice that steps 1 to 8 are performed relatively in order; you may have reached this point (step 11) without finding a muscle strain (step 8 directly to step 11). Contract-relax, contract-antagonist (PNF) with active assisted stretching is performed next. Performing the initial contract-relax technique incorporates a muscle resistance test prior to the stretch. This method can determine if there is an unsuspected muscle strain present. While contracting the muscle against resistance (contract-relax) to fatigue the muscle prior to the stretch the client may report pain in a specific area, which is a muscle strain. In such case, proceed in order from multidirectional friction (step 8) to pain-free movement (step 9), and finally to eccentric scar tissue alignment (step 10) until the client is pain-free. If there is no pain during the muscle contraction against resistance (contract-relax) before the stretch, continue to fatigue the muscle–tendon unit isometrically for 10 seconds. The client should take a deep breath to allow time for the proprioceptors to register the fatigue and create post isometric relaxation, and then proceed with the stretch (contract-antagonist with active assisted stretching) until the normal range of motion is achieved. The actual stretch, based on the work of Aaron Mattes, is held for only one to two seconds each time following postisometric relaxation.

Apply specific, isolated stretching techniques to the tight, contracted muscles restricting normal movement. Do *not* perform stretches on the weak, inhibited, or over-stretched muscles because these muscles need to be strengthened to restore structural balance (i.e., clients who stretch weak, painful muscle groups like the rhomboids may contribute to structural and postural imbalance). The technique you will use is a combination of two stretching techniques called contract-relax, contract-antagonist (PNF) and **active assisted stretching:**

- **Proprioceptive neuromuscular facilitation (PNF).** This is a stretching technique where a muscle is actively stretched, then contracts isometrically against resistance (contract-antagonist), then is actively stretched again to facilitate increased range of motion.[13]
- **Active assisted stretching.** This involves the therapist gently assisting a stretch with movement performed actively by the client. Active movements are recommended to provide a facilitated stretch and avoid potential injuries. When one muscle group contracts,

the antagonist is inhibited through reciprocal inhibition and the client will often avoid pain or a secondary injury if he or she is actively involved in the stretch.[14]

This type of stretching uses the nervous system to turn the muscles on and off, allowing the client's subconscious brain to remember the new pain-free movement so it does not undermine your work. If the client perceives pain, optimum stretching results may not occur. Common tendency is to not only stretch tissue before it can release, but also to stretch it for too long. Stretch the area for only 2 seconds each time, just enough to bring blood and oxygen to the area and to promote optimum results. If the tissue is already injured or ischemic, holding a stretch for more than 2 seconds can create a secondary **ischemia** and possible muscle spasm. If the restrictions in the muscle–tendon group being stretched have not been addressed prior to the stretch, the symptoms in the muscle–tendon junction and periosteal insertion could get worse as this is where the inflammation, calcification, and resultant tendonitis or tendinosis response is going on. Many people focus on the resultant symptoms of joint pain with ice and pain medications without first addressing the underlying cause.

TECHNIQUE FOR STRETCHING DURING THERAPY

Goal: to create normal muscle resting lengths in shortened or contracted muscle groups (Figure 1-41 ■).

- The therapist lengthens or stretches the agonist muscle (prime mover) to a comfortable point.
- Ask the client to contract the agonist isometrically (no movement occurs), contracting at 20 percent force for 5 to 10 seconds against your resistance. This action fatigues the agonist muscle.
- Ask the client to relax and inhale deeply to allow the **proprioceptors** to adjust to the change in the muscle tension and to create **post isometric relaxation.**

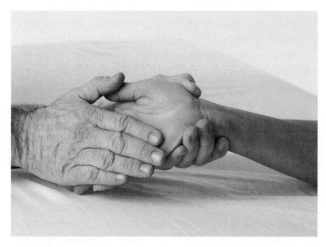

FIGURE 1-41
PNF Stretch, Wrist Flexors.

- On exhale, the client actively contracts the antagonist muscle to facilitate **reciprocal inhibition,** which inhibits the nerve impulses in the agonist and allows a greater range of motion to occur without tension or possible injury.
- Gently assist the stretch for about 2 seconds. At the new stretched position, repeat the sequence several times.

As you perform these stretches, remember several things:

- Make sure the client exhales during the contract-antagonist phase. Holding the breath may increase blood pressure.
- Gently traction the joint before and during stretching, as this increases joint space, which improves vascular circulation and may prevent excess pressure on articulating cartilage in that joint, preventing degenerative arthritis.
- It is critical not to increase range of motion past the normal range in all directions to avoid hypermobility. Your goal is to restore all muscle groups throughout the body to their normal resting lengths.

STRETCHING (CLIENT SELF-CARE)

 PRECAUTIONARY NOTE

In certain states, clinical massage therapists are not allowed to suggest stretches. If you are not competent, or feel that suggesting stretches is outside your scope of practice, do not suggest them to your clients. Be safe, refer out, or become certified as a personal trainer.

Emphasize client self-care! Client self-care is essential for the client to "keep" the new normal range of motion that was created during therapy. Clients *must* learn these techniques and perform them at home to accustom their minds and bodies to the new pain-free range of motion. Teach the clients active assisted stretching first. Once they understand the stretches and can correctly perform them for you, you can teach them the more advanced PNF stretches. To perform the stretches, the client needs a stretch rope, towel, or long belt.

TECHNIQUE FOR STRETCHING FOR CLIENT SELF-CARE

Goal: for the client to perform stretches suggested and demonstrated by you to create normal muscle resting lengths in shortened or contracted muscle groups (Figure 1-42 ■).

- Tell the client that the stretches will take only a few minutes a day to perform and are necessary for continued results.

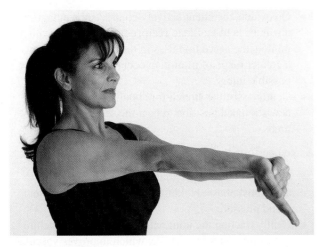

FIGURE 1-42
Forearm Flexors Stretch.

- The client should also stretch after exercise or a hot shower when the fascia and muscles are warm.
- Tell the client to *not* stretch into pain. He or she needs to differentiate between uncomfortable stretching due to tight muscles and painful stretching that can aggravate a condition.
- The client starts the stretches with the tightest side first until normal range of motion is achieved. Then he or she continues to stretch both sides for continued balance and symmetry.
- Suggest only two to four stretches or strengthening exercises, specific to his or her condition, each time you see a client. Make sure the client can perform these correctly before suggesting any additional exercises.
- Print copies of these exercises for your clients to take with them for reference.

Without client self-care, the client's therapy results will usually last less than 48 hours. As he or she returns to some of the same poor postural patterns and repetitive day-to-day motions, the result will be loss of range of motion. Even though clinical massage therapists can address proper posture and ergonomics of the workstation, as the client sits in a chair, drives a car, or works on the computer, he or she still returns to a flexed posture and the results of the therapy can be diminished.

Step 12: Strengthening (Client Self-Care)

 PRECAUTIONARY NOTE

In certain states, clinical massage therapists are not allowed to suggest strengthening exercises. If you are not competent, or if you feel that suggesting strengthening exercises is outside your scope of practice, do not suggest them to your clients. Be safe, refer out, or become certified as a personal trainer.

The final step in the twelve-step approach to pain management is strengthening the weak, inhibited, and sometimes overstretched muscles. These muscles lack blood flow and oxygen and need to be strengthened to allow complete structural integration throughout the body. Strengthening is essential to a client's continued improvement and recovery and prevention of injury. The client must stretch the tight, contracted muscles before strengthening the opposing weak, inhibited, or overstretched muscles.

Demonstrate the strengthening exercises for your clients and then instruct them on how to practice the movements at home. The only item needed is a Thera-Band (elastic resistance tubing). Research has proved that elastic resistance training (ERT) provides as much benefit as weight-training machines.[15]

- ERT can enhance strength, flexibility, speed, balance, gait, mobility, and agility.
- ERT can increase muscle mass and decrease body fat.
- ERT makes exercise functional and efficient by working single or multiple muscles at a time.
- The eccentric phase of the muscle contraction lays down new collagen and aligns the collagen that is softened during multidirectional frictioning. This makes recovery from muscle–tendon strains fast and permanent.

TECHNIQUE FOR STRENGTHENING FOR CLIENT SELF-CARE

Goal: to strengthen weak, inhibited muscle groups around a joint, creating muscle balance throughout the body and thus aiding in structural integration.

- Have the client stretch the tight antagonist muscles first.
- Show the client how to control and adjust the amount of resistance on the Thera-Band.
- Make sure the client's movements while performing the exercises are slow and controlled during both the concentric (muscle shortening phase) and eccentric (muscle lengthening phase) contractions, *placing more emphasis on the eccentric phase.* Since many injuries occur during eccentric activity, it is important to strengthen this phase for effective recovery.[16]
- Tell the client that only 5 to 10 minutes per day is needed to perform both stretching and strengthening exercises for any single clinical condition.
- After an injury, make sure the client is evaluated by a physician and wait 7 to 10 days or until the client is pain-free before beginning a strengthening program.
- Empower clients to take responsibility for reeducating their muscles, keeping their body aligned, and participating in their own wellness.

If you follow the twelve-step approach of assessment, treatment, and client self-care that is outlined in this chapter, it will lead you to breakthroughs in isolating the detailed issue of chronic pain and sports injuries.

ORIGINS OF THE TWELVE-STEP APPROACH

The twelve-step approach developed out of the author's study and teachings. In observing a presentation at an Australian Massage Therapy convention by a leading physiotherapist in that country, he was inspired by the physiotherapist's reference to work with patellar tendon pain.

This research project involved clients who had a clinical diagnosis of patellar tendonitis, and whose chief presenting complaint was anterior knee pain. Two different methods were used to treat these clients' symptoms:

- In one group of clients, techniques such as cross-fiber friction and sometimes electrical stimulation and ultrasound were applied to the area of the patellar tendon pain.
- In the other group, techniques such as massage and isolated stretching were employed to release and balance the tension in the quadriceps muscle groups.

The second method produced much better outcomes, with clients' knee symptoms either reduced or completely eliminated. The combination of massage and active isolated stretching techniques had reduced the unbalanced tension, thereby addressing the underlying cause of the symptoms in the area of muscle–tendon insertion, and eliminating the patellar tendon pain. These findings catalyzed the eventual development of the twelve-step approach in regard to balancing out muscle groups throughout the body prior to treating symptoms at joints. Their influence is evident in the descriptions of the steps presented earlier in this chapter.

TENDINOSIS TECHNIQUES AND SCAR TISSUE MOBILIZATION

The twelve-step approach differs from other methods of treating chronic pain, especially in its treatment of tendinosis and scar tissue mobilization.

Tendinosis Techniques

Tendinosis most often results from prolonged poor posture, repetitive motion, constant muscle overload, or musculoskeletal injury typically due to musculoskeletal imbalance. Conventional treatment has involved treating the strained fibers by performing 6 minutes of deep cross-fiber friction, often prior to treating the underlying muscle and skeletal imbalance, with ice applied afterward. The cross-fiber friction is intended to mobilize the collagen fibers, to allow movement to be less painful or pain-free, and to create a more functional scar. However, a number of factors suggest that 6 minutes of deep cross-fiber friction may not be an appropriate treatment method, especially in many types of tendon pain conditions.

Fascia is a form of connective tissue that wraps everything inside the body, including the muscles, like a web. When heat, pressure, and movement are applied, it becomes more fluid and more mobile. Thus, to enhance fascial mobilization, heat may be most effective on the muscle belly if there is not inflammation. Given that the cooling effect of ice restricts the fascia and reduces circulation, it seems logical to conclude that applying ice to the muscle belly may counteract the mobilizing effects of soft-tissue work. In regard to deep cross-fiber friction to the collagen fibers of a sprain or strain, in some clients, 6 minutes of deep cross-fiber friction can actually *induce* additional inflammation in the area of muscle–tendon or periosteal pain, and that inflammation in turn must be iced. Clients treated with traditional cross-fiber friction also frequently experience recurring tendon complaints, which also suggests that this method may not adequately address the problem based on cause and symptom.

In cases of tendon imbalance or opposing **tendon tension,** deep cross-fiber friction also is not appropriate. As suggested by the aforementioned Australian research project, a more effective approach would be to release and stretch the typically tight flexors to relax the typically weak, inhibited extensors and create balance in opposing groups of muscles and tendons around the joint. If muscles and tendons are left tight and out of balance, the result could be increased tendon pain, with resultant tendonitis or tendinosis, often referred to as muscle strain. Some health care practitioners do not even evaluate whether tendinitis or tendinosis is present, and inappropriately apply deep cross-fiber friction for 6 minutes to healthy, but tight and painful tendons.

To determine if there is an actual strain, the clinical massage therapist should perform muscle resistance testing by having the client contract the affected muscle group against the therapist's resistance. The client then identifies the exact area of torn fibers by pointing at it with one finger. If the results of this test indicate that there is no strain, then there is no reason to perform deep cross-fiber friction.

TENDINOSIS RESEARCH

There are many differing opinions on how to most effectively treat tendinitis and areas of scar tissue. In most instances, the term *tendinitis* itself is an inappropriate term. The suffix "-itis" refers to inflammation, but in most chronic cases of tendon pain, clients have no associated inflammation or accompanying redness and swelling. A more appropriate term would be *tendinosis:* the tearing of tendon fibers in the absence of an inflammatory process. Important research and information on tendinosis is both paraphrased and extracted in the following text primarily from two sources: Khan et al.[17] and Cook et al.[18]

> Overuse tendinopathies are common in primary care. Numerous investigators worldwide have shown that the pathology underlying these conditions is tendinosis or collagen degeneration. This applies equally in the Achilles, patellar, medial and lateral elbow, and rotator cuff tendons. Unfortunately, distinguishing

tendinosis from the rare tendinitis is difficult clinically. But because tendinosis is far more likely, our advice is to treat patients initially as if tendinosis were the diagnosis. An increasing body of evidence supports the notion that overuse conditions *do not involve inflammation.* The traditional approach to treating tendinopathies as an inflammatory "tendinitis" is likely flawed. If physicians acknowledge that overuse tendinopathies are due to tendinosis, they must modify patient management in at least 8 areas. [19]

These eight areas include:

- **Biomechanical deloading/correction:** "Tendinosis results from collagen degeneration and mechanical overload so determining why it occurred is important. Some of the reasons are muscular imbalances, training errors, faulty equipment and improper movement biomechanics."[20]
- **Load reduction and relative rest:** "Complete immobilization of an injured tendon is contraindicated because the tensile load stimulates collagen production and directs its alignment. Relative rest means the clients don't have to "stop everything" and may continue playing or training if elements of the activity or total weekly training hours can be reduced."[21]
- **Anti-inflammatory strategies:** "A review of the role of NSAIDS and corticosteroids in treating tendinopathy found little evidence that they were helpful. favor."[22]
- Given the known deleterious effect of corticosteroid injection into tendon and *inhibition of collagen repair* when the drug is injected around tendon, this treatment has lost favor.[23]
- **Appropriate strengthening:** "Eccentric strengthening programs have a long track record of clinical effectiveness[24,25] and recent research adds further scientific support.[26,27] It is likely that specific eccentric training result in tendon strengthening by stimulating mechanoreceptors in *tenocytes to produce collagen,* and thus help reverse the tendinosis *cycle.*[28] *Collagen production is probably the key cellular phenomenon that determines recovery from tendinosis.* Animal experiments have reve*aled that loading the tendon improves collagen alignment* and stimulates collagen cross-linkage formation, both of which improve tensile strength."[29]
- **Imaging:** "Tendinopathies are very well visualized with both magnetic resonance imaging (MRI) and diagnostic ultrasound. We use MRI to confirm our clinical diagnosis and to demonstrate to the patient that in tendinosis, tendon collagen has lost continuity."[30]
- **Patient education:** "The physician should take the time to explain and illustrate the pathology of tendinosis, especially since textbooks and Web sites have yet to embrace this pathology and its clinical implications."[31]
- **Surgery as a last resort:** Surgery has been considered the treatment of last resort for tendinosis as it has not been proven to stimulate collagen synthesis or maturation.

Physicians must shift their perspective and acknowledge that tendinosis is the pathology being treated in most cases and that treatment needs to combat collagen breakdown rather than inflammation because regimens that seek to minimize (nonexistent) inflammation would appear illogical. Tendinosis requires attention to strengthening with the aim of first breaking the tendinosis cycle. Once this is done, the client uses modalities that optimize collagen production and maturation so that the tendon achieves the necessary tensile strength for normal function. Although there have been few studies of massage, we believe this modality is essential for maintaining a compliant muscle during rehabilitation.

Scar Tissue Mobilization

When cross-fiber friction was revealed to be inappropriate in some cases, it became clear that a different approach was needed—hence the emergence of the multidirectional friction technique for mobilizing scar tissue. Scar tissue is dense, fibrous, contracted tissue that forms as a result of injury. Damaged tissue heals with scar tissue formation in multiple directions and multiple layers, resulting in limited movement and pain (Figure 1-43A ■). The use of the scar tissue mobilization technique frequently achieves the result of allowing the client to remain pain-free and the area of scar tissue to remain smooth to palpation after treatment. Long-term outcomes of patients treated with it support its effectiveness. Despite its practical success, however, it has been viewed as somewhat controversial because it runs counter to prevailing wisdom.

Conventional theory holds that it is the act of frictioning that reorients the direction of the injured fibers. However, this is a popular and persistent myth. It is not the friction technique itself but the movement *following* the friction that redirects the scar tissue matrix in the direction of the normal healthy fibers. This is the reason the therapist asks the client to lengthen and shorten the injured muscle after frictioning; this movement redirects the new functional scar formation and realigns the tissue in the direction of the movement or force (Figure 1-43B ■).

If the movement can be performed pain-free, then it would follow that a way to increase the number of fibers being redirected would be to increase the force involved in the movement process. Eccentric muscle contraction is a technique that can be used to recruit deeper scar tissue fibers, but only if performed pain-free.

Concentric contraction occurs when a muscle group shortens against mild resistance. In contrast, eccentric contraction occurs when a muscle group lengthens against mild resistance. Consider, for example, a biceps curl performed during weight lifting. When flexing the elbow, with

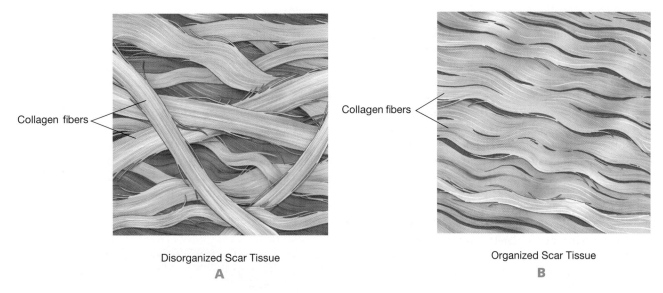

Collagen fibers

Collagen fibers

Disorganized Scar Tissue
A

Organized Scar Tissue
B

FIGURE 1-43
Comparison of Disorganized Scar and Organized Scar.

a weight held in the hand, the biceps are contracting concentrically. Eccentric contraction occurs when the elbow is slowly extended or straightened with the weight in the hand.

Consider another example of a therapist treating a client with muscle strain at the muscle–tendon junction of the wrist flexors at the elbow. After releasing the muscle belly, and following multidirectional frictioning, the client first fully flexes and extends the wrist. If that movement is pain-free, the client flexes the wrist and then resists very lightly, as the therapist extends the wrist back to neutral, creating an eccentric pain-free contraction. This is performed several times and the client resists a little more each time, but only if the eccentric force stays pain-free. The collagen matrix of the softened or frictioned fibers follows the direction of the eccentric contraction based on the forces of pull. Too much force in opposing directions can cause a new injury or reinjure the site. *The greatest error during the eccentric alignment procedure is being too aggressive and not keeping the technique pain-free each time.*

Since pain-free movement and eccentric contraction are the main factors responsible for reorienting injured muscle fibers, the theory of performing 6 minutes of cross-fiber friction for all cases of tendinitis comes into question. If a muscle resistance test were to determine that a muscle strain exists, there is no compelling reason to adhere to 6 minutes as a magic number, especially since this amount of time could exacerbate the client's inflammation.

Since the scar matrix is not only multidirectional but also multilayered, it seems reasonable to perform multiple rounds of multidirectional friction, from the superficial layers into the deeper layers, each lasting about 20 to 30 seconds, followed by pain-free movement and pain-free eccentric contraction. To lessen the likelihood of causing inflammation as a side effect of aggressive work, the friction

could be performed more slowly and deeply with each successive round. Experience has proved the effectiveness of this technique in clients treated at seminars throughout the world. Now that it is possible to realign the injured fibers in layers without causing inflammation, there is no longer any need to follow up friction with ice, except in isolated cases presenting with mild inflammation or stimulated pain receptors after the treatment. The application of Biofreeze is preferred at the end of any prolonged friction sessions to calm the activated pain receptors.

A NEW HYPOTHESIS

Once the evolutionary stages just described had been observed, tested, and successfully repeated, it was possible to formulate a new **hypothesis** of pain management, which forms the foundation of the twelve-step approach. Its main points may be summarized as follows:

- If a muscle group shortens enough times or over a long enough period, the fascia and shortened muscle groups must be stretched back to their normal resting state. If not, the tendons are likely to become painful or symptomatic, usually at the attachment areas.
- Each group of muscles has an antagonistic group of muscles. If the flexors become short and contracted, the extensors will often become weak, inhibited, or possibly overstretched.
- As opposing groups of muscles attempt to return to normal resting lengths, a myofascial or neuromuscular pain pattern may develop in either group of muscles and tendons, often without associated muscle strain or injury.

- Tendon tension may occur in both groups of tendons. Tendon tension may be defined as tight tendons in opposing muscle groups that are out of balance. The tendons may present with pain or tenderness and feel tight to palpation. That does not mean they are strained or injured.

- Most clients use their wrist flexors and pronators of the forearm more than their extensors and supinators. If the client complains of tendon pain in the extensors, the usually stronger and more contracted flexors should be released first. This brings the extensors out of a weak, inhibited, or overstretched position and relaxes both groups of opposing tendons. Many cases of tendon pain disappear simply by balancing out opposing muscle–tendon groups around each joint throughout the body.

- If tendon pain remains after performing this releasing and balancing, the next step is to (1) identify the different forms of tendon pain, such as tendon tension, tendinosis, and sheathed tendon adhesions; and (2) to distinguish them from muscle–tendon strains with inflammation. This helps ensure that the therapist applies the appropriate technique to each specific tendon pathology.

- The area of a strain is the weakest link in the chain because it is usually occurs in an area of transition of a muscle–tendon group, such as the muscle–tendon junction or periosteal junction. The weakest link should be treated last. Unfortunately, many therapists and clients go directly to the source of pain first, before releasing and balancing all of the opposing groups of muscles that lead to the area of the torn fibers.

- When performing frictioning, as the last part of the treatment protocol, the collagen matrix containing the injured fibers will follow the direction of movement and direction of the pain-free eccentric contractions based on the forces of pull.

EXPERT OPINION

This will be the most important piece of information a clinical massage therapist should live by: *Never treat a muscle–tendon strain unless the injured muscle group has first been brought back to its normal muscle resting length.*

CASE STUDY

The Pain Management Hypothesis Illustrated

A condition of the forearm, elbow, and wrist can serve as an excellent illustration of how to apply the hypothesis outlined in this chapter. This condition is generically called lateral epicondylitis, tendinitis, or tennis elbow because the symptoms occur in the areas of the lateral epicondyle where groups of muscles attach to the bones via tendons.

Let's consider the day-to-day activities of a clinical massage therapist as an example, using tendinitis of the elbow as a vehicle to explore musculoskeletal imbalance problems. A therapist who performs massage treatments all day uses the wrist flexors of his or her forearm and hand much more than the extensors.

Jane is a very successful massage therapist who sees six to eight clients per day. After her third client, her forearms begin to feel fatigued and extremely tight. The tendons of her wrist flexors are tender to palpation by lunchtime. Jane drove to work this morning, and due to heavy traffic she was squeezing the steering wheel tightly using her wrist and hand flexors. Jane then had to enter her client information into the computer for 30 minutes from yesterday's client load (Figure 1-44 ■). Jane does not realize it, but in addition to using her forearm, wrist, and hand flexors driving the car and working on the computer, she also shortened the forearm pronators during those activities. Jane is too busy to stretch the tight flexors and pronators at the end of her busy day. This may result in additional myofascial pain in the weaker and inhibited forearm extensors and supinator.

When Jane plays tennis that night she feels severe pain in the attachments of the extensors at the lateral epicondyle area. She realizes she was forced to return a lot of backhand shots using her overpowered weak, inhibited wrist extensors. She goes to her doctor and he diagnoses her with tendinitis or tennis elbow, and she takes her pain medications and ices the area for several days prior to coming to your office for treatment. What would you do? Here are some pointers:

- Your first step is to get a complete client history, some of which was just shared with you in this case study.

- This is followed by a thorough functional assessment and special orthopedic testing. You would note that

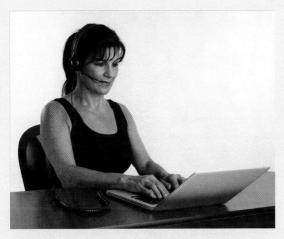

FIGURE 1-44
Working On Computer Shortens Forearm and Hand Flexors
and Pronators.

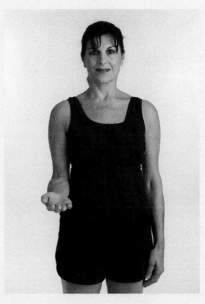

FIGURE 1-46
Limited Supination.

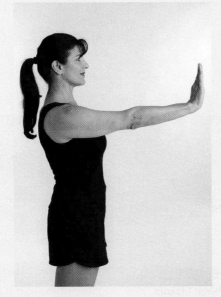

FIGURE 1-45
Limited Wrist Extension.

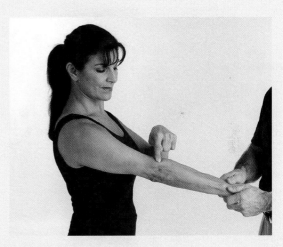

FIGURE 1-47
Muscle Resisted Test, Wrist Extensors.

Jane treated the acute inflammation with ice,
but still has chronic tendinosis in the extensors
of the wrist.

- Assessment shows limited range of motion in wrist
  extension and forearm supination due to tight
  wrist flexors and forearm pronators (Figures 1-45 ■
  and 1-46 ■). Muscle resistance testing reveals a
  strain in the wrist extensors at the attachments on
  the lateral epicondyle (Figure 1-47 ■). The use of
  ice for three days by the client has eliminated the
  possibility of inflammation in that area, making
  this a treatable condition of extensor tendinosis.
  Keep in mind there may not have even been any

inflammation in the extensors in the first place, as
is the case with tendinosis.

- Perform myofascial release to the muscle bellies of
  the contracted or shortened flexor groups, followed
  by compression, cross-fiber gliding strokes, then trigger point therapy if needed (Figures 1-48 ■, 1-49 ■,
  and 1-50 ■).

- Stretch and lengthen the flexors and pronators
  and relax the injured extensors and supinator
  (Figure 1-51 ■). The extensors were strained over
  time during the backhand of the tennis match,
  because they were weak and inhibited due to the
  tight flexors that Jane uses every day. If she had

(continued)

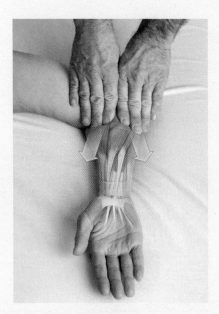

FIGURE 1-48
Myofascial Spreading, Wrist Flexors.

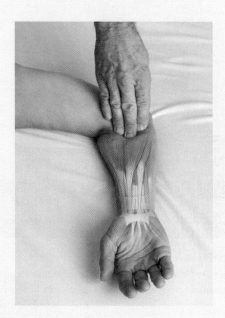

FIGURE 1-50
Cross-Fiber Gliding/Trigger Point Work.

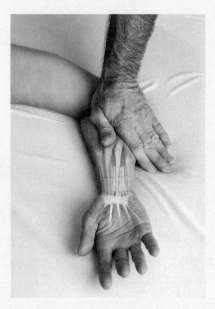

FIGURE 1-49
Compression Broadening, Wrist Flexors.

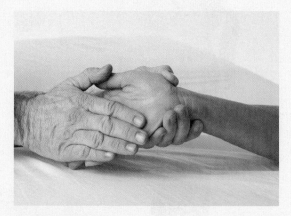

FIGURE 1-51
Stretch Wrist Flexors.

- Jane will then stretch her wrist flexors and pronators daily and strengthen her wrist extensors and supinators once the extensors can be strengthened pain-free. Eccentric strengthening of the extensors will lay down new collagen and realign the disorganized collagen created from the stress on the weak extensors during the tennis match. The goal is to eliminate tendon tension at the joints or the attachment sites of opposing muscle groups, and create balance based on restoring normal range of motion in opposing muscle groups.

Note: Multidirectional friction would not *be an appropriate technique to use on the wrist flexors or pronators, since they are not strained. This would be confirmed through muscle resistance testing in your assessment of those muscle groups.*

stretched the flexors and strengthened the extensors this injury most likely could have been avoided.

- Treat tendinosis in the extensors last, after all fibers leading to or feeding that area are brought to a neutral or relaxed position.
- Multidirectional friction followed by movement and eccentric contraction can be performed pain-free to create a functional scar (Figures 1-52 ■ and 1-53 ■).

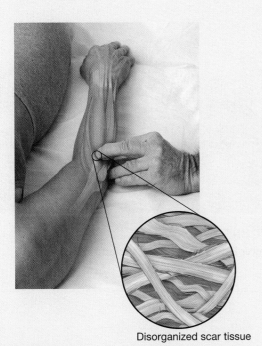

Disorganized scar tissue

FIGURE 1-52

Multidirectional Fiction, Wrist Extensors.

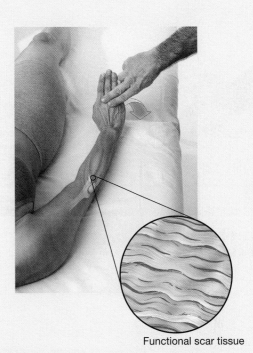

Functional scar tissue

FIGURE 1-53

Eccentric Muscle Contraction.

Many health care providers often treat tennis elbow or extensor tendinosis symptomatically, rather than balancing out opposing muscle groups and evaluating for tendinosis first. By getting a detailed history and doing a thorough evaluation, the clinical massage therapist is able to treat the underlying structural cause and be less aggressive and more specific when treating the resultant symptoms for all types of tendon pain. Tendonitis as a diagnosis is too generic and often inaccurate. Ice and pain medications are usually minimally effective in addressing the symptoms, especially if they do not address the underlying structural and postural cause.

Draping

Since this book is written for all clinical massage therapists, all of the work can be done without draping. Clients could wear shorts (males) and shorts and a sports bra (females), as is traditional in physical therapy settings. However, over the years there has been a huge demand to have clinical massage available in spa settings. Spas like Canyon Ranch and Cooper Aerobic Center set the pace for other top spas to follow. The author has had the opportunity to train therapists at Canyon Ranch, and has had requests to bring this to major hotels such as the Fairmont and Fours Seasons in Maui. It is likely that all spa environments will follow this trend by offering this work to their clientele. Therefore, it seems important to include a brief section on basic draping techniques, to evaluate and treat each part of the body. Massage therapists are encouraged to implement this into their relaxation massage protocols. This will certainly give spa therapists an edge in getting booked by more clients, because the majority of clients getting a massage have some sort of musculoskeletal complaint. Figures 1-54 ■ through 1-60 ■ show some basics about draping.

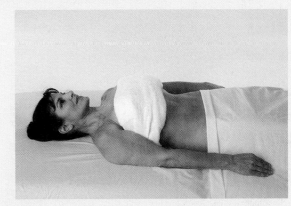

FIGURE 1-54

Pelvic, Abdominal, Head, Neck, Shoulder, and Arm Work.

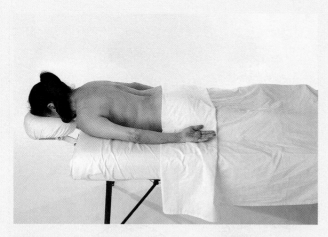

FIGURE 1-55
Pelvic, Back, Neck, Shoulder, and Arm Work.

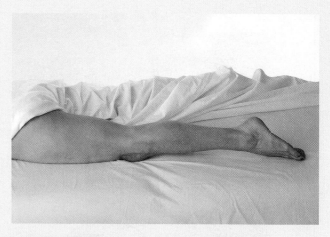

FIGURE 1-58
Lower Extremity Work (Posterior).

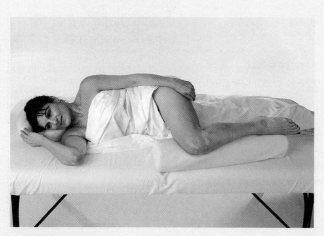

FIGURE 1-56
Neck, Shoulder, Arm, Thigh, and Lower Leg Work.

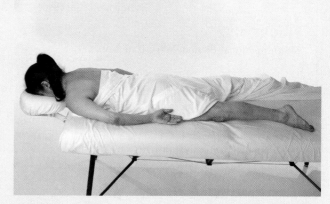

FIGURE 1-59
Neck, Shoulder, Back, Arm, and Lower Leg Work.

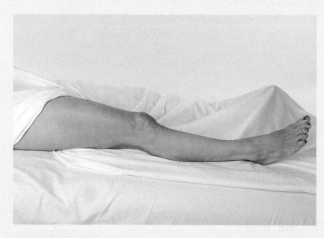

FIGURE 1-57
Lower Extremity Work (Anterior).

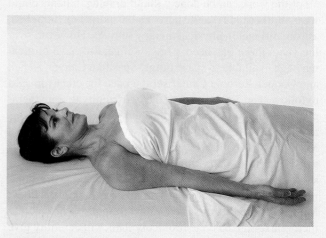

FIGURE 1-60
Head, Neck, Shoulder, and Upper Extremity Work.

CHAPTER SUMMARY

It is critical to realize that there are many different sources of musculoskeletal pain. In many clinical conditions, painful symptoms come from more than one area of the body. Clinical massage therapists should treat the underlying cause of musculoskeletal pain prior to addressing each clinical symptom. The twelve-step protocol for clinical massage allows the clinical massage therapist to sort out the various sources of pain and treat the different pathologies with the appropriate modality or technique. This system of assessments, special orthopedic testing, multidisciplinary and multimodality treatments along with precise client self-care protocols will facilitate structural balance, eliminate pain and injuries throughout the body, and optimize athletic performance. Clinical massage is an integral part of medical massage, which is an umbrella term that includes most forms of restorative and enhancement therapy techniques. This total system of clinical massage is directed at resolving a client's individual complaints to allow clients to live pain free and perform at their highest potential. It will take your manual therapy practice to a level you never imagined.

REVIEW QUESTIONS

1. Which statement is correct?
   a. Passive range of motion assesses if a muscle strain is present.
   b. Active range of motion is performed solely by the client.
   c. Passive range of motion is performed solely by the client.
   d. Resisted range of motion assesses if trigger points are present.

2. Tendinosis is described as _____.
   a. Inflammation of tendons or muscle–tendon attachments
   b. Inflammation of a tendon sheath
   c. Tearing of tendon fibers in the absence of an inflammatory process
   d. A ligament sprain

3. Your goals in applying the twelve steps are

   _____.
   a. To restore structural balance and postural alignment
   b. To create pain-free movement by balancing muscle groups
   c. To increase flexibility and joint space by increasing range of motion
   d. All of the above

4. A test to determine if a muscle strain is present is called _____.
   a. Resisted range of motion
   b. Passive range of motion
   c. Active range of motion
   d. Joint capsule work

5. What is step 6 called in the twelve-step protocol?
   a. Assess resisted range of motion
   b. Area preparation
   c. Trigger point therapy
   d. Myofascial release

6. What is performed immediately after multidirectional friction?
   a. Eccentric scar tissue alignment
   b. Stretching
   c. Pain-free movement
   d. Trigger point therapy

7. What is it called when the therapist gently assists a stretch performed actively by the client?
   a. Proprioceptive neuromuscular facilitation (PNF) stretching
   b. Active assisted stretching
   c. Isometric stretching
   d. Resistance stretching

8. What should be performed for 20 to 30 seconds?
   a. Trigger point therapy
   b. Multidirectional friction
   c. Myofascial release
   d. Stretching

9. Which of the following is a correct statement?
   a. The client must stretch tight muscles before strengthening opposing weak muscles.
   b. The client must always stretch all the muscles around a joint.
   c. The client must always stretch for 2 to 3 minutes.
   d. Using elastic bands is not an effective way to stretch.

10. At what angle should you perform myofascial release into the tissue?
    a. 30-degree angle
    b. 60-degree angle
    c. 45-degree angle
    d. 10-degree angle

2

Pelvic Stabilization—The Key to Structural Integration

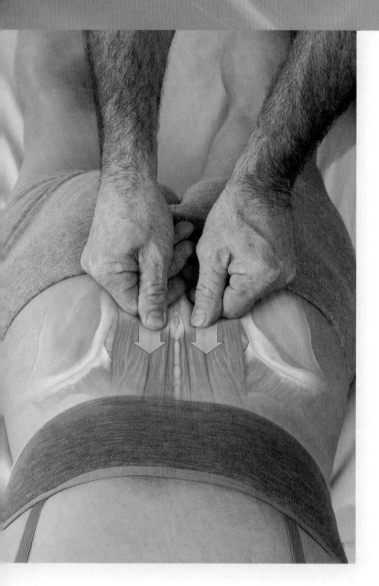

CHAPTER OUTLINE

Twelve-Step Approach to Pelvic Stabilization

Psoas Major, Iliacus (Iliopsoas), and Joint Capsule

Quadratus Lumborum (QL) and Erector Spinae

Lateral Hip Rotators or Medial Hip Rotators and
   Adductors

Lateral Hip Rotator Protocol

Medial Hip Rotators and Adductors

Quadriceps and Iliotibial Band (ITB)

Hamstrings

LEARNING OBJECTIVES

Upon completing this chapter the reader will be able to:

- Choose the appropriate massage modality or treatment protocol for each specific condition of the hip and lower back
- Restore normal range of motion throughout the body and normal muscle resting lengths by first working on short contracted muscle groups (iliopsoas and quadriceps) and then working the weak, inhibited antagonists (gluteals and hamstrings)
- Restore balance between other opposing muscle groups in the hip area such as internal and external hip rotators
- Assure myoskeletal balance; balance of the opposing muscle groups
- Assure that the therapist eliminates the underlying soft tissue cause of the lower back and hip conditions before addressing the symptoms
- Restore pain-free hip range of motion

- Create pelvic stability
- Differentiate between soft tissue problems caused by:
  - myofascial restrictions
  - joint capsule adhesions
  - muscle–tendon tension
  - trigger point tension
  - strained muscle fibers
  - sprained ligaments
  - nerve compression
  - bony fixations
- Teach the client self-care stretches and strengthening exercises (if needed) to perform at home to maintain musculoskeletal balance and pain-free movement, following therapy

KEY TERMS

Bulging disc *40*

Distal hamstring
  strain *77*

Eccentric muscle
  contraction *54*

Facet joints *53*

Herniated disc *40*

This chapter addresses pelvic stabilization techniques that should be a routine part of a massage protocol, prior to dealing with chronic pain in any other area of the body. The goal will be to ensure that each client achieves a balance between at least five basic muscle groups. This means each muscle group has the ability to release to the full range of motion on both the left and the right sides, and balance is achieved among all opposing muscle groups in the hip and back areas. Deep pelvic restrictions can cause distortions throughout the entire body, thus it is believed that pelvic stabilization may be the *key* to structural balance.

It is helpful to place a bolster under the client's hips or use a body cushion, when prone, during pelvic stabilization. This allows the ilium to rotate posteriorly and helps decompress the lumbar spine to reduce possible hyperlordosis and help relieve vertebral compression of the discs during therapy.

Be gentle and nonaggressive with all of your work. Assume the client could have preexisting clinical conditions including bulging or herniated discs, sacroiliac (SI) joint pain or dysfunction, and so on. High-velocity chiropractic manipulation to the SI joint on someone with a sprain or strain at the SI joint (also described as a tear) is *not* advised. The techniques in the book can often eliminate the cause of that pain and address clinical symptoms, without high velocity manipulation being needed.

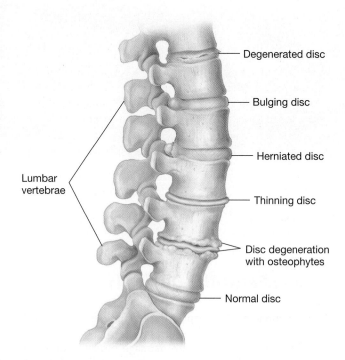

FIGURE 2-1
Examples of Disc Problems.

TWELVE-STEP APPROACH TO PELVIC STABILIZATION

Prior to going through the protocol for pelvic stabilization, you should learn a few important clinical terms:

Degenerative Disc Disease

Degenerative disc disease is not really a disease—it's the normal wear and tear process of aging on your spine. As we age, the intervertebral discs lose their flexibility, elasticity, and shock absorbing characteristics. When this happens, the discs change from a supple, flexible state that allows fluid movement, to a stiff and rigid state that restricts movement. Degenerative disc disease is relatively common in aging adults and seldom requires surgery. In fact, although 80% of adults will experience back or neck pain, only 1%–2% will need surgery.[1]

Bulging Discs and Herniated Discs

A **bulging disc** is formed when the soft, spongy center of the disc, the nucleus pulposus, pushes out and places pressure on the annulus fibrosis that contains the center. Unlike a herniated disc, the bulging disc still contains the nucleus material. A **herniated disc** is a disc that extrudes into the spinal canal. It is also referred to as a prolapsed disc, ruptured disc, or slipped disc (Figure 2-1 ■).

People between the ages of 30 and 50 are most at risk for herniation because the elasticity and water content of the nucleus pulposus decrease with age. Extended bed rest is no longer recommended for spine pain. Doctors now suggest exercise and mild activity, physical therapy, massage, chiropractic treatment, and acupuncture.[2]

Osteophytes

Osteophytes are also known as bone spurs. They are protrusions or enlargements of bone and cartilage that develop in a degenerative joint. Doctors believe they occur in reaction to changes in joints due to diseases and aging. The bone spurs themselves are not painful, but when they press or rub against nearby nerves and bones they can cause pain.[3]

Degeneration of the spine occurs in all persons to some degree. However, for 42 percent of the population, degeneration and development of bone spurs will lead to symptoms of neck and back pain, radiating arm and leg pain, and weakness in the extremities during their lifetime. Physical therapy, exercise, and manipulation may alleviate painful joint conditions. These modalities attempt to restore flexibility, balance, and strength to the neck and back, improving posture and possibly decreasing the compression on the nerves. However, nerve compression with radiating pain into an arm and leg should be clinically investigated before beginning any form of rehabilitation therapies.[4]

Clinical massage therapy can have an amazing effect on reducing or eliminating the pain associated with even these complicated clinical conditions by bringing the muscle groups throughout the body back into balance to help decompress and align the bones.

PRECAUTIONARY NOTE

Do not work on a client with a recent injury (acute condition), exhibiting inflammation: heat, redness, and/or swelling. RICE therapy; rest, ice, compression, elevation may be the appropriate treatment in this situation.

The specific order for releasing and balancing muscle groups is as follows, and are covered in this chapter:

- Psoas major, iliacus (iliopsoas), and joint capsule
- Quadratus lumborum (QL) and erector spinae
- Lateral hip rotators or medial hip rotators and adductors
- Quadriceps and iliotibial band (ITB)
- Hamstrings

Step 1: Client History

Ask the client when, where, and how the problem began. Have him or her describe the area of pain and what makes it better or worse. Make sure they have filled out the client intake form in Chapter 1.

Step 2: Assess Active Range of Motion (AROM)

Before you work through the specific order for releasing the muscle groups, ask the client to perform each of the six primary single-plane movements of the hip joint with zero discomfort. Determine if the range of motion is normal. Please understand that the normal degrees for each hip range of motion will vary with different references. The degrees listed in this text are accurate estimates for clients with healthy hips. If the range of motion is less than average, identify which muscle groups are restricted and therefore preventing normal movement (Figures 2-2 ■ through 2-8 ■).

HIP JOINT SINGLE-PLANE MOVEMENTS—PRIMARY MUSCLES

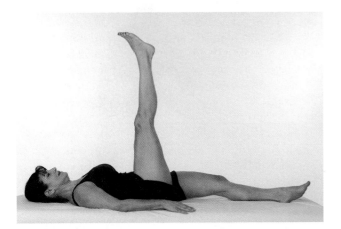

FIGURE 2-2
Hip Flexion, 90 Degrees.

Flexion, 90 Degrees (Knee Extended)

- Iliacus
- Psoas
- Rectus femoris
- Sartorius
- Tensor fasciae latae

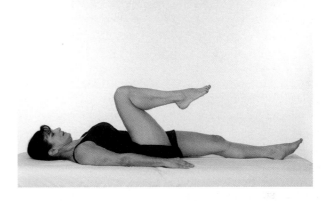

FIGURE 2-3
Hip Flexion (Knee Flexed), 120 Degrees.

Flexion, 120 Degrees (Knee Flexed)

- Iliacus
- Psoas
- Rectus femoris
- Sartorius
- Tensor fasciae latae

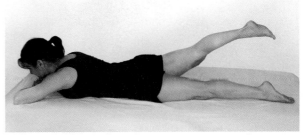

FIGURE 2-4
Hip Extension, 35–45 Degrees.

Extension, 35 to 45 Degrees

- Biceps femoris (long head)
- Gluteus maximus
- Semimembranosus
- Semitendinosus

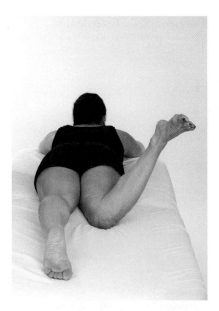

FIGURE 2-5
Internal Hip Rotation, 30–45 Degrees.

Medial/Internal Rotation, 30 to 45 Degrees

- Adductor brevis
- Adductor longus
- Adductor magnus
- Gluteus medius
- Gluteus minimus
- Tensor fasciae latae

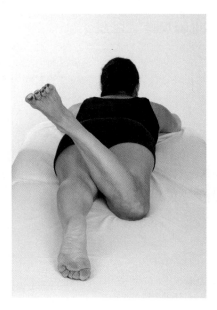

FIGURE 2-6
External Hip Rotation, 60 Degrees.

Lateral/External Rotation, 60 Degrees

- Gemellus inferior, superior
- Gluteus maximus

- Obturator externus, internus
- Piriformis
- Quadratus femoris
- Sartorius

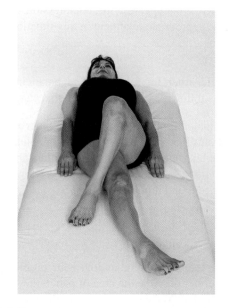

FIGURE 2-7
Hip Adduction, 30 Degrees.

Adduction, 30 Degrees

- Adductor brevis
- Adductor longus
- Adductor magnus
- Gracilis
- Pectineus

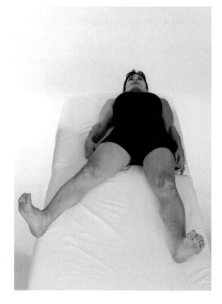

FIGURE 2-8
Hip Abduction, 45 Degrees.

Abduction, 45 Degrees (Pelvis Stationary)

- Gluteus maximus
- Gluteus medius
- Gluteus minimus
- Sartorius
- Tensor fasciae latae

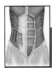

CORE PRINCIPLE

To simplify how to correct a limited movement, the clinical massage therapist should work on the opposite, group of muscles listed here for each movement (i.e., if hip extension is limited to less than 35 to 45 degrees, the therapist should work on the following muscles to restore normal hip extension; iliacus, psoas, rectus femoris, sartorius, and tenser fasciae latae). These are the muscles that are not releasing to allow normal hip extension. It is recommended that therapists should focus more on identifying muscle groups that limit a normal movement in the body, than those that create each movement.

Step 3: Assess Passive Range of Motion (PROM)

Gently evaluate the end feel of the previous movements. This is done passively. All movements should have a tissue stretch or soft and leathery end feel, except for extension, which will feel more ligamentous and abrupt.

Step 4: Assess Resisted Range of Motion (RROM)

The client attempts each of the hip joint single-plane movements using 20 percent of their strength, while you apply resistance. If the client experiences pain or discomfort, ask him or her to point to the specific spot. This is most likely a muscle–tendon strain Work this area last.

PSOAS MAJOR, ILIACUS (ILIOPSOAS), AND JOINT CAPSULE

The psoas major attaches to the transverse processes of lumbar vertebrae 1 to 5 and the intervertebral disks above each vertebra. The iliacus attaches to the iliac fossa. Both insert on the lesser trochanter of the femur (Figure 2-9A ■). Together they are called the iliopsoas and they are strong hip flexors and lower back stabilizers.

Restricted, dense connective tissue where the iliacus and psoas major join on the inside rim of the iliac crest can be a major cause of pain in the lower back.[5] Tight psoas major muscles compress the lumbar spine downward and forward onto the nerve roots causing pain, and can also

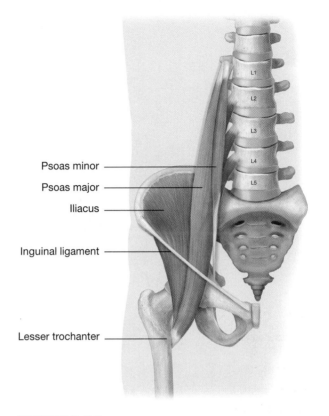

Psoas minor
Psoas major
Iliacus
Inguinal ligament
Lesser trochanter

FIGURE 2-9A
Iliopsoas.

herniate and rupture the lumbar discs. Tight iliacus muscles can rotate the ilium anteriorly because they are directly attached to the ilium (Figure 2-9B ■).

Think about the psoas major for lumbar compression, bulging and herniated discs, nerve compression, and excessive lumbar lordosis. Think about the iliacus for anterior pelvic tilt and sacroiliac (SI) joint pain.

Typically, the client's dominant side will have more anterior ilium rotation, which may also elevate the iliac crest on that side. This creates stress between the articulation of the sacrum and the ilium, which can cause SI joint pain to occur. When this happens the sacrum can be pulled onto the vertebrae, which are then pulled onto the nerve roots, causing lower back pain. Imbalance in these two muscle groups in the pelvis can affect the entire body and should be corrected *first* before any other orthopedic massage is performed.

PRECAUTIONARY NOTE

As you pin down the psoas, be cautious. If you feel a pulsation in this area, immediately reposition your hand and consider the possibility of an aneurysm. If for any reason you expect a possible aneurysm, refer the client to a physician and do not perform pelvic stabilization.

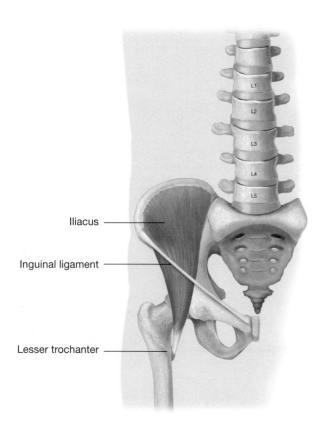

Iliacus

Inguinal ligament

Lesser trochanter

FIGURE 2-9B
Iliacus.

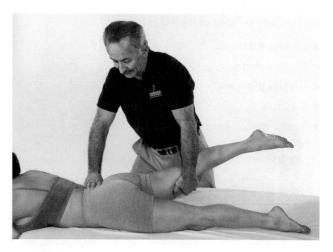

FIGURE 2-10
Assessment for Hip Extension.

Step 2: Assess Active Range of Motion (AROM)

The client is prone with the knee straight, especially if he or she has tight quadriceps. Ask the client to lift his or her leg off the table and explain that this step is to be performed with zero discomfort. Thus he or she should lift the leg only to the point where it feels comfortable. Normal range of motion is 35 to 45 degrees. If the client cannot achieve this, then the hip flexors, psoas, and iliacus, and quadriceps are contracted and tight and need to be released.

Step 3: Assess Passive Range of Motion (PROM)

The client is prone with the knee straight. Place one hand under the knee. Place the other hand on the client's hip to stabilize it as the ilium must stay on the table. Monitor the ilium with your stabilizing hand, to make sure it does not move as the femur extends during this evaluation. This will prevent stirring up preexisting conditions like bulging disc pain and SI joint sprains or strains. Move your index finger over the SI joint, inferior of the iliac crest, to better assess if the ilium is moving with femoral extension. The client's lower leg can rest on your supporting knee if your leg is on the table. Gently lift the leg only to the restrictive barrier, pain-free, and assess the end feel of the hip joint (Figure 2-10). It should feel soft and leathery. If it has a bone-on-bone-like end feel, the hip needs joint capsule work.

HIP JOINT CAPSULE WORK

Joint capsule work is one of the author's trademark techniques. An imbalance of the muscles around the hip joint can set up a neuromuscular response attempting to restore balance. This also creates tension in the joint, which may eventually lead to joint degeneration and arthritis as the cartilage wears down. Progressive hip imbalance, discomfort or injury may also limit range of motion contributing to a formation of fascial adhesions inside the joint capsule itself. Fascial adhesions inside the hip capsule are more predominant in the anterior capsule due to excessive or prolonged hip flexion. The deepest level of articulating fascia thickens and acts as "superglue" and limits range of motion in the hip.

✋ PRECAUTIONARY NOTE

It is the author's experience that what is typically thought of as true adhesive capsulitis is a late stage and more aggressive fibroblast formation. It is also the author's opinion, based on 20 years of experience with adhesive capsulitis, that aggressive manual therapy that tries to stretch the early onset inner capsule myofascial restrictions can play a contributing role in creating more aggressive capsular adhesions involving the joint capsule itself. This common error occurs when the manual therapist does not pick up on the bone-on-bone-like end feel, and proceeds to stretch tissue even though there is not a soft tissue or leathery end feel in the hip.

These deep fascial adhesions, however, can be softened and mobilized much like you would soften and mobilize fascia anywhere else in the body. The head of the femur can be used as a massage tool to soften and mobilize the deep investing fascia inside the hip joint capsule using very gentle pressure,

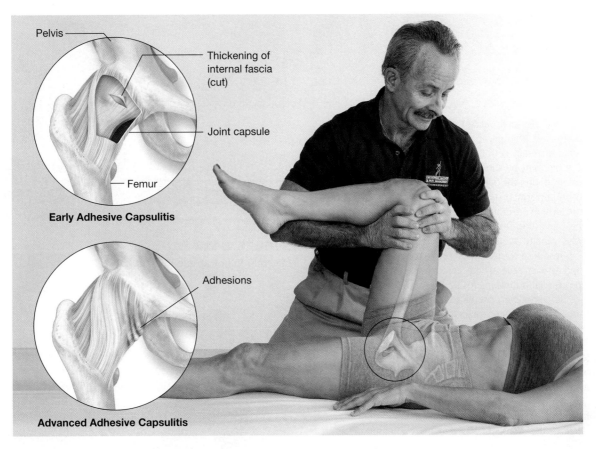

Pelvis

Thickening of internal fascia (cut)

Joint capsule

Femur

Early Adhesive Capsulitis

Adhesions

Advanced Adhesive Capsulitis

FIGURE 2-11
Neutral Position Femur–Hip Fascial and Joint Capsule Mobilization.

pain-free movements, and slow-velocity fascial and capsular stretch. Perform joint capsule work if any hip ROM end feel is bone-on-bone-like (Figure 2-11 ■). Pressure, movement, and gentle, slow-velocity stretch facilitates myofascial mobilization and myofascial release. The hypothesis also exists that gentle compression and then decompression of the hip capsule can play a role in mobilizing and eccentric loading of the disorganized collagen in the hip capsule. This is like a "mortar and pestle," and as you gently compress the head of the femur into the hip socket it is like a strain-counterstrain technique. It allows the fibrin formation in the hip capsule to shorten and relax. As you gently decompress the ball and socket joint, or come out of the hip capsule it is believed that the resistance created by the fascial and collagen adhesions may create an eccentric force to help realign or better mobilize the collagen adhesions.

The client is supine with one hip flexed 90 degrees and the knee flexed 90 degrees. Having the hip flexed 90 degrees is important, as this allows the slow, but firm compression to be performed straight down toward the table so that the lumbar spine is not compromised. Cartilage of the femoral head must be compressed pain-free to the cartilage inside the ilium to access the deep fascial adhesions that are inside the joint capsule. Place both hands around the client's thigh. The lower leg can rest on your forearm, but should not be used as a lever to facilitate the stretch. Gently move and rock the leg to make sure the client is fully relaxed. Push down on the thigh gently so that the femur goes into the hip socket, rotate it into lateral (external) rotation, and then pull it out (Figure 2-12A ■). Compress, rotate, decompress—this is a plunging type of technique, cartilage on cartilage, to soften and mobilize the fascial adhesions inside the joint capsule. It mimics a mortar and pestle effect.

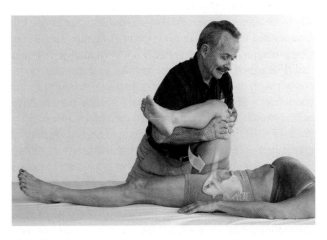

FIGURE 2-12A
External Joint Capsule Stretch.

EXPERT OPINION

Tell the client to visualize the joint capsule "softening, releasing, and letting go." Ask him or her if this is uncomfortable. It usually is not, as you are taking the pressure off the hip joint by shortening and softening the fascial adhesions during the compression and rotation phase. This *must* be performed pain-free, and slowly as even minor muscle tension prevents the depth necessary to address the deepest investing fascia, for effective joint capsule work. So you want to avoid causing the muscles to splint the area in response to discomfort. Repeat the gentle plunging and rotation several times, progressively mobilizing the deeper fascial adhesions inside the hip. Then compress firmly, but very slowly once into the joint capsule, making sure the femoral head contacts the ilium, rotate it laterally (externally) to the restriction, and then give a deep, slow, pain-free fascial and capsular stretch. Back off the stretch, return to neutral, and then pull back out of the joint capsule. Watch the ilium; if it moves with the femur, you are not stretching the deep inner fascia and joint capsule. Your goal is to achieve 60 degrees of pain-free external femoral rotation, and 45 degrees of internal femoral rotation.

Watch the client's facial expressions and look for any changes in breathing to indicate discomfort. Making your plunges nonsynchronized and stretching the capsule when the client least expects it prevents him or her from guarding or helping during this work. It should always be pain-free.

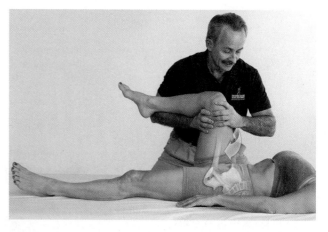

FIGURE 2-12B
Internal Joint Capsule Release.

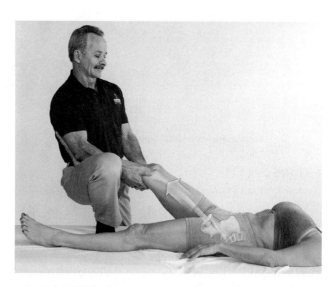

FIGURE 2-13
Traction Hip After Releasing Joint Capsule Adhesions.

Next, repeat this sequence, rotating and stretching the femur medially (internally) (Figure 2-12B ■). On joint capsule work, lateral rotation usually moves more freely on most clients. If internal rotation causes the client to guard against your work, perform capsule work laterally first to gain a sense of trust with clients who have had a painful iliopsoas or painful manipulation experience. Medial rotation is usually more adhesive due to prolonged shortening of lateral hip rotators and this is where your focus of therapy should be. Compress and rotate the femur deep, slow, and gentle several times, then compress once into the joint capsule, make contact with the ilium, rotate it medially (internally) to the restriction, and then give a slow, deep capsular stretch. Back off the stretch, return to neutral, and then pull back out (Figure 2-13 ■). Repeat this sequence again, if needed. Your goal is to achieve 45 degrees of internal hip rotation.

You must rotate the hip both ways, as there could be multiple adhesions in different directions. You should usually start with external rotation. Medial rotation is typically more adhesive and restricted, therefore it should be worked second after you have gained the client's trust. However, this will vary with each client, and may even differ from the right to the left hip.

On a large client you can perform the same technique by placing the leg over your knee and then leaning into the leg, plunging and rotating the thigh and then leaning back to pull out (Figure 2-14 ■). Proceed carefully if the client has SI joint pathologies. This work must be performed *totally pain-free.*

CORE PRINCIPLE

You *must* change the protocol and return to joint capsule work anytime that you find a bone-on-bone-like end feel during the rest of the hip session.

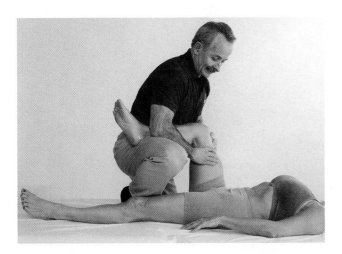

FIGURE 2-14
Femur–Hip Joint Capsule Work on Large Client.

ILIACUS RELEASE

To perform the iliacus release, the client is supine with the hip flexed 90 degrees. Lay the bent leg over your leg so the muscles are shortened and completely relaxed. Palpate the anterior superior iliac spine (ASIS) and to make sure the client is completely relaxed, distract the client by gently moving or rocking the leg. Have the client take a deep breath, and on exhale go in using your finger pads, *very slowly*. Do not go in too far or too fast toward the psoas. Lead with your little finger, with your hand at a slight angle. Come back to the iliacus and pin the fascia directly onto the inside of the ilium. Conform the pads of your fingers to the shape of the inside of the ilium. Then lift and lengthen the fascia superior toward the same shoulder and pin it there (pin and stretch) (Figures 2-15 ■ and 2-16 ■). You want to create an upward traction on the fascia. See video clip on www.myhealthprofessionskit.com.

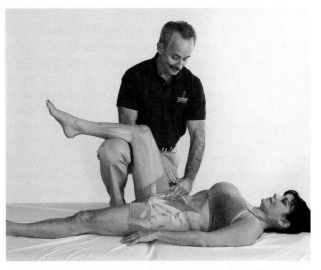

FIGURE 2-15
Iliacus Release (Body Mechanics).

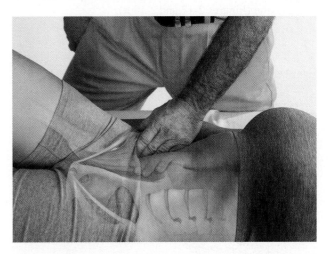

FIGURE 2-16
Iliacus Release (Hand Placement).

CORE PRINCIPLE

Always get the client's permission before you treat this area. Use a visual aid, if needed, to explain where you are going to be working. This can be a very personal, emotional area of the body.

Now, while keeping your finger pads on the iliacus, place your other hand under the client's knee. Help the client drop the heel down onto the table and allow him or her to actively drag the heel toward hip extension. As the client engages the extensors (hamstrings and glutes), he or she inhibits the hip flexors. As described in Chapter 1, this is called *reciprocal inhibition*. Have the client dorsiflex the foot at the end of hip extension, and place your hand that is not on the iliacus just below the ilium. Use that hand to press down

on the upper fibers of the rectus femoris, to gently decompress the femur. This will get more length in the iliacus and psoas muscles, and decompress the articulating cartilage of the hip (Figure 2-17 ■). Repeat this procedure several times, going in a little deeper onto the iliacus, sweeping, scooping, pinning, and stretching the connective tissue upward each time. This will stretch the fascia so you can gently isolate and deactivate any tight bands and trigger points in the iliacus.

CORE PRINCIPLE

You must continually "check in" with the client—is he or she guarding? Pay attention to the client's face, voice tonality, and breathing. What is his or her comfort or discomfort level? The iliacus release *must* be performed pain-free.

PSOAS RELEASE

The client is in the same position as for the iliacus release. As the client exhales after taking a deep breath, go in using your finger pads, very slowly toward the psoas, at a 45-degree angle toward the spine. Enter just lateral to the rectus abdominal muscle. To find the psoas have the client attempt to bring the knee toward the chest. The psoas will pop up under your fingers. Gently pin it down with the finger pads, not the fingertips, as they can be painful. Give it a gentle stretch by passively moving the client's hip from the flexed position towards slight extension. If your knee is under the client's leg, gently move and rock the client's knee on your knee toward extension. Repeat this psoas pin and stretch several times. These are very subtle movements.

Next, go in and again pin the psoas with your finger pads and then help the client drop the heel onto the table and have them push their heel down the table from the flexed hip position toward hip extension. When the client's knee is fully extended, have the client *gently* bring the foot into dorsiflexion (Figures 2-17 and 2-18 ■).

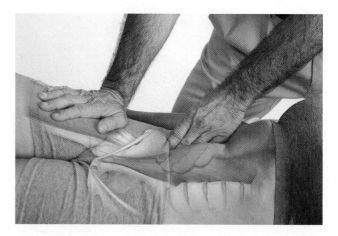

FIGURE 2-18
Psoas Release (Hand Placement).

Tight psoas can create compression and rotation of the lumbar spine.

Go to the end of the table. Grasp the client's ankle, lean back, and give a gentle stretch and traction to the hip, knee, and ankle for 5 seconds. Release very slowly.

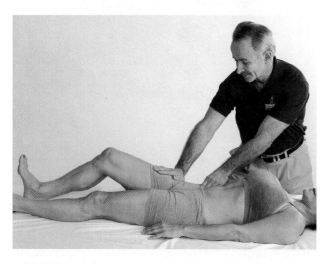

FIGURE 2-17
Psoas Release (Body Mechanics).

 PRECAUTIONARY NOTE

Be cautious when pressing directly downward on the psoas, as there could be an underlying medical condition. If you ever feel a pulsation in this area, consider the possibility of an aneurysm, or you may be pressing on the wrong structure. Immediately reposition your hand. If you suspect an aneurysm do not perform this work. Refer the client to a physician immediately.

Step 11: Stretching (During Therapy)

To stretch the iliacus and psoas, the client is prone with the knee straight. Place one hand under the knee, just above the patella. Place the other hand on the client's hip, pulling the hip inferiorly and laterally and then stabilizing it. The ilium must stay on the table and not go into flexion during the stretch.

 CORE PRINCIPLE

Place your hand that is not on the psoas on the upper fibers of the rectus femoris. Gently rock the femur and press into the upper quadriceps at a 45-degree angle, pushing distally toward the knee to decompress the hip. This will distract the client and enhance the psoas stretch and release. Repeat this sequence several times working up the psoas (superiorly) toward the attachments.

 CORE PRINCIPLE

The hand on the hip can also monitor if the ilium is moving into flexion as the femur goes into extension, indicating a joint capsule problem or unresolved restrictions in the iliopsoas.

The client's lower leg can rest across your forearm. Remind him or her to do nothing that is uncomfortable. Then ask the client to gently press the knee into the table with 20 percent force for 5 to 10 seconds as you provide resistance. The client relaxes, takes a deep breath, and on exhale lifts the leg only to where he or she is comfortable while you assist the stretch for about 2 seconds (Figure 2-19 ■). Keep the leg at this new height and put your knee under the leg as a restrictive barrier. Repeat this contract-relax, contract-antagonist with active assisted stretching two or three times or until the client attains the normal range of motion of 35 to 45 degrees. Do *not* stretch past a pain-free end feel. Only continue to stretch if there is a tissue stretch end feel. If it becomes a bone-on-bone-like end feel do additional joint capsule work.

Next, ask the client to actively lift the leg several times only to where he or she is comfortable, for neuromuscular reeducation.

CORE PRINCIPLE

To isolate the psoas, have the client move the leg into 30-degree abduction and perform the stretch. To isolate the iliacus, have the client keep the leg adducted (knees closer together) during the stretch.

If you found a bone-on-bone-like end feel during the previous stretch or you could not achieve the full 35- to 45-degree range of motion, perform the following technique. This releases the anterior portion of the hip joint capsule. Place one hand under the client's knee, just above the patella, and place your other hand just below the gluteal fold on the upper hamstrings. Lift the client's knee (hip extension) as you press straight down anteriorly on the upper hamstrings, gently pumping the femur into the anterior joint capsule (Figure 2-20 ■). Repeat this several times. This is performed passively and will increase fascial release inside the joint capsule, gap the hip joint, and could create an increased synovial fluid response back into the hip joint, You also need to bring the hip into abduction in 15-degree increments, out to 45 degrees, to release multiple angles of the anterior hip capsule.

Finally, go to the end of the table and grasp the client's ankle. Lean back and give a gentle stretch and traction to the hip, knee, and ankle for 5 seconds and release very slowly (Figure 2-21 ■).

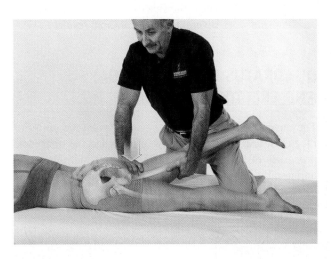

FIGURE 2-20
Anterior Joint Capsule Release.

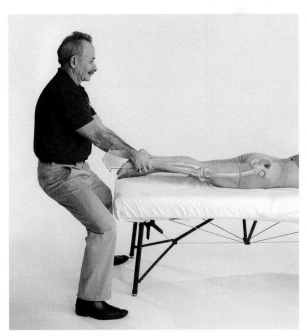

FIGURE 2-21
Decompress Superior Hip Capsule.

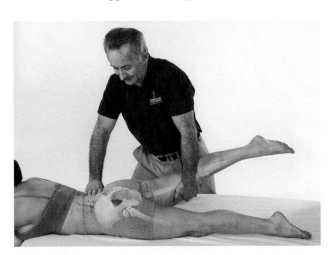

FIGURE 2-19
Iliopsoas Stretch.

CORE PRINCIPLE

The SI joint may spontaneously align during the stretch. When the ilia are back into their proper balanced position the SI joint symptoms may completely disappear.

Step 2: Assess Active Range of Motion (AROM)

To restore normal active range of motion for hip extension, you may need to repeat the iliacus and psoas release and joint capsule work several times for optimal results.

QUADRATUS LUMBORUM (QL) AND ERECTOR SPINAE

The quadratus lumborum (QL) originates on the posterior iliac crest and inserts on the twelfth rib and the transverse processes of L1 to L4 (Figure 2-22 ■). Its actions are to unilaterally elevate, or hike, the hip and laterally flex the

vertebral column. The QL can often be dominant side tight with the other side weak, inhibited, or overstretched. The erector spinae is a group of muscles that run from the sacrum to the occiput along the spine (Figure 2-23 ■). They extend and laterally flex the vertebral column and can contribute to SI joint symptoms, if they are not balanced in the lower back.

Step 3: Assess Passive Range of Motion (PROM)

The client is prone. Make sure he or she is straight on the table. Perform a visual posture assessment of the client both when standing and when prone on the table. Does he or she have a low shoulder or the appearance of a shorter leg while lying on the table? Traction both ankles for a few seconds to ensure the client is straight on the table. When you let go slowly, the dominant or tight QL can function as a hip hiker. Palpate the QL and erectors with your thumbs coming onto the iliac crest superiorly (Figure 2-24 ■). Assess which iliac crest is elevated. This will indicate which side is contracted and short. This is the side you will release first, regardless of on what side the client reports the pain. If you have advanced palpation skills, palpate the posterior, superior, iliac spine (PSIS) and assess which side is elevated (Figure 2-25 ■).

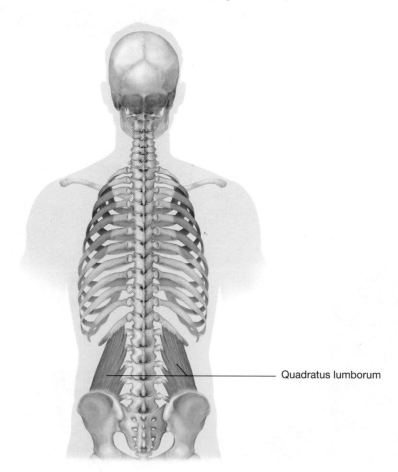

Quadratus lumborum

FIGURE 2-22
Quadratus Lumborum.

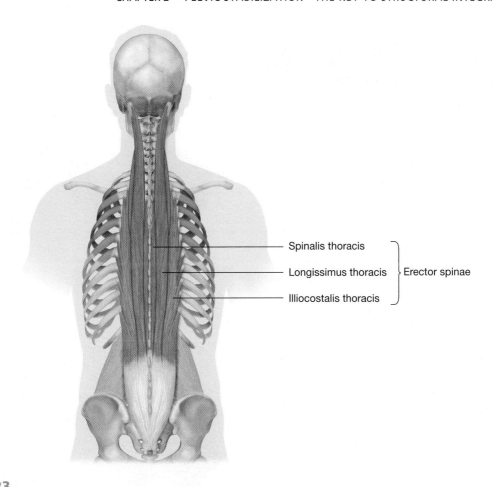

Spinalis thoracis
Longissimus thoracis } Erector spinae
Illiocostalis thoracis

FIGURE 2-23
Erector Spinae.

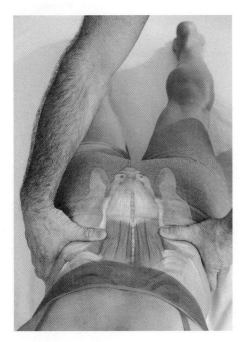

FIGURE 2-24
Palpate Iliac Crests.

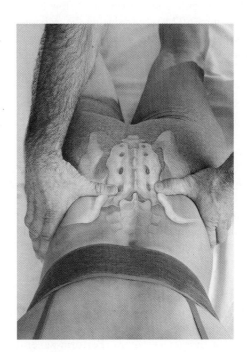

FIGURE 2-25
Palpate PSIS.

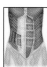

CORE PRINCIPLE

Remember, pain is an unreliable sign of where the problem is. Equally balancing the QL and erectors ensures that the lumbar spine is not unilaterally out of balance and compressed on one side.

Step 6: Myofascial Release

With the client prone and your hands on the client's back, start with gentle rocking motions to relax him or her. Next, perform myofascial spreading of the shortened or contracted QL and the erector spinae. Start at the base of the spine on the shortened QL side, with one hand on the ilium to stabilize it, and your other hand moving superiorly, toward the upper back to about the twelfth rib. Repeat this several times.

Have the client move into a side-lying position. Provide support under the neck and upper bent leg so he or she is comfortable. This allows the muscles to be as relaxed as possible before you begin. Have the client place an arm over his or her head if a shoulder problem does not exist, and keep the spine in alignment—not rolled forward or backward. Perform myofascial release with your forearm, up the erectors, to lift and lengthen them. With your other hand, stabilize the client's hip and pull downward toward the foot of the table (Figure 2-26 ■).

Next, do cross-fiber gliding strokes through the erectors longitudinally, working medial to lateral in the lumbar region, to loosen them and to maximize blood flow to the underlying QL (Figure 2-27 ■). By reducing the ischemia and restoring normal muscle resting length in the short tight QL you will be less likely to find muscle belly trigger points.

Step 7: Trigger Point Therapy

If the client does have trigger points, they are usually found at the attachments of the QL: the ilium, or the twelfth rib. If present, release these with direct pressure for 10 to 12 seconds. As the trigger point softens, compress the tissue several times and then gently stretch it. Tease through any tight bands if found. Strum and stretch to release them. Remember that your goal is to combine different modalities to restore normal muscle resting lengths. It is suggested that you do not treat trigger points first and do not get too caught up in trigger point work alone.

Step 6: Myofascial Release

Then, using two fingers or your thumb perform myofascial spreading on the erectors, working up the spine while gently rocking the client. Work along the spine to approximately the twelfth thoracic vertebra. Perform several strokes in the *lamina groove* to check for rotated vertebrae (Figure 2-28 ■). The lamina groove should feel smooth

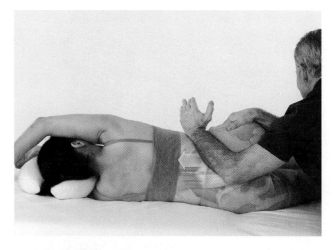

FIGURE 2-26
Myofascial Release, Erectors/QL.

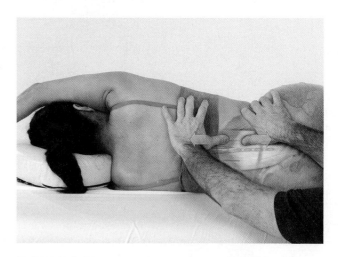

FIGURE 2-27
QL/Erector Cross-Fiber Gliding Strokes.

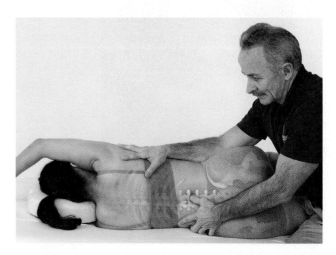

FIGURE 2-28
Evaluate for a Smooth Lamina Groove.

when the bones are in alignment. If it is not, return to the two-finger myofascial strokes, working a little deeper while gently rocking the client.

CORE PRINCIPLE

Rock the spine to let the discs decompress and possibly spontaneously realign.

The **facet joints** may also spontaneously align. If the erectors are still tight, you can also perform cross-fiber friction gliding strokes up the erectors.

Step 11: Stretching (During Therapy)

Stand behind the side-lying client. Reposition him or her at a 45-degree angle on the table, bringing the hip closer to you, allowing the client to stretch the leg below the table. Have the client place his or her arm over the head to lengthen the back. Hold the upper straight leg above the knee. Place your other hand below the twelfth rib. Ask the client to hike up the hip toward the shoulder with 20 percent force for 5 to 10 seconds while you provide resistance (Figure 2-29 ■). The client then relaxes, takes a deep breath, and on exhale you lean back and assist while the client adducts the leg down toward the floor for about 2 seconds (Figure 2-30 ■). Make sure the client keeps the hip in line with the rest of his or her body. The spine is straight with no hip extension. At this new position, repeat the contract-relax, contract-antagonist with active assisted stretching two or three times if needed to achieve between 30 to 45 degrees of adduction.

PRECAUTIONARY NOTE

Be very cautious of SI joint dysfunction or pain. If there is any discomfort, stop immediately and go to the next step, or return to the myofascial work, as needed.

Step 8: Multidirectional Friction

If the client complains of discomfort or pain when he or she contracts against your resistance during the previous stretch, stop the stretch and ask the client to point to the specific spot (Figure 2-31A ■). Put your finger on the spot and ask if the pain is directly under your finger. If so, and pain increases to that specific area when the client contracts that muscle group against your resistance, this is a muscle strain (which may also be described as a tear) most likely at the attachment of the QL on the ilium (Figure 2-31B ■).

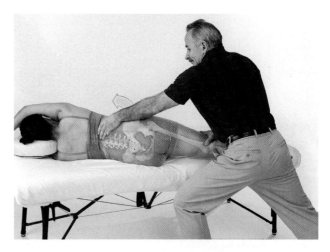

FIGURE 2-29
Right QL PNF Stretch.

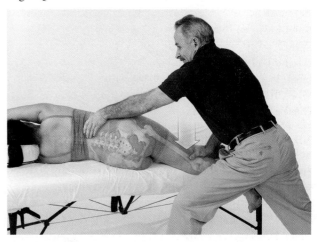

FIGURE 2-30
Right QL Stretch.

Disorganized scar tissue

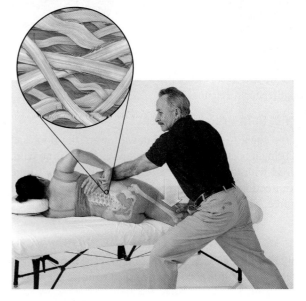

FIGURE 2-31A
Muscle Resistance Test, Right QL.

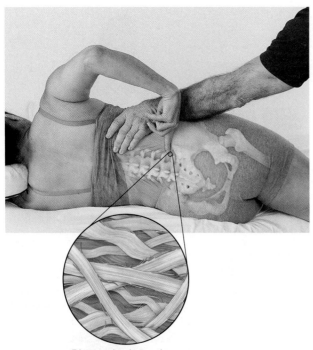

Disorganized scar tissue

FIGURE 2-31B
Muscle Strain, Right QL.

Perform multidirectional friction to the specific area to soften the disorganized collagen or scar tissue that is causing the pain. Use a supported finger and work for only 20 to 30 seconds so you don't create inflammation (Figure 2-32 ■). Go to the next step.

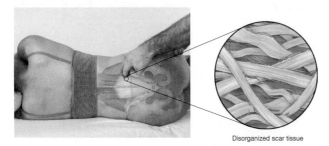

Disorganized scar tissue

FIGURE 2-32
Multidirectional Friction.

Step 9: Pain-Free Movement

Ask the client to lower the leg down toward the floor and then bring it back up again several times. If there is no pain, proceed with the next step. If there is pain, return to the multidirectional friction working a little deeper, but still pain-free. Then repeat the movement again.

Step 10: Eccentric Scar Tissue Alignment

Apply **eccentric muscle contraction** to realign the scar tissue. Remember, this *must* be performed pain-free.

1. Stand behind or in front of the side-lying client and have him or her move close to you. Place two fingers above the client's knee to apply moderate downward force. Press the client's leg slowly down below the table telling the client to "barely resist, but let me win." Start with a resistance of only two fingers and then have the client increase resistance only if there is zero discomfort. Repeat this several times (Figures 2-33A ■ and 2-33B ■).

2. This can also be performed in the prone position, but it is not as effective as in the side-lying position shown in number 1. The client is prone with the knee bent and

Disorganized scar tissue

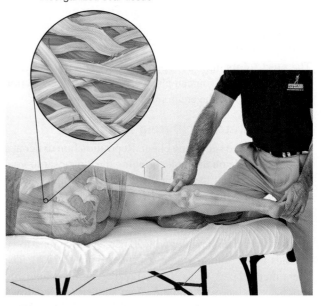

FIGURE 2-33A
QL Eccentric Muscle Contraction (Start).

Functional scar tissue

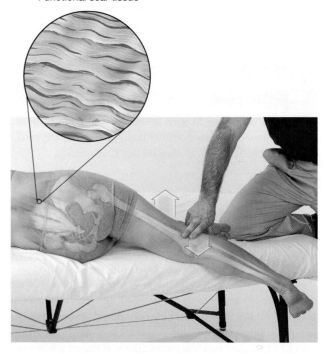

FIGURE 2-33B
QL Eccentric Muscle Contraction (Finish).

the hip laterally rotated. Stand at the end of the table and grasp the ankle. Have the client create mild resistance while you slowly traction the ankle to straighten the leg. Make sure he or she keeps the hip on the table (or body cushion) in slight lateral rotation. Lean back and traction the leg, telling the client to "barely resist, but let me win." Begin with a resistance of only two fingers. Repeat this several times, pain-free.

Step 4: Assess Resisted Range of Motion (RROM)

To reassess RROM, repeat the resisted test by hiking up the hip against resistance—either prone or side lying (Figure 2-34 ■). If there is still pain, return to the multidirectional friction working even slower and deeper and then repeat the eccentric work. If there is no pain, the scar tissue has been functionally realigned (Figure 2-35 ■). Now you can perform the stretch.

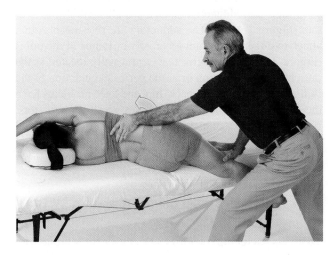

FIGURE 2-34
Repeat Muscle Resistance Test for QL.

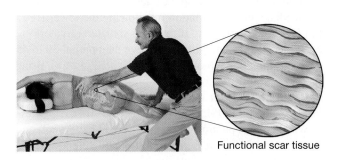

Functional scar tissue

FIGURE 2-35
Right QL Stretch.

Step 6: Myofascial Release

After the right and left side are in balance, finish the work on the QL and erectors with the following myofascial strokes. Move to the side of the table and perform deep-tissue release using your thumbs and knuckles, upward, on both sides of the spine. First, have the client tuck his or her sacrum and

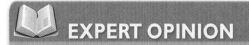

EXPERT OPINION

If you don't feel a smooth lamina groove there may be a rotated vertebra. If so, refer to Erik Dalton's *Myoskeletal Alignment Techniques* (see the "Suggested Readings" in Appendix C), or refer out to a chiropractor.

try to extend the ilia. This will eliminate any lumbar hyperlordosis and prevent the next technique from compromising any existing problems with lateral or anterior bulging discs. Have the client take a deep breath and then exhale. As he or she relaxes, give an upward lift and slowly push superiorly (Figure 2-36 ■). This will stretch the erectors and connective tissue and take the pressure off the discs of the lower back. Start from the sacrum and repeat the strokes, to approximately the twelfth thoracic vertebra, on the deep intrinsic muscles. Lift and lengthen the tissue. This can create spontaneous alignment of the vertebrae, as the facet joints may open up. Next, have the client take a deep breath and exhale. As he or she relaxes, use the back of your hands or your knuckles on the erectors, with your thumbs as a guide going deeper into the lamina groove (Figure 2-37 ■). Repeat this several times, working toward the middle back. This will clear out fibrosis in the lamina groove and decompress the discs of the lumbar spine.

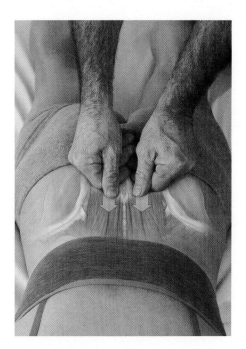

FIGURE 2-36
Decompress Lumbar Spine.

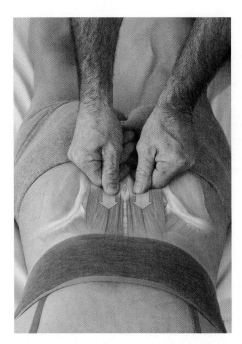

FIGURE 2-37
Evaluate for a Smooth Lamina Groove Using Thumbs.

Step 3: Assess Passive Range of Motion (PROM)

To reassess PROM, with the client prone, go to the end of the table and grasp his or her ankle. Lean back and give a gentle stretch and traction to the body for 5 seconds and then release very slowly (Figure 2-38 ■). Alternate gently pulling (not jerking) each leg to allow each ilium to move separately. You may create a balance of the SI joint as spontaneous alignment may occur. Reevaluate by palpating the iliac crests, after the stretch, to make sure the QL and erectors are balanced on both the left and right sides.

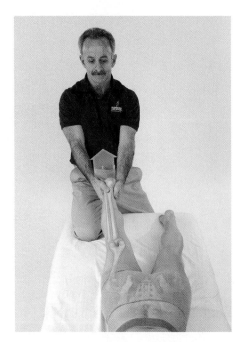

FIGURE 2-38
Traction to Mobilize the Ilium.

LATERAL HIP ROTATORS OR MEDIAL HIP ROTATORS AND ADDUCTORS

The deep six lateral hip rotators are a group of small muscles located beneath the gluteus maximus: gemellus inferior, gemellus superior, obturator externus, obturator internus, piriformis, and quadratus femoris. They all insert on the greater trochanter and attach to various aspects of the sacrum and pelvis (Figures 2-39A ■ and 2-39B ■). The piriformis lies above the large *sciatic nerve,* whereas the other five lateral rotators are deep to it. The sciatic nerve can get compressed beneath a contracted or tight piriformis, but some clinical studies say it is more likely compressed as it passes over the quadratus femoris, causing sciatica and lower back pain. However, occasionally the sciatic nerve passes through the piriformis muscle and these individuals will be more prone to piriformis syndrome (Figure 2-40 ■).

The gluteus medius, gluteus minimus, tensor fasciae latae, and the adductor muscles are all medial hip rotators (Figure 2-41 ■). The adductors are five muscles that attach to either the ischial tuberosity or ramus of the pubis (Figure 2-42 ■). Adductor tears are usually located at the muscle–tendon junction or at the periosteal junction of the ischial tuberosity. Many back, hip, and knee problems have their origin in muscle imbalances between the hip rotators. It is essential to achieve balance between the lateral and medial hip rotators on both legs. Ideal range of motion at the hip is 45 degrees of internal hip rotation and 60 degrees of external hip rotation.

Step 3: Assess Passive Range of Motion (PROM) for Lateral Hip Rotation

To assess lateral hip rotator PROM, the client is prone with the knees together, one knee bent 90 degrees. Stand at one side of the table and place one hand on the client's hip to stabilize it. Make sure the ilium does not move while evaluating femoral rotation. Grasp the client's lower leg and check the medial (internal) rotation by allowing the lower leg to fall laterally toward you. If the deep six lateral rotators are contracted, the client will not achieve the optimal 30 to 45 degrees of internal femoral rotation (Figure 2-43A ■). Bring the leg out at 30-degree abduction and test again for the lower five hip rotator muscles. If both sides of the hip are less than normal ROM, work the tighter side first, regardless of which side is painful. Both sides should have a soft and leathery end feel. If it is a bone-on-bone-like end feel, go immediately to joint capsule work.

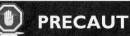

✋ PRECAUTIONARY NOTE

If the client is hypermobile, with more than 45 degrees of internal hip rotation, do not lengthen the lateral hip rotators.

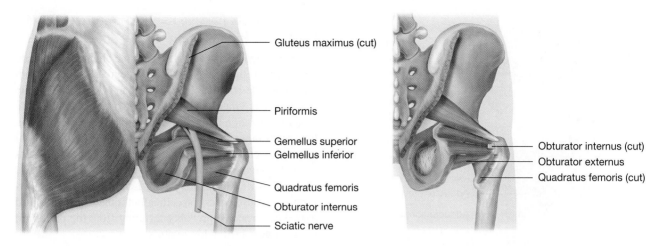

FIGURE 2-39A
Sciatic Nerve.

FIGURE 2-39B
Muscles of the Hip.

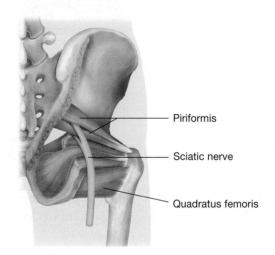

FIGURE 2-40
Sciatic Nerve May Run Through Piriformos.

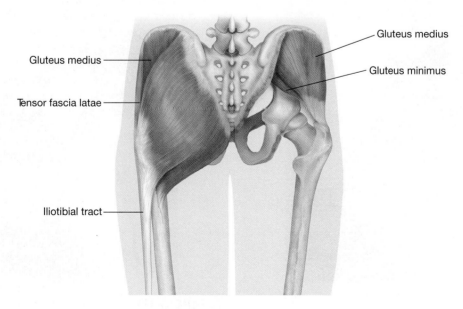

FIGURE 2-41
Internal (Medial) Hip Rotators.

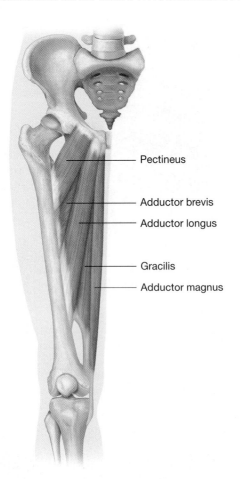

FIGURE 2-42
Adductors.

Labels in figure: Pectineus, Adductor brevis, Adductor longus, Gracilis, Adductor magnus

Step 3: Assess Passive Range of Motion (PROM) for Medial Hip Rotation

To assess medial hip rotator PROM, the client is prone with the knees together, one knee bent 90 degrees. You are standing at the side of the table with one hand on the client's hip to stabilize it. Grasp the client's ankle and check the lateral (external) rotation by pressing the bent leg away from you, toward the other leg. If the medial rotators are tight and contracted the client will not achieve the optimum 60 degrees of external femoral rotation (Figure 2-43B ■). The end feel should be soft and leathery. If it is not, immediately perform joint capsule work, specifically for the inner fascial and capsular adhesions, probably resulting from the prolonged tension in the medial hip rotators.

 CORE PRINCIPLE

You must evaluate both the lateral and medial hip rotators, as this will determine what protocol to follow. Focus on treating the tight, restricted muscle groups first. If the client cannot achieve 30 to 45 degrees of medial hip rotation and has a tissue-stretch end feel, the problem is most likely tight lateral hip rotators. If the client cannot achieve 60 degrees of lateral hip rotation with a tissue-stretch end feel, the problem is most likely tight medial rotators. If there is a bone-on-bone-like end feel in either direction, the problem is probably inner fascial and capsular adhesions and that changes the treatment technique completely.

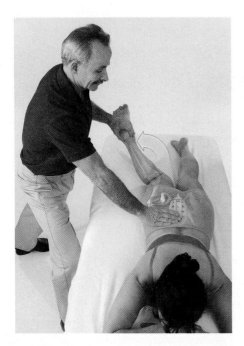

FIGURE 2-43A
Evaluate Internal Femoral Rotation.

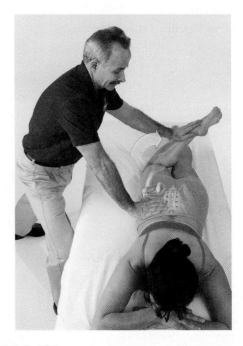

FIGURE 2-43B
Evaluate External Femoral Rotation.

LATERAL HIP ROTATOR PROTOCOL

Step 4: Assess Resisted Range of Motion (RROM)

The client is prone with the knee bent 90 degrees. Place one hand on the inside of the client's leg to protect and support the knee. Your other hand stabilizes the hip. Ask the client to attempt lateral rotation by bringing the ankle toward the midline while you provide resistance. If he or she experiences pain, have the client point to the specific spot. If there is a strain, work this area last.

PRONE JOINT CAPSULE WORK

The prone joint capsule work is usually performed when balancing the medial and lateral hip rotators. Use this technique to free up whatever direction hip rotation is restricted, if there is a bone-on-bone-like end feel. The client is in the prone position with the legs straight. Place your hands around the thigh and push the femur *gently* into the hip joint, rotate it, and then pull it back out. Be extremely cautious, and avoid any aggressive pressure directed toward the lumbar spine, especially if there is a possibility of a bulging disc. Contact, rotate, decompress. Do not lift the leg off the table; just glide it along the table. Continue massaging the deep inner fascial and capsular adhesions while rotating gently to the restriction. Then perform a deep fascial and capsular stretch either laterally (Figure 2-44 ■) or medially (Figure 2-45 ■), depending on which direction is restricted. Stretch just until the ilium starts to move and then stop. Repeat this sequence several times.

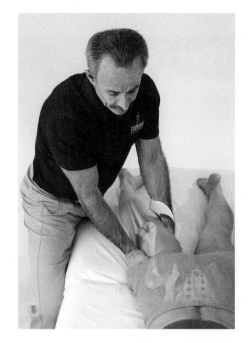

FIGURE 2-45
Internal Joint Capsule Work.

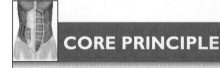

CORE PRINCIPLE

This work *must* be performed *totally pain-free*.

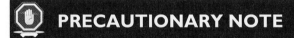

PRECAUTIONARY NOTE

If the client has any joint pathology (degenerative discs, SI joint dysfunction, etc.), push the femur into the hip joint just until you make contact with the ilium (about 1/8 inch). This is a subtle movement. Pushing forcefully may create pain or discomfort in the lower back and could severely compromise the lumbar spine!

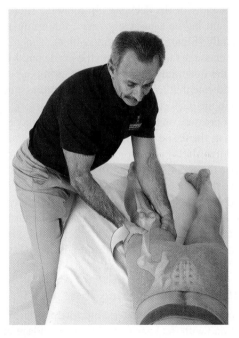

FIGURE 2-44
External Joint Capsule Work.

Step 6: Myofascial Release

With the client prone, release the gluteals by pushing and warming up the edges around the sacrum. Start with gentle compression, broadening to bring blood and oxygen to the area. If the lateral rotators are tight and not allowing full range of motion, perform myofascial work to the gluteal attachments all around the circumference.

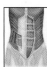

CORE PRINCIPLE

Always ask the client for permission before you work directly on the gluteal area.

You can drape the glutes with a towel for client comfort and modesty, or you can work directly through the clothing. Place one hand on the hip to stabilize the sacrum. Then use the back of a closed fist and work away from the sacrum, *superior* to *inferior* and medial to lateral (Figure 2-46 ■). Repeat this several times. Also, apply compressions to the glutes and deep six to enhance blood flow. Do *not* work directly on the tendon attachments on the lateral side of the hip; only work up to them as they are rarely injured.

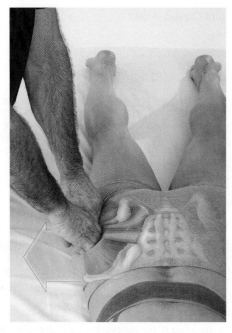

FIGURE 2-46
Deep Six Lateral Hip Rotator Myofascial Release.

Step 7: Cross-Fiber Gliding Strokes/Trigger Point Therapy

CROSS-FIBER GLIDING STROKES

Then, come off the lateral side of the sacrum and strum and stretch all of the deep six lateral rotator muscles using a cross-fiber gliding stroke, with your thumbs, working medial to lateral (Figure 2-47 ■). Work *origin* to *insertion*, from the sacrum to the femur (superior to inferior). Repeat this several times.

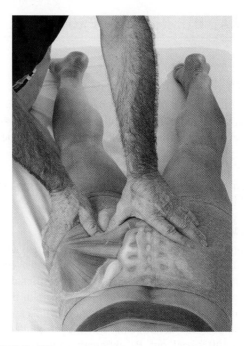

FIGURE 2-47
Cross-Fiber Gliding/Trigger Point Work to Deep Six Lateral Hip Rotators.

TRIGGER POINT THERAPY

Tease through tight bands and treat any trigger points with direct pressure for 10 to 12 seconds, compress, and then gently stretch the tissue. Finally, perform compressions over the entire area to increase blood flow to these large muscles.

Step 6: Myofascial Release

Come off the edge of the sacrum and place the back of your fist on the belly of the deep six hip rotators. Then hold the client's bent leg and passively rotate the femur medially and laterally (Figures 2-48 ■ and 2-49 ■). This allows the femur to massage the muscle from the inside out. Make sure to work the quadratus femoris muscle. Some new clinical studies indicate that it is more likely to compress the sciatic nerve than the piriformis muscle.

Your pressure on the lateral hip rotators is moderate, but increases as the tissue warms up and softens. Remember to keep this pain-free.

Move the client's knee to 30 to 45 degrees hip abduction and move the back of your fist inferiorly, to affect the lower lateral hip rotators (Figure 2-50 ■). With moderate pressure on these muscles, again passively rotate the femur medially and laterally. If the client has knee problems, place your hand on the medial side of the knee (to protect it) as you are rotating the hip.

Step 11: Stretching (During Therapy)

1. This stretch is for the lateral hip rotators. The client is prone with the knee bent 90 degrees. Place one hand on the inside of the leg to protect and support the knee. This is important, especially for clients with

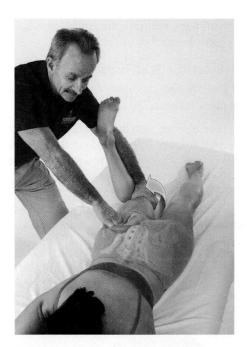

FIGURE 2-48
Internal Femur Rotation to Massage Deep Six.

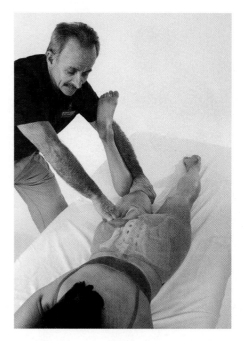

FIGURE 2-50
Compress More Inferior/Repeat.

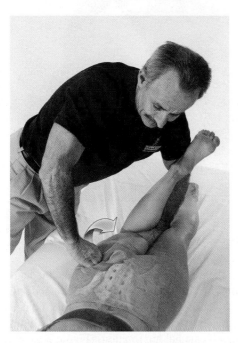

FIGURE 2-49
External Femur Rotation to Massage Deep Six.

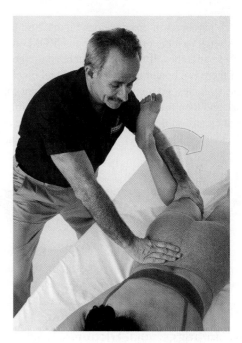

FIGURE 2-51
Deep Six Lateral Hip Rotator Stretch.

knee problems. Place your other hand on the hip to stabilize it. Have the client's ankle fall toward you, to the restriction. The foot can rest on your shoulder. Ask the client to pull the ankle toward the midline (lateral rotation) for 5 to 10 seconds at 20 percent force while you resist (Figure 2-51 ■). He or she relaxes, takes a deep breath, and on exhale actively moves the ankle laterally (medial hip rotation) toward you, and you assist the stretch for about 2 seconds. At this new

position, repeat the contract-relax, contract-antagonist with active assisted stretching two or three times, or until the client attains the normal range of motion of 30 to 45 degrees of medial rotation.

2. This stretch is for the lower lateral hip rotators. The client is prone with the knee bent 90 degrees. Bring the client's leg out to 30-degree abduction. Place one hand on the inside of the leg to protect and support the knee. Place your other hand on the hip to stabilize it. Repeat

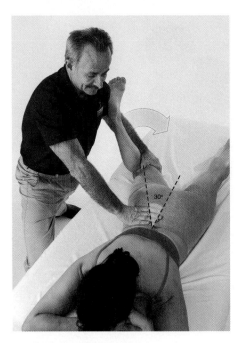

FIGURE 2-52
Deep Six Stretch.

stretch number 1 in this position (Figure 2-52 ■). Do not stretch past the optimal 45-degree ROM on either of these stretches. If the client cannot attain the ROM, or if there is a bone-on-bone-like end feel on either of these stretches, go immediately to prone joint capsule work and then back to the myofascial spreading. If the client cannot achieve the normal ROM and the end feel is leathery, go back and rework the muscle group.

CORE PRINCIPLE

Anytime there is a bone-on-bone-like end feel, perform joint capsule work rather than focusing on tight muscle groups.

Step 8: Multidirectional Friction

If the client complains of pain when the previous stretches are attempted, stop and ask him or her to point to the specific area of discomfort. Have the client contract that muscle group against your resistance and ask if that increases pain to that specific area. If so, perform multidirectional friction to the specific area for only 20 to 30 seconds. Then go to the next step.

Step 9: Pain-Free Movement

Ask the client to move the femur through the hip's full range of motion of both lateral and medial rotation. There should be about a 90- to 105-degree arc between the two motions (60-degree lateral rotation, 30- to 45-degree medial rotation). If there is no pain, proceed with the eccentric work.

If there is still pain, return to the multidirectional friction working a little deeper, but still pain-free.

Step 10: Eccentric Scar Tissue Alignment

Apply an eccentric muscle contraction, performed pain-free, to realign the scar tissue.

1. The client is prone with the knee bent 90 degrees. Place your forearm on the inside of the tibia. Have the client gently resist while you gently pull the ankle toward yourself (medial hip rotation) (Figure 2-53 ■). Ask the client to "barely resist, but let me win." Start with a pull using only two fingers, and then have the client increase resistance only if there is no discomfort. Repeat this several times, pain-free.

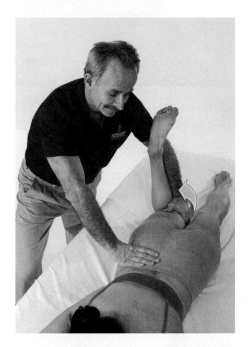

FIGURE 2-53
Deep Six Eccentric Muscle Contraction.

2. The client is prone with the knee bent 90 degrees. Bring the client's leg out to 30-degree abduction. Place your forearm on the inside of the tibia. Have the client gently resist while you pull the ankle toward yourself (medial hip rotation) (Figure 2-54 ■). Tell him or her to "barely resist, but let me win." Start with a pull using only two fingers. Have the client increase resistance if there is zero discomfort. Repeat this eccentric work several times, pain-free.

Note: This is performed only if there was a muscle strain in the deep six hip rotators.

Step 4: Assess Resisted Range of Motion (RROM)

To reassess RROM, repeat the resisted test again. If there is pain, return to the multidirectional friction working slower and deeper, but still pain-free, and then repeat the eccentric work. If there is no pain, perform the stretch.

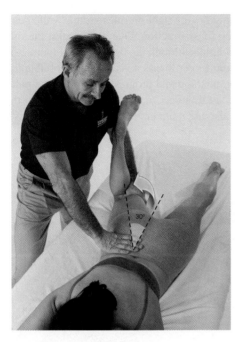

FIGURE 2-54
Lower Deep Six Eccentric Contraction.

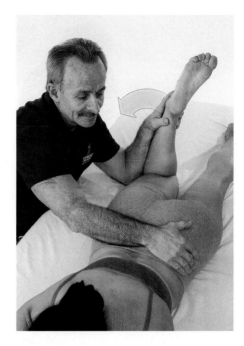

FIGURE 2-55
Assess for Strain, Medial Hip Rotators.

Step 3: Assess Passive Range of Motion (PROM)

To reassess PROM, the client should achieve a minimum of 30 degrees of internal femoral rotation, with a tissue stretch end feel, if you created length in lateral hip rotators of the left and right sides; 45 degrees is optimal.

MEDIAL HIP ROTATORS AND ADDUCTORS

Step 4: Assess Medial Hip Rotation Resisted Range of Motion (RROM)

To assess medial hip rotator RROM, the client is prone with the knee bent 90 degrees. Grasp the ankle with one hand while your other hand stabilizes the hip. Ask the client to attempt medial hip rotation (bring the ankle toward you) while you provide resistance. If he or she experiences pain, have the client point to the specific spot (Figure 2-55 ■). Work this area last.

Step 3: Assess Adductor Passive Range of Motion (PROM)

To assess adductor PROM, the client is seated or supine on the table. Grasp and support one leg and slowly move it to abduction. The client should attain the normal 45-degree ROM without pain. The end feel should be soft and leathery.

Step 4: Assess Adductor Resisted Range of Motion (RROM)

To assess adductor RROM, the client is seated with one leg straight and the other off the side of the table, to anchor the body. Stand on the side of the table next to the straight leg. Grasp and support that leg at the knee, at the distal end of the femur, to protect the knee. Ask the client to abduct only

to where he or she is comfortable, and then have the client perform adduction against your resistance. If there is pain, have the client point to the specific spot (Figure 2-56 ■). Work this area last.

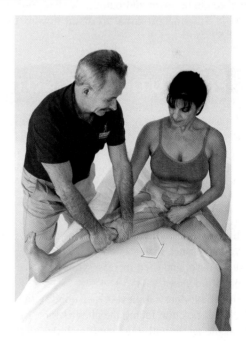

FIGURE 2-56
Assess for Strain, Adductors.

Step 6: Myofascial Release

To release the adductors, the client is side lying, in a comfortable position, with support to the shoulders and neck and with a bolster under the top leg. The hip should be flexed at

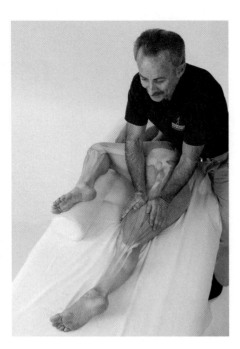

FIGURE 2-57
Myofascial Release, Adductors.

least 90 degrees. The bottom leg is the one you will be working on and it is straight. For draping, you can use a sheet or a towel between the client's legs.

Start with myofascial release on the medial thigh at a 45-degree angle down and out, on the leg. Start as high as possible, moving proximal to distal toward the knee (Figure 2-57 ■).

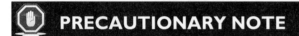

PRECAUTIONARY NOTE

Avoid massage directly to any areas where you see distended varacosities, and consult with the client's physician in regard to working away from the heart in these areas. Also consult with their physician if they have any history of lymphatic problems.

When you get to the medial side of the knee, lighten up on your pressure if you continue your stroke onto the lower leg. Pause, and then increase your pressure again to decompress the knee.

If the client does not have hypermobility of the knee, get in a lunge position facing the client's foot. Make a "c" clamp on the ankle with one hand; stabilize the hip with the other. Gently apply in-line traction, pressing the ankle toward the end of the table, moving the tibia away from femur to open up the knee joint (Figure 2-58 ■).

Use compressions on the inner thigh to bring blood flow, oxygen, and heat to the area to help release the deep investing fascia. Next, use your palm and finger pads and roll them over the inner thigh, gently and slowly stretching, pulling,

and pushing on any tight muscles groups while gently rocking the leg for distraction. One hand rocks, the other hand pushes and pulls through the tight bands (Figure 2-59 ■). Do not use your fingertips, as it is too uncomfortable for the client. Rock the thigh and progressively push and pull through the fibers until there is no longer any tension in the tissue. You can also use counterstretches with your palms working

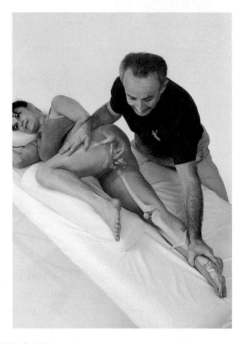

FIGURE 2-58
Traction Hip and Knee.

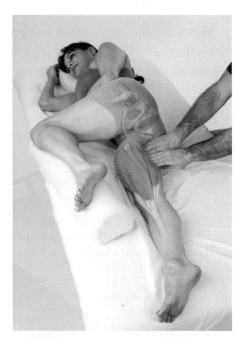

FIGURE 2-59
Use Muscles to Stretch the Intermuscular Septums and Deep Investing Fascia.

in opposite directions. *Use the muscles to release the supporting and surrounding fascia.* As you work deeper, go slower and really tune in and get present with your hands. Palpate the tissue like you are kneading dough. As muscle fibers and fascia soften, the ischemia will be reduced and the trigger points may disappear. This noninvasive technique also uses the muscle groups to soften and stretch the intermuscular septums and deep investing fascia from the inside out.

Step 7: Trigger Point Therapy

Treat any remaining trigger points using direct pressure for 10 to 12 seconds, compress, and then gently stretch the tissue. Very few or no active muscle myofascial trigger points will remain after doing the myofascial mobilization techniques, to restore normal muscle resting lengths, outlined in this chapter. Repeat the compressions over the entire area, if needed.

Finally, grasp the client's ankle to traction and gently decompress the leg (Figure 2-60 ■). Hold for 5 seconds and then slowly release.

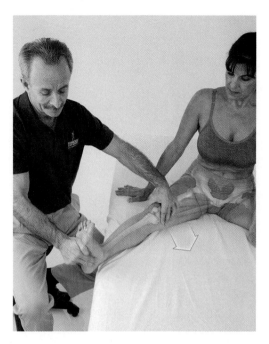

FIGURE 2-61
Adductors Stretch.

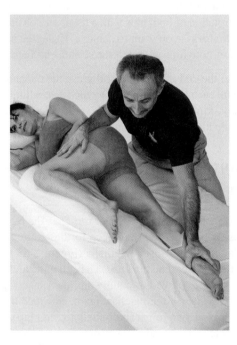

FIGURE 2-60
Traction Hip, Knee, and Ankle.

Step 11: Stretching Adductors (During Therapy)

To stretch the adductors, the client is sitting on the table with one leg straight, the other off the side of the table to anchor the body. You can drape a towel between and over the upper thighs and hip, if needed. Stand on the side of the table next to the straight leg. Grasp and support that leg at the knee, on the distal end of the femur, to protect the knee with both hands. Keeping the foot and knee in line (the hip is not externally or internally rotated), ask the client to abduct the hip only to where he or she is comfortable. The client then performs adduction at 20 percent force for 5 to

10 seconds as you provide resistance (Figure 2-61 ■). The client relaxes, takes a deep breath, and exhales as he or she actively moves the leg to abduction. You assist the stretch for about 2 seconds, bringing the leg toward you. At this new position, repeat this contract-relax, contract-antagonist with active assisted stretching two or three times, or until achieving the normal 45-degree range of motion.

Step 11: Stretching Medial Hip Rotators (During Therapy)

To stretch the medial rotators, the client is prone with the knee bent 90 degrees. Grasp the ankle with one hand while the other hand stabilizes the hip. Have the client move the ankle toward the other leg (lateral femoral rotation) only to where it is comfortable. Then ask the client to move the ankle toward you (medial femoral rotation) for 5 to 10 seconds at 20 percent force while you resist (Figure 2-62 ■). The client relaxes, takes a deep breath, and exhales as he or she moves the ankle away from you (lateral rotation) and you assist the stretch for about 2 seconds. At this new position, repeat the contract-relax, contract-antagonist with active assisted stretching two or three times, or until achieving the normal range of motion of 60-degree lateral femoral rotation.

🖐 PRECAUTIONARY NOTE

If the client has knee problems, place your forearm on their entire lower leg so there is not excessive torque on the lateral side of the knee.

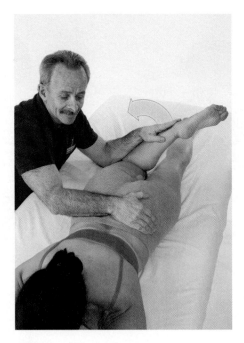

FIGURE 2-62
Medial Hip Rotator P.N.F. Stretch.

Step 8: Multidirectional Friction

If the client complains of pain when they contract against resistance or during the previous stretches, it is most likely that there is a muscle strain. For the adductors it may be at the attachment, on the base of the pelvis. Ask the client to place a finger on that tender area. With *permission,* match your finger to the client's and perform multidirectional friction for 20 to 30 seconds. If the client is too modest to allow this, you can also ask him or her to perform the friction. You *must* receive the client's permission to friction this area.

Step 9: Pain-Free Movement

1. For the adductors, the client is in the same position as the stretch. Ask him or her to move the leg through abduction and adduction several times. The client can slide the back of the leg across the table.
2. For the medial rotators, the client is in the same position as the stretch. Ask him or her to move the hip through medial and lateral rotation several times.

If there is no pain during these movements, proceed with the eccentric work. If there is pain, return to the multidirectional friction working a little slower and deeper, but still pain-free.

Step 10: Eccentric Scar Tissue Alignment

Next, have the client perform eccentric contraction to realign the scar tissue. This must be performed pain-free.

1. For the adductors, the client is in the same position as for the stretch. Have him or her gently resist as you abduct the leg. Tell the client to "barely resist, but let

me win." Start with a pressure using only two fingers and have the client increase resistance only if there is no discomfort. Repeat this several times.
2. For the medial rotators, the client is in the same position as for the stretch. Have the client gently resist as you laterally rotate the femur. Gently push the ankle toward the other leg. Tell the client to "barely resist, but let me win." Begin with a resistance using only two fingers. Have the client increase resistance if there is zero discomfort. Repeat this several times.

Step 4: Assess Resisted Range of Motion (RROM)

To reassess RROM, repeat the resisted tests for both the adductors and the medial rotators. If the client still experiences pain, return to the multidirectional friction working a little slower and deeper, but still pain-free. Return to the stretch and repeat all of the steps, as needed, until the pain is gone.

Step 3: Assess Passive Range of Motion (PROM)

To reassess PROM:

- **Medial Rotators**—you want to achieve a 60-degree lateral rotation of both hips with a tissue stretch end feel.
- **Adductors**—you want to achieve 45-degree abduction of both hips with a tissue stretch end feel.

Go to the end of the table and grasp the client's ankles. Gently pull each leg one at a time to allow each ilium to move separately. Finish by leaning back and pulling both legs to traction the hips, knees, and ankles. Release very slowly.

QUADRICEPS AND ILIOTIBIAL BAND (ITB)

The quadriceps are a group of four muscles: the rectus femoris, vastus intermedius (lies deep to the rectus femoris), vastus lateralis, and vastus medialis (Figure 2-63 ■). Their main action is to extend the knee. They all unite and become a single tendon above the patella and then insert onto the tibial tuberosity via the patellar ligament. Since the rectus femoris crosses two joints (both the knee and hip), it is the only muscle in the quadriceps group that flexes the hip. It originates on the anterior inferior iliac spine. The superficial, thick iliotibial band (ITB) runs down the lateral side of the leg over the vastus lateralis. It inserts on the tibial tubercle

CORE PRINCIPLE

In most cases you should work the quadriceps before the hamstrings to restore balance between these two opposing muscle groups. Typically, the iliopsoas and quadriceps are short and tight and the glutes and upper hamstrings are weak and inhibited.

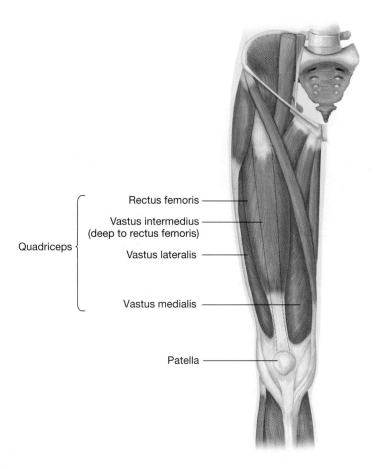

Quadriceps
- Rectus femoris
- Vastus intermedius (deep to rectus femoris)
- Vastus lateralis
- Vastus medialis

Patella

FIGURE 2-63
Muscle Review.

and is a stabilizer for both the hip and knee joints. The TFL (tensor fascia latae) and gluteus maximus both attach to the proximal IT band. Excessive stress or a tight, contracted condition of the ITB can cause pain on the lateral side of the knee. This is called *iliotibial band friction syndrome*. The client typically reports pain during activity, usually enhanced going down steps and kneeling. The pain then diminishes with rest.

QUADRICEPS

Step 3: Assess Passive Range of Motion (PROM)

The client is prone. Go to the end of the table and grasp the client's ankles. Lean back and give a gentle stretch to traction and decompress the knees before you check the range of motion. Release very slowly. This will increase knee space, increasing quadriceps range of motion up to 30 degrees. Have the client bend one knee. Bring the foot toward the hip. Traction the tibia away from the femur and again bring the foot toward the hip. Lean back and perform another gentle traction of the hip, knee, and ankle. Again release very slowly.

Normal ROM is 135 degrees or optimal ROM is touching the glutes with the foot. This will be a tissue-on-tissue or leathery end feel. If it feels springy, or bone-on-bone-like, do *not* force it; the knee joint could have damaged cartilage, damaged ligaments, or abnormal knee rotation problems.

Step 4: Assess Resisted Range of Motion (RROM)

The client is prone. Bring the knee into flexion. Have the client attempt to extend the knee as you provide resistance. If he or she experiences pain, have the client point to the specific spot. Work this area last.

ASSESS ANTERIOR SUPERIOR ILIAC SPINE (ASIS)

The client is supine. Palpate the ASIS on the client's left and right sides. Determine if they are at the same height, which is normal. If so, proceed with the quadriceps work. If one ASIS is lower than the other, this indicates that the ilium is anteriorly rotated (forward) on that side. To rotate the ilium backward, stand next to the client. Have him or her flex the hip and bend the knee so that the back of the lower leg rests on your shoulder. Place one hand on the lateral side of this hip. Ask the client to attempt to extend the hip (toward

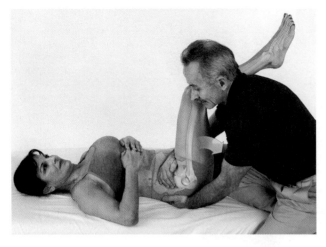

FIGURE 2-64
Correcting Flexion in the Ilium (Resisted Hip Extension).

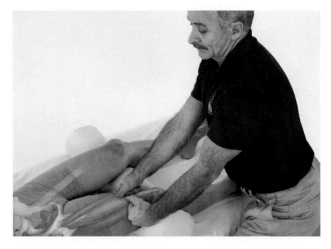

FIGURE 2-66
Myofascial Release up Quadriceps.

the table) for 5 to 10 seconds at 20 percent force while you resist (Figure 2-64 ■). He or she relaxes, takes a deep breath, and exhales while bringing the knee toward the chest (hip flexion) for about 2 seconds as you assist the stretch. Your hand on the lateral side of the hip also assists by rotating the ilium posterior (Figure 2-65 ■). At this new position, repeat the contract-relax, contract-antagonist with active assisted stretching until the ASIS are at the same height.

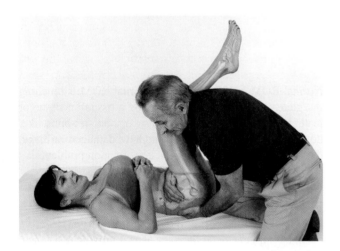

FIGURE 2-65
Correcting Flexion in the Ilium (Assisted Hip Flexion).

Step 6: Myofascial Release

The client is supine with the leg slightly abducted. Perform myofascial spreading at a 45-degree angle on the quads, working from the knee progressively to the hip (Figure 2-66 ■). This is done very slowly with fists, palms, knuckles, hands, or fingers. Make sure you work through the upper attachments. Then use slow, rhythmical compressions over the entire quads, pinning and moving the tissue at a 45-degree angle inferiorly toward the knee. This will unload the forces

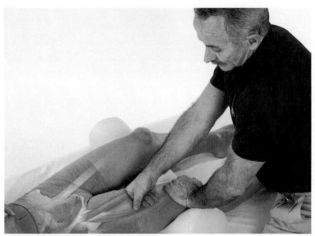

FIGURE 2-67
Myofascial Release up Rectus Femoris.

on the patellar ligament and help decompress the femoral head in the hip joint.

Next, "iron" up the rectus femoris using your forearm or the back of your fist. Pin or traction the skin with your lower hand, while the upper hand performs the stroke (Figure 2-67 ■). This will increase blood flow to the area and lengthen the rectus femoris. Repeat the compressions.

Step 7: Cross-Fiber Gliding Strokes/Trigger Point Therapy

CROSS-FIBER GLIDING STROKES

Goal: to tease apart tight quadriceps muscle bands (tight, contracted muscle)

Use cross-fiber gliding strokes to tease through and gently spread any tight quadriceps muscle bands. This will loosen up tight muscle fibers that often feed and contribute to trigger points, allowing tissue to move more freely and independently.

- Tight muscles, with tenderness located directly under your pressure?
- This requires cross-fiber gliding strokes working from insertion to origin (distal to proximal) on the quadriceps.

TRIGGER POINT THERAPY

Goal: to release trigger points in the muscle belly of the quadriceps, if found.

You should first and primarily perform trigger point work on the contracted, tight muscles.

If there is a specific area of pain that radiates or refers to a predictable area or site, based on Travell's trigger point theories, apply trigger point therapy.

- Use direct, moderate pressure for 10 to 12 seconds.
- As the trigger point softens, compress the tissue several times.
- Gently stretch the fascia that feeds the ischemic tender area.

After performing cross-fiber gliding strokes and trigger point therapy (if needed), you may need to return to the myofascial spreading, working even slower and deeper, but still pain-free to release any tissue that is still restricted.

ILIOTIBIAL BAND (ITB)

Step 6: Myofascial Release

To release the ITB, think of it as a tight tendon even though it is a ligamentous structure. You need to release the ITB to affect the underlying vastus lateralis. Proximally, this band comes off the fibers of the gluteus maximus and the tensor fasciae latae (TFL) and when it is tight or restricted it can cause lateral knee pain.

Start by working the gluteus maximus and medius with compressions. Bend the client's knee to bring the hip into flexion. Then, over his or her clothing perform gentle cross-fiber gliding strokes, compressions, and trigger point work if needed to the TFL. To locate the TFL, palpate the ASIS and drop laterally off it. Have the client medially rotate the hip against your resistance and you will feel the TFL contract and broaden under your fingers. Use your fingers or thumbs to work the fibers from the hip toward the IT band. Be careful, as this area is likely to be tender.

Next, using the heel of your hands and thumb, hook the inferior angle of the ITB and rotate it from lateral to medial as you draw it distally toward the knee. Use the other hand on the other side of the leg to help create a rotational

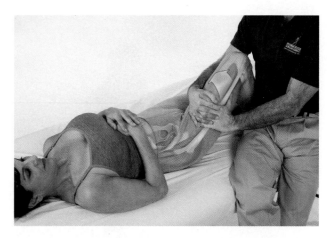

FIGURE 2-68
Iliotibial Band Mobilization.

movement (Figure 2-68 ■). Do not slide over the skin. Begin at the broader fibers at the hip first and work toward the knee. You can use your thumb as a guide along the lateral border of the ITB. This will free up the fascial binding to allow the ITB to move more independently of the vastus lateralis. See video clip on www.myhealthprofessionskit.com.

Next, pin your elbow into your side (as additional pressure) and work the ITB several times with the palm of your hand. This will help release adhesions between the ITB and the vastus lateralis. Alternate with compression strokes with intention to lengthen the vastus lateralis. The compressive strokes into the vastus lateralis should start at the hip and enter the vastus lateralis at a 45-degree angle, as you move from the hip to the knee, to create length in the lateral quadriceps. If the vastus lateralis is tender during the compressions, you haven't fully released the ITB. Go back to the rotational stroke. It is usually a tight vastus lateralis and a weak vastus medialis that cause lateral tracking of the knee cap, leading to clinical conditions such as patellar femoral pain, chondromalacia, and patellar tendinosis. Next, go to the attachment of the ITB on the tibial tubercle, at the lateral side of the knee. Make sure everything is moving and there are no "crunchies" (fibrotic tissue) in the ligamentous structures here.

Step 7: Cross-Fiber Gliding Strokes/Trigger Point Therapy

Use cross-fiber gliding strokes working from origin to insertion (proximal to distal) to tease through and gently spread muscle fibers in the gluteus maximus, and TFL. Release any muscle belly trigger points, if found, with direct pressure for 10 to 12 seconds, compressions, and a gentle stretch of the surrounding area. Finally, go to the end of the table, grasp the client's ankle, and lean back and give a gentle traction of the leg for 5 seconds to decompress the client's hip, knee, and ankle (Figure 2-69 ■). Release very slowly.

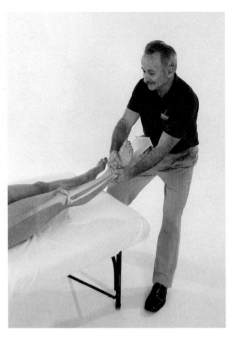

FIGURE 2-69
Hip, Knee, and Ankle Traction.

Step 11: Stretching (During Therapy)

The ITB is relatively avascular and relatively noncontractile, therefore you actually stretch the TFL muscle and the lateral fibers of the gluteus maximus to keep the IT soft and released.

1. **TFL stretch #1:** The client is supine with the uninvolved leg bent and crossed over the other leg, which is straight and laterally rotated, to also affect the TFL. Bring (adduct) the straight leg toward you, to the restriction, lengthening the TFL. Stabilize the pelvis on that side with your other hand, so it doesn't move, or you are stretching only the QL (Figure 2-70 ■). Ask the client to perform abduction at 20 percent force for 5 to 10 seconds as you provide resistance with your hand under the knee to protect it. He or she relaxes, takes a deep breath, and on exhale, the client actively

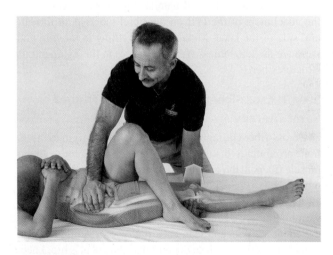

FIGURE 2-70
TFL Stretch.

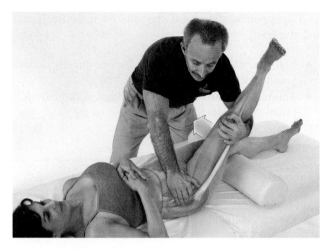

FIGURE 2-71
Optional TFL Stretch.

moves the leg to adduction for about 2 seconds while you assist the stretch. At this new position, repeat this contract-relax, contract-antagonist with active assisted stretching two or three times, or until achieving the normal 30-degree range of motion. Then lean back and traction the client's leg. Release very slowly.

2. **TFL stretch #2:** This stretch can be performed if the client is physically unable to cross one leg over the other as in stretch number 1. The client is supine with the leg straight and laterally rotated. That same hip is flexed about 30 degrees. Stabilize the hip on that side with one hand. Compress the TFL muscle with your finger pads, and do not allow the ilium to move. Bring this leg toward you (adduction), to the restriction, lengthening the TFL (Figure 2-71 ■). Ask the client to attempt abduction at 20 percent force for 5 to 10 seconds as you provide resistance with your hand under the knee to protect it. He or she relaxes, takes a breath, and on exhale actively moves the leg to adduction for about 2 seconds while you assist the stretch. Have the client keep the leg being stretched low and as close to the other leg as possible. At this new position, repeat this contract-relax, contract-antagonist with active assisted stretching two or three times, or until achieving the normal 30-degree range of motion. Then lean back and traction the client's leg. Release very slowly.

3. **Gluteus Maximus stretch:** The client is supine with their knee bent 90 degrees. Stand on the opposite side of the table. Place one hand on the outside of the client's thigh, on the distal quads. The other hand is placed over the lateral fibers of the glute max, pressing it down toward the table. Have the client actively bring their knee toward you; hip adduction, as you assist the stretch for about 2 seconds. Make sure you pin down the glute max during the stretch; the hip must stay on the table. Do not press down on the ilium.

Step 8: Multidirectional Friction

If the client experiences pain when performing the ITB stretch isolate the exact spot by having the client put a finger directly on it. This will most likely be on the lateral side of the knee. This condition is known as iliotibial band friction syndrome, as indicated earlier in this chapter. According to recent clinical studies, there is rarely damage to the fibers that pass over the lateral condyle of the knee, needing the next part of this protocol to be done. Usually after you release and stretch the lateral fibers of gluteus maximus, and the TFL muscle, the pain on the lateral side of the knee goes away. You have treated the cause of ITB friction syndrome to eliminate the symptom in the area of the lateral condyle of the knee. However, in that rare situation where there is damage to those fibers due to prolonged frictioning over the lateral femoral condyle, place your finger on the spot and ask the client if he or she feels the pain directly under your finger. If so, it is probably damaged fibers, also described as a tear by other health care practitioners. Perform multidirectional friction to the area for 20 to 30 seconds. If the area is tender, use only feather-light pressure. Proceed with the next step.

Step 9: Pain-Free Movement

The client is in the same position as the TFL stretch. Have him or her move the leg on top of the table into adduction (toward the middle of the table) and back to neutral several times to redirect the scar tissue. If there is no pain, proceed with the eccentric contraction. If there is pain, return to the multidirectional friction working a little deeper, but still pain-free.

Step 10: Eccentric Scar Tissue Alignment

The client is supine with the leg straight and the hip flexed 45 degrees. Stabilize the hip with one hand. The client gently resists as you perform adduction (bringing the leg toward you). Tell him or her to "barely resist, but let me win." Start with a resistance of only two fingers. If there is zero discomfort the client can increase resistance. Repeat the eccentric contraction several times, then repeat the resisted test. If the client still experiences pain, return to the multidirectional friction again. After the eccentric contraction go back and finish the stretches. It is rare you will ever have to do this (Figure 2-72 ■).

QUADRICEPS

Step 11: Stretching (During Therapy)

 PRECAUTIONARY NOTE

Stretching is not suggested for the muscle groups around a hypermobile joint. Strengthening would be more appropriate to stabilize any joint that has excessive movement due to ligamentous laxity.

This is the only *passive stretch* in the body. It is performed passively to prevent the hamstrings from cramping due to dehydration, imbalance of electrolytes, or poor nutrition.

With the client in the prone position, go to the end of the table and grasp both of the ankles. Lean back and give a gentle stretch and traction to the lower extremity for 5 seconds, then release very slowly. Bring the client's knee into 90-degree flexion and place one hand behind the knee and gently traction the tibia away from the femur to decompress the knee. Then, passively bring the foot toward the hip, folding the lower leg over your hand behind the knee. With the knee flexed 90 degrees, ask the client to attempt to gently extend the leg while you provide resistance at 20 percent force for 5 to 10 seconds. He or she relaxes, takes a deep breath, and on exhale you traction the tibia away from the femur. Fold the lower leg over your hand as a pivot as you move the foot to the hip for about 2 seconds (Figure 2-73 ■). This stretch *must* have a tissue stretch or tissue compression end feel, and be pain-free. Normal range of motion for knee flexion is 135 degrees. Repeat this sequence two or three times, then move to the end of the table. Grasp the client's ankle, lean back, and stretch to decompress the hip, knee, and ankle. Release very slowly. If the client has a hypermobile knee, or ligament laxity, do not traction the knee. Strengthening would replace stretching.

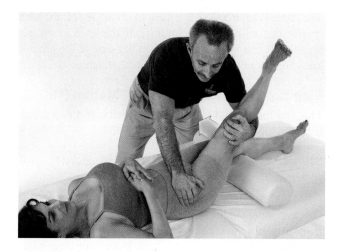

FIGURE 2-72
Eccentric Contraction, ITB.

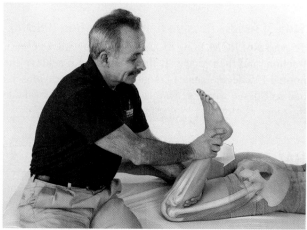

FIGURE 2-73
Quadriceps Stretch.

Step 8: Multidirectional Friction

If the client reports a specific spot of pain during the quadriceps stretch, have him or her isolate it by pointing to it. Usually this will be on the medial side of the patellar ligament, just below the patella. Oftentimes, however, the symptoms of patellar tendinosis do not surface until they perform a weight-bearing test to the quadriceps. If the initial history indicates that pain is produced in the patellar ligament while walking down a flight of steps, but pain does not surface when the client is prone and contracting the quadriceps against resistance, you can have the client stand up and do a one-legged knee flexion test. If pain increases around the patella, perform multidirectional friction on the exact spot for only 20 to 30 seconds. Use only enough pressure to soften the collagen matrix. Do not overwork the area. Proceed with the next step. This will be addressed in detail in Chapter 3.

Step 9: Pain-Free Movement

The client is in the same position as for the quadriceps stretch. Have him or her actively bend and straighten the knee several times. If there is no pain, proceed with the eccentric contraction. If there is pain, return to the multidirectional friction working a little deeper, but still pain-free.

Step 10: Eccentric Scar Tissue Alignment

The client is prone with the knee flexed 90 degrees. Traction the tibia away from the femur. Ask the client to create mild resistance as you gently flex the knee toward the glutes. Tell the client to "barely resist, but let me win." Start with a resistance using only two fingers and then have the client increase resistance only if there is zero discomfort. Repeat this several times.

Step 4: Assess Resisted Range of Motion (RROM)

To reassess RROM, repeat the resisted test. If the client still experiences pain, return to the multidirectional friction and eccentric contraction again. After the pain is gone, perform the stretch.

Step 3: Assess Passive Range of Motion (PROM)

To reassess PROM, bring the client's foot toward the glutes, traction, and then repeat. If the client cannot achieve the normal 135-degree range of motion, return to the myofascial and soft-tissue work on the quadriceps and then reevaluate the range of motion.

HAMSTRINGS

The hamstrings are comprised of the biceps femoris, semitendinosus, and semimembranosus (Figure 2-74 ■). All three muscles extend the hip, flex the knee, and posteriorly rotate the pelvis. The biceps femoris laterally rotates the hip and the flexed knee. The semitendinosus and semimembranosus medially rotate the hip and the flexed knee. They all

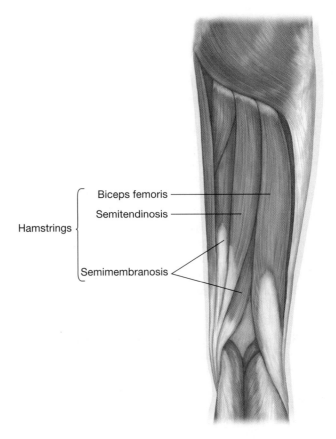

FIGURE 2-74
Hamstrings.

originate at the ischial tuberosity and extend down the back of the thigh and over the posterior knee. The only time the hamstrings should be worked before the quadriceps would be for a client with posterior pelvic tilt, which is much less common than an anterior pelvic tilt. An example is long-distance or marathon runners with short strides that shorten the hamstrings over time.

Step 2: Assess Active Range of Motion (AROM)

The client is supine. Ask the client to lift the leg off the table (performed with zero discomfort). If the knee is straight (extended), the normal ROM is 90 degrees. If the hip and knee are flexed, the normal ROM is 120 degrees.

Step 3: Assess Passive Range of Motion (PROM)

This end-feel should feel soft and leathery. If it is not, perform the hip joint capsule work.

Step 4: Assess Resisted Range of Motion (RROM)

1. This will test the upper hamstrings attachments for a muscle–tendon strain. The client is prone with the knee bent 90 degrees. Place your palm on the distal hamstrings just above the knee. Place your other hand on the hip to stabilize it. Ask the client to attempt to gently extend the hip by lifting the straight leg off the

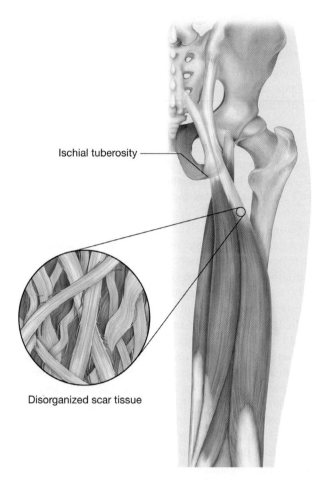

Ischial tuberosity

Disorganized scar tissue

FIGURE 2-75
Hamstring Strain.

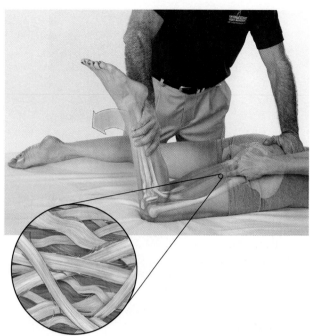

Disorganized scar tissue

FIGURE 2-76
Hamstring Muscle Belly Strain Test.

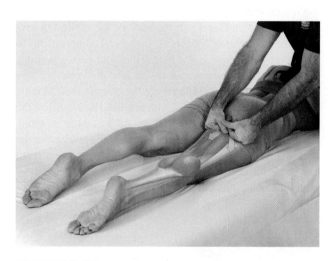

FIGURE 2-77
Myofascial Release, Hamstrings.

table as you provide resistance. Have him or her point to any area of increased pain with one finger. There may be a tear at or near the ischial tuberosity. Work this area last (Figure 2-75 ▪).

2. This will test the muscle belly of the hamstrings and distal hamstrings for a muscle–tendon strain. The client is prone with the knee bent 90 degrees. He or she gently resists as you attempt to extend the knee. Start the test very gently using only two fingers, but if there is no pain on the initial test, use your entire hand with progressively increased strength to recruit the deeper fibers. If the client experiences pain, have him or her point to the specific spot. This is the location of the tear or scar tissue formation (Figure 2-76 ▪). This area will be worked last. If the client points directly behind the knee, it could be a popliteus, plantaris, or distal hamstring strain. Review Chapter 3 on knee conditions for testing the popliteus and plantaris muscles.

Step 6: Myofascial Release

The client is prone. Perform myofascial spreading 45 degrees down and out on the hamstrings from the glutes to the knee (Figure 2-77 ▪). This is done very slowly using your palms, back of your hands, fists, knuckles, or fingers. When you get to the knee, use your finger pads over the back of the knee and perform several gentle myofascial strokes.

CORE PRINCIPLE

The vascular structures behind the knee are very deep and it is not likely that you will harm them using moderate pressure.

Continue the 45-degree myofascial spreading onto the gastrocnemius. Increase your pressure and then momentarily stop, pushing the gastrocnemius away from the hamstrings (Figure 2-78 ▪). This will decompress the tibia away from

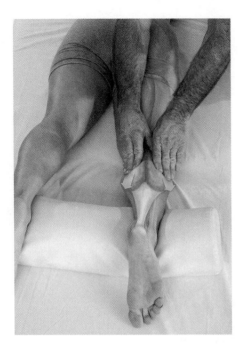

FIGURE 2-78
Myofascial Release, Gastrocnemius.

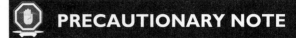

the femur, creating space around the knee joint. Repeat the myofascial spreading down the back of the entire leg several times alternating with slow, rhythmical compressions to maximize blood flow to the hamstrings and gastrocnemius. Do not do compressions over the back of the knee.

Get in a lunge position facing the client's foot. Make a "c" clamp on the client's heel with one hand and stabilize the hip with the other. Press the heel toward the end of the table, stretching and further decompressing the tibia away from the femur (Figure 2-79 ■). If you have a tall client, this stretch can be performed with one hand on the client's heel and the other just below the gluteal fold on the upper hamstrings.

Next, separate each of the hamstring muscles. Find the three tendons that insert on the back of the knee. There will be one on the lateral side and two on the medial side. You can have the client flex the hamstrings to pop up the tendons to help you locate them. Once you identify the distal hamstring tendons, it will be easier to identify the individual hamstrings. At this point, with the knee bent 90 degrees, and the femur in neutral, observe the foot for abnormal internal or external rotation of the knee. If the foot is rotated externally, work on the lateral hamstrings first to create length, and correct the external tibia–fibular rotation. If the foot is medially rotated, work on the medial hamstrings first. There should not be any more than 10 degrees of external tibial rotation. If there is abnormal external or internal tibial rotation, that must be corrected before working on damaged structures of the knee such as the medial or lateral collateral ligaments, the medial or lateral meniscus, or the popliteus. Abnormal rotational patterns of the knee will put unnecessary stress on the inert structures of the knee making your treatment of those structures temporary at best. It can also cause conditions such as fixated posterior fibular head pain. That is commonly found in the right foot of over 50 percent of clients due to the rotation and shortening in the biceps femoris, resulting from the position of the knee to press on the gas peddle of the car (Figure 2-80 ■). It is critical to work

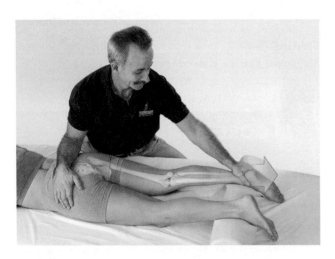

FIGURE 2-79
Decompress Hip and Knee.

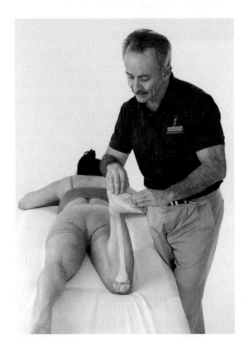

FIGURE 2-80
Evaluate External Tibial Rotation.

on the lateral hamstrings first, with intent to lengthen the biceps femoris, to correct this abnormal knee rotation. Fixated posterior fibular head pain will mimic ITB pain, lateral meniscus pain, and even lateral collateral ligament pain.

Chapter 3 will show you how to differentiate each of these complicated knee conditions. Too often the health care provider classifies these multifaceted knee conditions into the catchall term *runner's knee*. In the less common case of internal tibial rotation, start with the two medial hamstrings—semimembranosus and semitendinosus, with intent to lengthen those muscles to correct knee rotation. If the knee is abnormally rotated, spend more time working the hamstrings that are shortened to eliminate that rotation. Using your thumbs, knuckles, or finger pads work through these muscles, from the ischial tuberosity to the insertion behind the knee. Place one hand behind your working hand and pin and traction the tissue as you work distally. You can gently rock the leg for distraction. Repeat the stroke several times, working progressively deeper, alternating with compressions.

To correct excess lateral knee rotation, spend most of your time lengthening the biceps femoris muscle (lateral hamstring). Perform strokes from the ischial tuberosity toward the knee. Pin and traction the skin as you repeat this stroke several times, (Figure 2-81 ■).

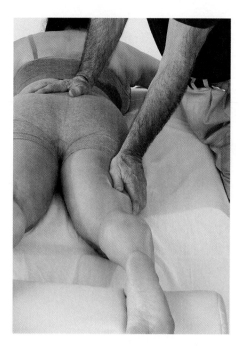

FIGURE 2-82
Trigger Point Work Biceps Femoris.

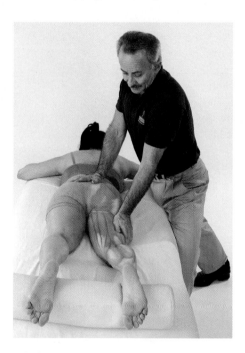

FIGURE 2-81
Lengthen Biceps Femoris.

Step 7: Cross-Fiber Gliding Strokes/Trigger Point Therapy

After you release and balance the hamstring muscles perform cross-fiber gliding strokes, moving medial to lateral to separate tight bands. If needed, repeat the myofascial strokes and compressive broadening to increase blood flow to the area. Release any trigger points, if found, with direct

pressure for 10 to 12 seconds. As the trigger point softens, compress the tissue several times and then gently stretch through it (Figure 2-82 ■).

Step 11: Stretching (During Therapy)

This will stretch the distal hamstrings. If the client is not able to attain 90 degrees of hip flexion and extend the knee back to zero degrees of knee extension, or if he or she starts to bend the knee to attain it, the problem is usually with tight distal hamstrings and the proximal gastrocnemius. To specifically stretch this area, have the client lift the leg to the restriction and then bend the knee. Stabilize the femur, in neutral, with one hand just proximal to the knee while holding the ankle with the other hand (Figure 2-83 ■). Then have the client extend the leg and lock out the knee while you lift up on the leg creating traction, decompression, and space around the knee joint for about 2 seconds (Figure 2-84 ■). The femur does not move. This is an active assisted isolated stretch; the client *must* actively bend and extend the knee. Repeat this several times.

You may also need to stretch either the medial or lateral distal hamstrings. Quite often, the biceps femoris muscle shortens, rotating the tibia and fibula into excess lateral rotation. This usually coincides with internal femoral rotation. If this is not corrected, it can create a shearing force on the knee, resulting in damage to the ligaments, cartilage, and meniscus. This is discussed in much greater detail in Chapter 3.

1. To specifically stretch the lateral distal hamstrings, medially (internally) rotate the client's tibia while the knee is bent. Stabilize the femur, in neutral, with

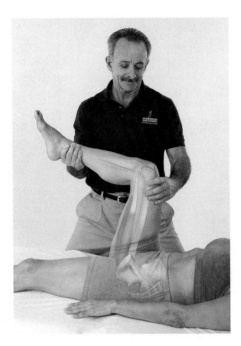

FIGURE 2-83
Active Assisted Stretch Distal Hamstrings (Start).

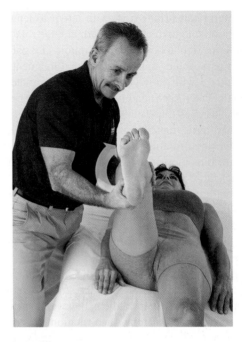

FIGURE 2-85
Distal Lateral Hamstring Stretch (Start).

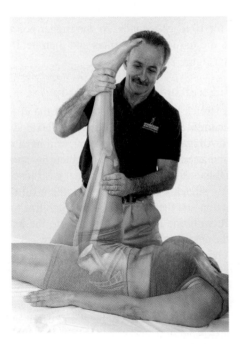

FIGURE 2-84
Active Assisted Stretch Distal Hamstrings (Finish).

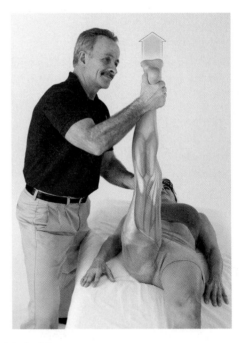

FIGURE 2-86
Distal Lateral Hamstring Stretch (Finish).

one hand just proximal to the knee while holding the ankle with the other hand (Figure 2-85 ■). Then have the client extend the knee while you lift up on the tibia creating traction, decompression, and space around the knee joint for 2 seconds (Figure 2-86 ■). Only the tibia/ fibula rotates medial during the stretch, not the femur. Repeat this several times,

if needed, to correct abnormal lateral rotation of the knee. Remember, the client *must* actively extend the knee during this stretch.

2. To specifically stretch the medial distal hamstring muscle, externally rotate the client's tibia while the knee is bent. Repeat the bend and extend active assisted stretch, as done previously. The femur does

not move, only the tibia. Rotate the tibia first before the client extends the knee. This is not as common as the need to correct external rotation.

PRECAUTIONARY NOTE

Do not rotate the tibia during this distal hamstring stretch, unless it is needed to correct abnormal or excessive knee rotation.

CORE PRINCIPLE

Stretching the distal hamstrings will also stretch the popliteus, which is located behind the knee. For more information on the popliteus muscle, refer to Chapter 3.

Step 8: Multidirectional Friction

If the client feels a specific area of pain during the stretch, or had pain in a specific spot during the previous muscle resisted test, have him or her place one finger on the exact problem area. You may repeat the muscle resistance for a muscle belly or **distal hamstring strain,** by having the client flex the knee against your resistance in this supine position. If the muscle resistance test is positive for a strain, perform multidirectional friction for 20 to 30 seconds to the specific area.

Step 9: Pain-Free Movement

Ask the client to flex the hip and extend the knee several times. If there is no pain, proceed with the eccentric work. If the client still has pain in the hamstrings, return to the multidirectional friction working a little deeper, but still pain-free.

Step 10: Eccentric Scar Tissue Alignment

Next, realign the scar tissue with eccentric contraction performed pain-free. The client is prone or supine with the knee bent 90 degrees. (For larger clients it is easier and allows better control of the leg to do this technique prone.) He or she creates light resistance as you gently extend the knee back to full extension. Use only two fingers on the back of the ankle for resistance at first (feather-light pressure). Tell the client to "barely resist, but let me win." (See Figure 2-83 [start] and Figure 2-84 [finish].)

Repeat several times having the client progressively increase resistance, while the therapist uses the entire hand to extend the knee, only if there is no pain.

Step 4: Assess Resisted Range of Motion (RROM)

To reassess RROM, repeat the resisted test. If there is still a specific point of pain, return to the multidirectional friction working a little slower and deeper and then repeat the eccentric work. Continue to reevaluate until the client is pain-free, which would indicate the scar tissue is functionally realigned.

Step 2: Assess Active Range of Motion (AROM)

To reassess AROM, you want the client to achieve 90-degree ROM for hip flexion with the leg straight, 120-degree ROM with the hip flexed and the knee bent.

Note: Additional distal hamstring stretching, to resolve abnormal knee rotation and resultant shearing forces in the knee, will be covered in greater detail in Chapter 3.

To finish the pelvic stabilization and structural balancing, go to the end of the table and grasp the client's ankles. Lean back and perform a gentle stretch and traction to decompress the client's hips, knees, and ankles to create joint space and to better balance the body.

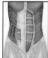

CORE PRINCIPLE

On all of the five major hip muscle groups, make sure you learn the difference between soft-tissue restrictions and joint capsule adhesions so you can perform the appropriate protocol.

Step 11: Stretching (Client Self-Care)

PRECAUTIONARY NOTE

In order to stretch tissue there should be a tissue stretch end feel. The stretch must also be done pain-free to make sure the therapist is not compromising a pre-existing clinical condition such as a strain, sprain, or any unresolved capsular adhesions.

All the client needs is a stretch rope, towel, or even a long belt. The stretches will take the client only 5 minutes per day to perform and are necessary for continued results. The stretches will allow neuromuscular repatterning and reeducation to occur and are critical for keeping the body in balance and out of pain.

The best time to stretch is after a warm shower when the fascia and muscles are warm or after moving the involved area through a comfortable range of motion to increase blood flow. Make sure the client understands that he or she should *not* stretch into pain. The client needs to learn to differentiate between uncomfortable stretching due to tight muscles, and painful stretching that can tear muscle fibers and lead to injury. He or she will start the stretches with the tightest side of the body until attaining balance, and then continue to stretch both sides for symmetry. Empower the client to reeducate his or her muscles, keep the body in alignment, and be a part of his or her own wellness.

The client must stretch the tight, contracted muscles before strengthening the opposing weak, inhibited, over-stretched muscles. Suggest only two to four stretches or strengthening exercises each time you see a client. Make sure he or she can perform these correctly before suggesting any additional exercises.

PSOAS AND ILIACUS

The client takes one long step forward into a lunge and bends both knees until the back knee rests on the floor. The legs are almost in a straight line with each other. You can place a pad under the knee for comfort or if the client has knee problems. Make sure the front knee does not pass forward of the plane of that ankle. In other words, do not bend the front knee more than 90 degrees. Have the client place either one or both hands on a table, chair, or exercise ball for support (Figure 2-87 ■). He or she exhales and slowly leans forward, keeping the upper body upright; this isolates the upper fibers of the psoas. Cue the client to draw in the navel and activate the glutes to stabilize their core. Then, if there is no discomfort, the client should engage the glutes and the hamstrings and extend the back leg lifting the knee slightly off the floor (Figure 2-88 ■). Have him or her hold for about 2 seconds and then lower the knee back to the floor. Then the client inhales, relaxes, leans forward, and extends the leg again, exhaling during the stretch. He or she repeats the stretch

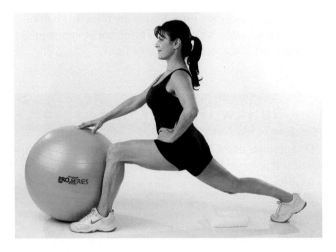

FIGURE 2-88
Iliopsoas Stretch (Finish).

8 to 10 times, or until 35 to 45 degrees of hip extension is achieved, and then repeats the sequence on the other leg.

QUADRATUS LUMBORUM AND ERECTOR SPINAE

The client is standing and lifts both arms overhead. One is straight and the other arm is bent, grasping the straight arm just above the elbow. He or she then lifts the straight arm up and turns shoulders 10 degrees toward that side, exhales, and bends sideways for about 2 seconds (Figure 2-89 ■). He or she bends away from the tight side. The client then inhales, relaxes, and repeats the stretch 8 to 10 times. Tell the client he or she needs to keep the hips square to the front.

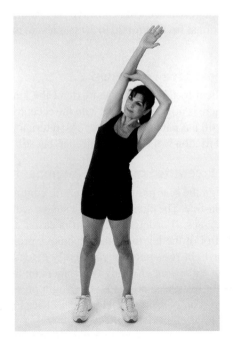

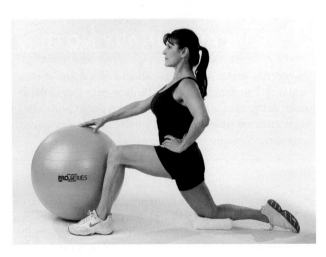

FIGURE 2-87
Iliopsoas Stretch (Start).

FIGURE 2-89
Right QL Stretch.

This also stretches and opens up the psoas and the pectorals, which will benefit clients with thoracic outlet syndrome. If the client's hip is lifting up during the stretch, have him or her cross one leg behind the other. If the client is turning and bending to the left, he or she would cross the right leg behind the left. Advise the client to stretch only the tight side until you reevaluate him or her.

LATERAL HIP ROTATORS

1. Have the client sit with both legs straight. Using the hands above the knee, he or she actively medially rotates the hip at the thigh (turning it inward), assisting the stretch with the hands for about 2 seconds (Figure 2-90 ◼). He or she repeats 8 to 10 times. Then the client abducts the leg 30 degrees, moving it away from the other knee, repeats the stretch 8 to 10 times, then repeats both stretches on the other leg, if needed.

CORE PRINCIPLE

Determine which of the two opposing muscle groups— lateral hip rotators or medial hip rotators—are tight and stretch only the short, tight muscle group.

2. Once the client masters the kinesthetic sense of this stretch you can teach him or her how to perform it using the contract-relax, contract-antagonist method. The client laterally rotates the hip, turning it outward against his

or her own resistance with the hands above the knee for 5 to 10 seconds. He or she relaxes, takes a breath, and then while exhaling medially rotates the hip for about 2 seconds while assisting with the hands. At this new position, the client repeats the stretch two or three times, then repeats the stretch on the other hip, if necessary.

QUADRICEPS

1. The client is prone with one knee bent and with a towel behind the knee. This creates leverage of the knee joint and tractions the tibia away from the knee, to decompress the knee. He or she reaches back and grasps the ankle and attempts to extend the knee against his or her own resistance with 20 percent force for 5 to 10 seconds. The client relaxes, takes a deep breath, and then on exhale pulls the ankle to the glutes for about 2 seconds. This is a passive stretch; the client does *not* engage the hamstrings, in order to prevent a muscle cramp of the hamstrings in this shortened position. He or she repeats the stretch 8 to 10 times, then repeats it on the other leg, if needed.

2. If the client is not flexible enough to perform stretch number 1, he or she can substitute this one. The client is prone with one knee bent, with a stretch rope looped around the ankle, coming up over the back to hold it. The client extends the knee against his or her own resistance with 20 percent force for 5 to 10 seconds. He or she relaxes, takes a deep breath, and then while exhaling gently pulls on the stretch rope bringing the ankle toward the glutes for about 2 seconds (Figure 2-91 ◼). At this new position, the client repeats the stretch 8 to 10 times and then repeats it on the other leg, if needed. This is a passive stretch; the client does *not* engage the hamstrings.

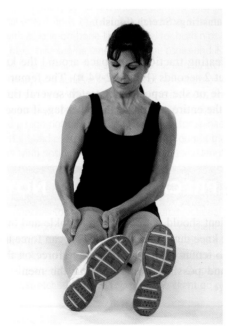

FIGURE 2-90
Lateral Hip Rotator Stretch.

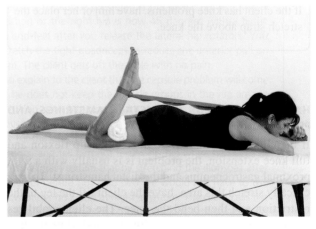

FIGURE 2-91
Quadriceps Stretch.

ILIOTIBIAL BAND: STRETCHING THE TFL MUSCLE

The client is supine with the uninvolved leg straight and medially rotated (turned in). He or she places a stretch rope

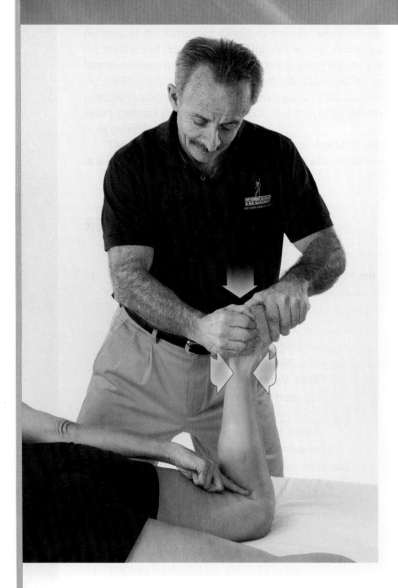

CHAPTER

3   Knee and Thigh Conditions

CHAPTER OUTLINE

Twelve-Step Approach to Knee and Thigh Conditions

Anterior Cruciate Ligament (ACL) and Posterior Cruciate Ligament (PCL) Instability

Patellar Tendinosis and Chondromalacia

Quadriceps Protocol

Plantaris Strain

Popliteus Strain

Medial Meniscus Injury and Medial Collateral Ligament (MCL) Sprain

Iliotibial Band Friction Syndrome

Lateral Meniscus Injury and Lateral Collateral Ligament (LCL) Sprain

LEARNING OBJECTIVES

Upon completing this chapter the reader will be able to:

- Choose the appropriate massage modality or treatment protocol for each specific clinical knee condition
- Release all the forces surrounding the knee, and eliminate the underlying cause of the knee conditions before addressing the clinical symptoms
- Determine if there is an imbalance among the muscle groups that surround the knee
- Restore pain-free knee joint normal range of motion
- Differentiate between soft-tissue problems caused by
  - instability or hypermobility of the knee
  - myofascial restrictions

- muscle–tendon tension
- muscle imbalance
- myoskeletal alignment problems
- trigger point tension
- strained muscle or sprained ligament fibers
- scar tissue
- Teach the client self-care stretching and strengthening exercises (if needed) to perform at home to maintain muscle balance, joint alignment, and pain-free movement following therapy

KEY TERMS

Anterior cruciate ligament (ACL) sprain 86

Anterior drawer test 86

Apley compression test 104

Apley distraction test 104

Chondromalacia 91

Fixated fibular head dysfunction 88

Iliotibial band friction syndrome 104

Lateral collateral ligament (LCL) 88

LCL sprain test 88

Ligament sprain 94

MCL sprain test 102

Medial collateral ligament (MCL) 88

Meniscus 90

Muscle strain 95

Patellar tendinitis 91

Patellar tendinosis 91

Patello femoral compression test 91

Posterior cruciate ligament (PCL) sprain 86

Posterior drawer test 86

SAG test 86

This chapter addresses a muscular and skeletal balancing approach to treating specific clinical conditions of the knee. Muscle groups are worked superficial to deep with the focus on the short, contracted muscles *limiting* movement before working on the actual injury or condition. This will ensure balance of the muscles surrounding the knee joint, optimal alignment of the knee, and adequate joint space in the knee. That alone will reduce many of the knee symptoms.

It is highly recommended to perform pelvic stabilization (see Chapter 2) prior to the knee protocol, because many muscle groups that originate in the pelvic area affect the knee. Imbalances in the hips due to tight muscles can create additional joint tension and rotational forces of the femur and tibia, which can result in degeneration of the knee joint structures. It then must be determined if the knee problem is due to myofascial restriction, muscle–tendon tension, trigger point tension, strained fibers, scar tissue, or damage to structures in the joint such as the ligaments or meniscus. The treatment focuses on the contracted structures that limit pain-free movement and create tension and imbalance in the knee. *Keep in mind that this chapter is really an extension of Chapter 2 on pelvic stabilization.*

 PRECAUTIONARY NOTE

Do not work on a client with a recent injury (acute condition) exhibiting inflammation, heat, redness, or swelling. RICE therapy (rest, ice, compression, elevation) may be the appropriate treatment in this situation. Clients with a hypermobile knee, due to excess ligament laxity, should consult with their physician. If in doubt, refer out!

TWELVE-STEP APPROACH TO KNEE AND THIGH CONDITIONS

The following conditions and their treatments are covered in this chapter:

- Anterior cruciate ligament (ACL) and posterior cruciate ligament (PCL) instability
- Patellar tendinosis and chondromalacia
- Plantaris strain
- Popliteus strain
- Medial meniscus injury and medial collateral ligament (MCL) sprain
- Iliotibial band friction syndrome
- Lateral meniscus injury and lateral collateral ligament (LCL) sprain

ANTERIOR CRUCIATE LIGAMENT (ACL) AND POSTERIOR CRUCIATE LIGAMENT (PCL) INSTABILITY

Step 1: Client History

Goal: to obtain a thorough medical history including precautions and contraindications for treatment of the client's knee condition.

Taking a complete client history will offer you valuable information regarding a client's condition. Also, ask the client when, where, and how the problem began, and to describe the area of pain and what makes it better or worse. This will give you a starting point from which to assess the client's active range of motion.

Before you start your assessment and special tests, it is suggested that you rule out hypermobility situations of the knee, especially moderate to extreme injuries to the **anterior cruciate ligament (ACL)** and **posterior cruciate ligament (PCL)**. Following trauma a client with a positive **SAG test** indicating extreme knee instability should be referred out to an orthopedic physician. A posterior SAG Sign is present with either a rupture of the posterior cruciate ligament, or when there is substantial posterior ligament laxity. The SAG sign reveals posterior displacement of the tibial tuberosity, when the distal quadriceps and hamstrings are relaxed and the knee is flexed at 90 degrees.

If there is a positive SAG test, refer the client out to an orthopedic surgeon. If you just suspect hypermobility of the knee, but there is not a positive SAG test, you need to gently perform the Lachman test to evaluate for damage to the ACL and the posterior drawer test to evaluate for damage to the PCL. A positive sign for ACL or PCL damage is a soft or mushy end feel, pain, and excess movement. *There should be minimal movement, no pain, and a ligament end feel.*[1]

ANTERIOR DRAWER TEST AND LACHMAN TEST

The ACL prevents anterior movement of the tibia in relation to the femur. Perform the **anterior drawer test** with the client in the sitting or supine position, the hip flexed to 45 degrees and the knee bent at 90 degrees. Place both hands behind the upper gastrocnemius and attempt to gently pull the proximal tibia forward. You do not want to feel excessive movement or elicit pain (Figure 3-1 ■). This test can be inaccurate due to the position of the knee and the fact that the hamstrings can often be splinting the injured area. A second test that can be performed to evaluate the stability of the ACL is the Lachman test. This is done with the knee straight or in only slight flexion, so the hamstrings do not affect the test. See video clip on www.myhealthprofessionskit.com.

POSTERIOR DRAWER TEST FOR PCL INSTABILITY

The PCL is responsible for preventing posterior movement of the tibia in relation to the femur. Perform the **posterior drawer test** with the client in the sitting or supine position, the hip flexed

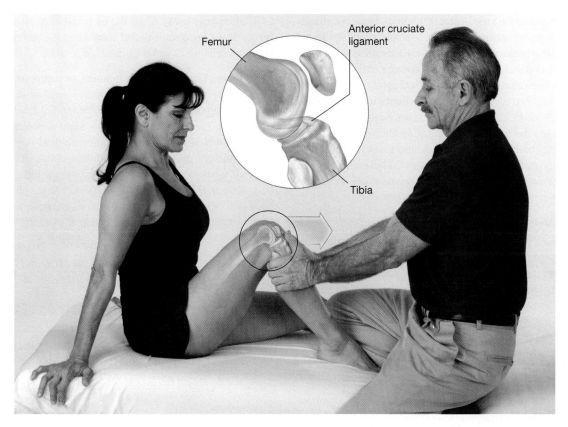

FIGURE 3-1
ACL Stability Test.

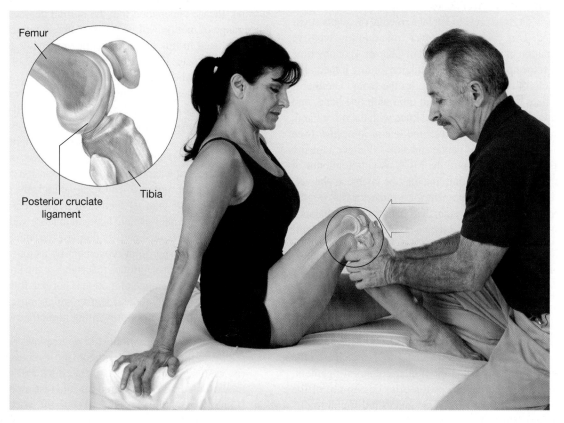

FIGURE 3-2
PCL Stability Test.

to 45 degrees and the knee bent at 90 degrees. Place both hands around the upper gastrocnemius and attempt to gently push the proximal tibia backward. If there is pain and excess movement or a mushy end feel it is indicative of damage to the PCL (Figure 3-2 ■). See video clip on www.myhealthprofessionskit.com.

It is highly recommended that clients with instability to the ACL or PCL are referred out for further evaluation. Surgery may be necessary. Releasing the muscle groups such as the quadriceps, hamstrings, and gastrocnemius will most likely make this condition worse. These clients need bracing, taping, strengthening, and even possibly surgery to restore knee stability. If in doubt, refer out.

VALGUS AND VARUS STRESS TESTS

This is also a good time to test for sprains of the **medial collateral ligament** or the **lateral collateral ligament.** Keep in mind these tests will be repeated after you balance out the muscle groups around the knee and correct abnormal rotational patterns of the knee. In many cases when you correct rotational patterns of the knee to bring the MCL and LCL into their resting positions, pain in those structures will disappear.

Note: The Valgus stress test (MCL sprain test) is done to determine damage to the medial collateral ligament (MCL).

Valgus Stress Test   The distal medial collateral ligament attaches to the tibial and is also called the tibial collateral ligament. "It has a fibrous attachment on the medial meniscus. As a result, tensile stress injuries on the MCL often cause tearing of the outer edge of the medial meniscus."[2] The major role of the MCL is to prevent lateral to medial or valgus stress to the knee. This can come on over time due to excessive hyperpronation of the foot (covered in Chapter 4) or any time there is a force applied to the lateral knee forcing it medially.

The client is supine or sitting on the table. The therapist stabilizes the proximal medial tibia with one hand, and applies a valgus force to the lateral knee with the other hand. This hand is placed directly over the lateral joint line. (See Figure 3-26). The force is gentle and slow. "Pain or a mushy end feel indicates damage to the MCL. A small amount of gapping over the medial joint line may be visible as the valgus force is applied."[3] Treatment for a minor or first degree MCL sprain will be addressed in this chapter after we balance all the muscle groups around the knee. If in doubt, refer out!

Note: The Varus stress test (LCL sprain test) is performed to determine damage to the lateral collateral ligament (LCL).

"The lateral collateral ligament is the least frequently injured of the four primary stabilizing ligaments of the knee. The most common cause of LCL sprain is a direct blow to the inside of the knee, which can occur in contact sports like football or rugby."[4] Because the distal LCL attaches to the fibular head it is also called the fibular collateral ligament. The hamstrings tendon (biceps femoris) lies on top of the distal attachment of the LCL. This makes it difficult to differentiate conditions like a **fixated fibular head dysfunction** from pain in the LCL (addressed later in Chapter 3). The primary function of the LCL is to resist medial to lateral forces on the knee also known as varus load. The pain in the LCL often goes away when the therapist corrects rotational forces of the knee such as that seen when the biceps femoris shortens causing external tibia/fibula rotation.

Varus Stress Test   The client is supine or sitting on the table. The therapist stabilizes the proximal lateral tibia with one hand, and applies a varus force to the medial knee with the other hand. (See Figure 3-36). This hand is placed directly over the medial joint line. The force applied is gentle and slow. "Pain or a mushy end-feel indicates damage to the LCL. A small amount of gapping over the lateral joint line may be visible as the varus force is applied."[5] Keep in mind this book will only address the treatment of a minor or first degree sprain of the LCL later in this chapter. *If in doubt, refer out!*

Note: Flexing the knee approximately 15 to 20 degrees will increase the accuracy of the tests to the MCL and LCL. This will limit the role of the ACL in stabilizing the knee.[6]

Step 2: Assess Active Range of Motion (AROM)

Goal: to assess range of motion of knee single-plane movements performed solely by the client to identify tight or restricted muscle groups.

To assess the client's AROM of the knee joint, have the client lay prone. Ask him or her to perform with zero discomfort both of the primary single-plane movements of the knee: flexion and extension. Determine if the range of motion is normal. Please understand that the normal degrees for each knee range of motion will vary with different references. The degrees listed in this text are accurate estimates for clients with healthy knees. For flexion, the normal range of motion is 135 degrees or when the muscles of the lower leg press against the muscles of the posterior thigh (Figure 3-3 ■). For extension, the normal range of motion is 0 to 10 degrees. Full extension takes the knee from the flexed position back to zero degrees (Figure 3-4 ■). In a number of clients, due to slight ligament laxity, even in a healthy knee, most practitioners say that the extra 10 degrees of what is actually hyperextension can be normal knee range of motion. Genu recurvatum is the term used when there is more than 10 degrees of hyperextension of the knee due to abnormal ligament laxity of anterior and posterior cruciate ligaments of the knee.[7] In this case the author does not recommend increasing joint movement by using techniques that lengthen the muscle groups that stabilize the knee.

Determine if the range of motion is normal. If the client's AROM is less than average, identify which muscle groups are restricted and therefore preventing normal movement.

- If knee flexion is less than 135 degrees, work on releasing the extensors (antagonists)—rectus femoris, vastus intermedius, vastus lateralis, and vastus medialis—to restore normal muscle resting lengths.
- If knee extension is less than 0 degrees, work on releasing the flexors (antagonists)—biceps femoris, gastrocnemius, plantaris, popliteus, semimembranosus, and semitendinosus—to restore normal muscle resting lengths.

KNEE JOINT SINGLE-PLANE MOVEMENTS—PRIMARY MUSCLES

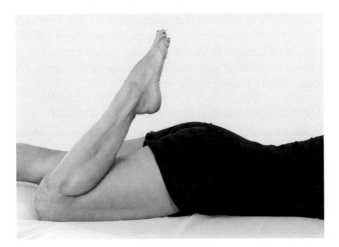

FIGURE 3-3
Knee Flexion, 135 degrees.

Flexion, 135 Degrees

- biceps femoris
- gastrocnemius
- plantaris, popliteus
- semimembranosus
- semitendinosus

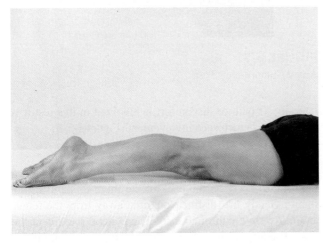

FIGURE 3-4
Knee Extension, 0–10 degrees.

Extension, 0 to 10 Degrees.

- rectus femoris
- vastus intermedius
- vastus lateralis
- vastus medialis

Medial Tibial Rotation

- semitendinosus
- semimembranosus
- popliteus
- gracilis
- sartorius

Lateral Tibial Rotation

- biceps femoris

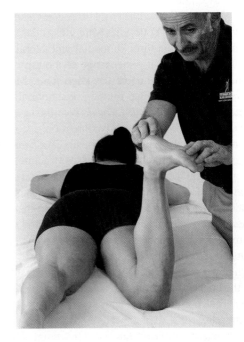

FIGURE 3-5
Abnormal External Tibial Rotation.

- Also, assess if there is balance between the knee tibial medial rotators—semitendinosus, semimembranosus, popliteus, gracilis, and sartorius—and the knee tibial lateral rotator—biceps femoris. Often you will observe an externally rotated foot, with the knee flexed at 90 degrees due to a short biceps femoris, resulting in a posterior fixated fibular head (Figure 3-5 ■). This will give you a springy end feel, rather than a tissue stretch or tissue compression end feel for knee flexion. This must be corrected in your treatment by lengthening the biceps femoris and getting the fibula moving again.

Step 3: Assess Passive Range of Motion (PROM)

Goal: to assess range of motion and the end feel of knee single-plane movements performed on the client. When performing PROM the joint is moved passively by the therapist all the way through normal and accessory motion. The sensation felt at the end of accessory motion of the joint is called the end feel.[8]

You can determine the end feel of each of the primary two single-plane movements of the knee joint by performing passive PROM tests.

- **Flexion:** The normal end feel will either be a tissue stretch, also known as soft and leathery, or tissue-on-tissue, as the calf presses on the hamstrings.
- **Extension:** The end feel will be more abrubt due to the limitations of the ligaments. This is known as a ligamentous end feel. Ligaments have less capability to stretch than muscle and tendons.

Also, evaluate for abnormal medial and lateral tibial rotation. With the client's knee bent 90 degrees, stabilize the femur with one hand. Your other hand grasps the ankle and gently moves the tibia through medial and lateral rotation (Figure 3-6 ■). Assess if either range of motion is present and creating an imbalance of the knee joint. More than 10 degrees of external tibial rotation is abnormal and will stress the structures of the knee. *You do not want to see excess knee rotation.* It is believed that compression, accompanied with abnormal knee rotation, is responsible for a majority of clinical symptoms of the knee. It stresses structures like the medial and lateral meniscus, and medial and lateral collateral ligaments. It also can contribute to fixated posterior fibular head pain and abnormal patella tracking. In many cases, once you release the muscle groups that surround the knee, and correct abnormal knee rotation, the knee pain goes away without even treating the structures of the knee.

When performing PROM, you should always be sensitive to the client's breathing and patterns of guarding. Your overall confidence, combined with a calming voice, can help the client relax.

Evaluate for **meniscus** damage at this point: The lateral and medial menisci are cartilage discs that are in the knee joint, between the tibia and the femur. Their primary role is shock absorption and maintaining a proper gliding surface for the femoral condyles on the tibial plateau. Excessive compressive or rotational forces or severe traction forces on the knee may cause damage to the meniscus. Minor surface tears are addressed in this chapter, but with deep tears or if a loose fragment of the meniscal cartilage is floating in the joint, surgery is most likely necessary.

APLEY COMPRESSION TEST FOR MENISCUS DAMAGE

When performing the **Apley Compression Test,** the client is prone with the knee bent 90 degrees. Gently compress the tibia straight down and slowly rotate the tibia medially and

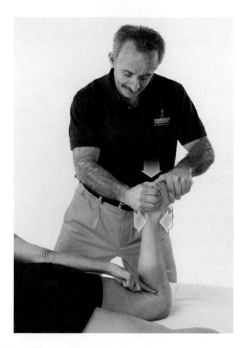

FIGURE 3-7
Apley Compression Test.

laterally. If pain or discomfort is involved in this test it is likely there is meniscus involvement (Figure 3-7 ■).

APLEY DISTRACTION TEST

The client is prone with the knee bent at 90 degrees. Place your knee gently on the back of the thigh to stabilize the femur. Gently lift (distract) the tibia away from the femur and move slowly through medail and lateral rotation of the tibia. If pain increases that means the injury is more likely the medial or lateral collateral ligaments, rather than the medial or lateral meniscus. Often the injury will involve both the MCL and meniscus, with pain on the medial side, because the fibers are interconnected (Figure 3-8 ■).

Step 4: Assess Resisted Range of Motion (RROM)

Goal: to assess if there is a muscle–tendon strain present and exactly where it is located.

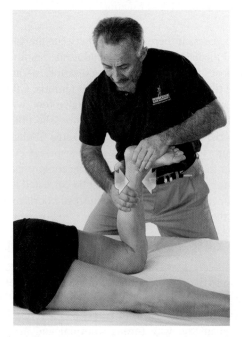

FIGURE 3-6
Gentle Passive Evaluation for Abnormal Knee Rotation.

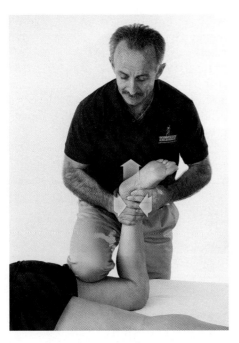

FIGURE 3-8
Apley Distraction Test.

If there is a torn muscle or tendon, treat it *last,* after you have balanced out opposing muscle groups and addressed the problems in the muscle belly leading to the muscle tear. Do not move too fast or use too much force while performing a resisted test

- Have the client attempt both flexion and then extension of the knee joint while you gently apply reverse resistance.
- Pain? Ask the client to point to the specific spot. This indicates a muscle–tendon strain and will be worked last.

PATELLAR TENDINOSIS AND CHONDROMALACIA

Patellar tendinitis is rare and not a typical "-itis" because in many cases it does not produce redness, swelling, or inflammation. A better term would be *tendon pain* or *tendinosis,* which is tearing of tendon fibers in the absence of an inflammatory process.[9]

Patellar tendinosis is usually caused by overuse of the quadriceps, which place an excessive amount of upward pressure on the patella. This then stretches and irritates the patellar ligament, which attaches to the tibia. Lack of balance between the quadriceps and hamstring muscle groups is the common cause of injury to the patellar ligament.[10] Pain is usually felt below the knee or even described as coming from around the knee joint. With hypermobile knee joints, you must strengthen the muscles surrounding the knee to help support the ligaments and reduce tear problems.

CORE PRINCIPLE

Having an imbalance between a strong vastus lateralis and a weaker vastus medialis can also exacerbate this condition and lead to lateral tracking of the knee and chondromalacia.

Chondromalacia is described as degeneration of cartilage on the underside of the patella, resulting in pain and a grating sensation. To test for chondromalacia perform the **patello femoral compression test.** Have the client sit down and then press on the patella while he or she flexes and extends the knee. If the client experiences grating sounds, he or she has chondromalacia. Follow the same protocol for patellar tendinosis in step 4 (Figure 3-9 ■).

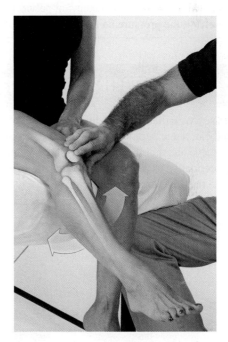

FIGURE 3-9
Patello Femoral Compression Test.

QUADRICEPS PROTOCOL

Step 4: Assess Resisted Range of Motion (RROM)

Goal: to assess if there is a patellar tendon strain present and exactly where it is located.

- The client is seated on the edge of the table. You can place support under the knee using a large bolster or your thigh.
- Place one hand on the client's distal anterior tibia.
- Grasp the client's lower leg and have the client gently attempt knee extension using 20 percent of his or her strength as you resist extension or gently flex the knee.
- You control the intensity of the test.
- Pain? Ask the client to point to the specific spot (Figure 3-10A ■). This indicates a muscle–tendon strain and will be worked last.
- Often the client will not test positive unless this test is done using a weight-bearing model that simulates going down a flight of steps. Have the client stand up and do a squat on both legs (Figure 3-10B ■).
- If the test is still not positive, have the client do a one-legged squat (Figure 3-10C ■). This puts more load on the patellar ligament to test for even a minor tear.

Step 5: Area Preparation

Goal: to follow the steps for the myofascial work on the quadriceps (also outlined under step 4 of pelvic stabilization) to release the pressure on the patella.

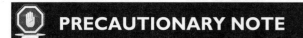

PRECAUTIONARY NOTE

Do *not* use ice on the muscle belly unless there is inflammation (heat, redness, or swelling). Ice can cause the fascia to become less mobile and restricts movement. This is counterproductive to the mobilizing and healing process, which the therapy work is promoting.

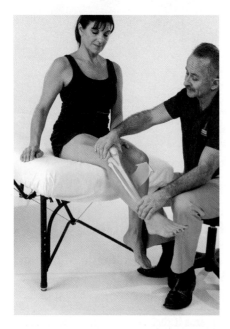

FIGURE 3-10A
Patella Tendinosis Test.

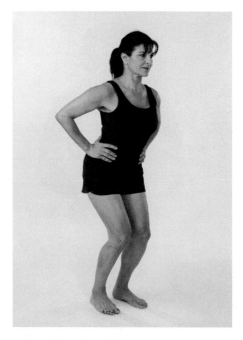

FIGURE 3-10B
Patellar Tendinosis Knee Flexion Test.

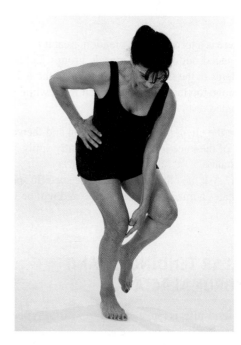

FIGURE 3-10C
Patellar Tendinosis One-Legged Knee Flexion Test.

Step 6: Myofascial Release

Goal: to warm up, soften, and mobilize the quadriceps and to move the fascial layers back to normal resting positions.

- The client is supine with the leg slightly abducted.
- Perform myofascial spreading at a 45-degree angle into the tissue on the quads, working from the knee to the hip (distal to proximal). Work very slowly with

fists, palms, knuckles, or fingers. Make sure you work through the upper attachments (Figure 3-11 ■).

- Use slow, rhythmical compressions over the entire quads.
- Next, "iron" up the rectus femoris using your forearm or the back of your fist. Pin or traction the skin with your lower hand, while the upper hand performs the stroke. This will increase blood flow to the area (Figure 3-12 ■).
- Repeat the compressions.

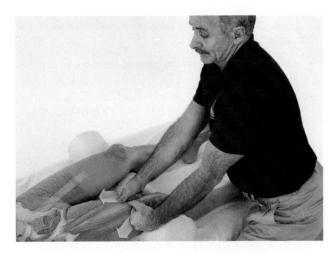

FIGURE 3-11
Myofascial Release Up Quadriceps.

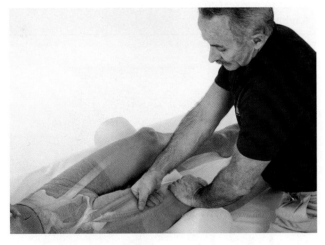

FIGURE 3-12
Myofascial Release Up Rectus Femoris.

Step 7: Cross-Fiber Gliding Strokes/Trigger Point Therapy

CROSS-FIBER GLIDING STROKES

Goal: to tease apart tight quadriceps muscles bands (tight, contracted muscle).

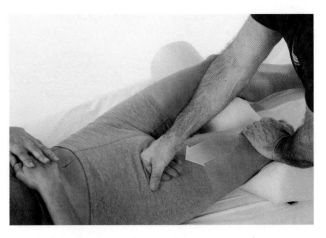

FIGURE 3-13
Quadriceps Compression.

Use compression broadening and cross-fiber gliding strokes to broaden, tease through, and lengthen any tight quadriceps muscles bands. This will loosen up tight muscle fibers that often feed and contribute to active trigger points, allowing tissue to move more freely and independently (Figure 3-13 ■).

- Tight muscles, with tenderness located directly under your pressure?
- This requires cross-fiber gliding strokes working from insertion to origin (distal to proximal) on the quadriceps.

TRIGGER POINT THERAPY

Goal: to release trigger points in the muscle belly of the quadriceps, if found.

First perform trigger point work on the contracted, tight muscles. If there is a specific area of pain that radiates or refers to a predictable area or site, based on Travell's trigger point theories, apply trigger point therapy.

- Use direct, moderate pressure for 10 to 12 seconds.
- As the trigger point softens, compress the tissue several times.
- Gently stretch the fascia that feeds the ischemic tender area.

After performing cross-fiber gliding strokes and trigger point therapy (if needed), you may need to return to the myofascial spreading, working even slower and deeper, but still pain-free to release any tissue that is still restricted.

Step 8: Multidirectional Friction

Goal: to soften the collagen matrix by working in multiple directions to prepare for a more functional mobilization of scar tissue fibers.

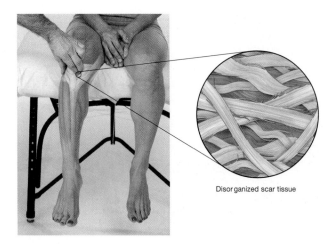

Disorganized scar tissue

FIGURE 3-14
Multidirectional Friction, Patellar Tendon.

If there is not a muscle–tendon strain or **ligament sprain,** multidirectional friction would *not* be part of the treatment.

Perform the resisted test: Have the client gently attempt extension as you flex the knee and have him or her point to the exact area of pain. Perform multidirectional friction, with a supported finger, to the specific area for 20 to 30 seconds to soften or free up the scar tissue that is causing the pain (Figure 3-14 ■). Ease up on your pressure if the area is too uncomfortable. Proceed with the next step.

Step 9: Pain-Free Movement

Goal: to determine if the client can actively perform knee flexion and extension without pain. If so, this gives permission to proceed with pain-free eccentric scar tissue alignment techniques.

- Ask the client to actively flex and extend the knee through full pain-free range of motion several times. This begins the process of realigning collagen fibers (scar tissue).
- Pain-free? Proceed to step 10.
- Pain? Repeat step 8, working slower and deeper, but still pain-free. Repeat step 9 and then proceed to step 10 when there is no pain.

Step 10: Eccentric Scar Tissue Alignment

Goal: to apply pain-free eccentric contraction by lengthening an injured patellar tendon against mild resistance to realign or redirect the scar tissue.

PRECAUTIONARY NOTE

After surgery, do not disrupt the proper healing of scar tissue by beginning this protocol too soon. Consult the client's physician before treatment.

The greatest error during the eccentric alignment procedure is being too aggressive and not keeping the technique pain-free each time. Too much force in opposing directions can cause a new injury or reinjure the site.

Now, realign the deeper layers of scar tissue with eccentric contraction.

- The client is sitting on the edge of the table with the leg extended.
- With a two-finger pressure on the front of the client's ankle, ask him or her to gently resist knee flexion (Figure 3-15 ■).
- Tell the client to "barely resist, but let me win."
- Start with a pressure of two fingers and have the client increase resistance only if it is pain-free.
- Repeat several times, pain-free. This will create functional scar tissue (Figure 3-16 ■).

Step 4: Assess Resisted Range of Motion (RROM)

Goal: to reassess to determine if there is still a patellar tendon strain present.

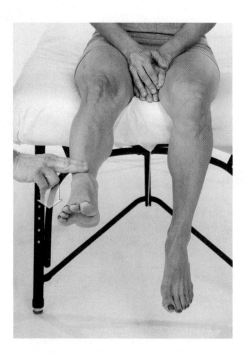

FIGURE 3-15
Eccentric Contraction, Patellar Tendon.

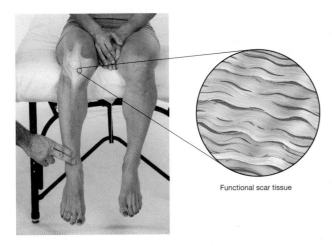

FIGURE 3-16
Eccentric Muscle Contraction, Patellar Ligament.

Do not move too fast, or use too much force while performing a resisted test. To perform the test:

- Have the client gently attempt knee extension using 20 percent of his or her strength as you resist or gently attempt to flex the knee.
- Pain? Repeat steps 8 through 10. Then perform the resisted test again.
- Pain-free? Finish with step 11 when there is no longer any pain.

Step 11: Stretching (During Therapy)

> ### ✋ PRECAUTIONARY NOTE
>
> Stretching is not suggested for the muscle groups around a hypermobile joint. Strengthening would be more appropriate to stabilize any joint that has excessive movement due to ligamentous laxity.

Goal: to create the normal range of motion of 135-degree knee flexion.

Contracting the muscle against resistance to fatigue the muscle prior to the stretch becomes a muscle resistance test and the client may report pain in a specific area, which is a **muscle strain.** If so, proceed to multidirectional friction (step 8), pain-free movement (step 9), and eccentric scar tissue alignment (step 10) until the client is pain-free.

> ### ✋ PRECAUTIONARY NOTE
>
> This is the only passive stretch recommended in the body. The client does not engage the hamstrings, as this may result in a hamstrings cramp.

Bring the client's knee into 90-degree flexion and traction the tibia away from the femur.

- Ask the client to attempt to extend the knee while you provide resistance at 20 percent force for 5 to 10 seconds. No movement should happen. This is an isometric contraction.
- He or she relaxes, takes a deep breath, and on exhale you traction the tibia away from the femur and move the foot toward the hip for about 2 seconds (Figure 3-17 ■).
- Repeat several times, or until you achieve the normal range of motion of 135 degrees of flexion.

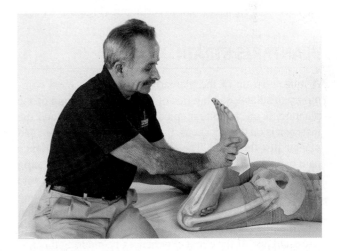

FIGURE 3-17
Quadriceps Stretch.

> ### ✋ PRECAUTIONARY NOTE
>
> The end feel during the quadriceps stretch should be tissue stretch or leathery. If it is abnormal, springy, abrupt, or a bone-on-bone-like end feel, do *not* continue. If it is a springy end feel, it could be a fixated posterior fibular head due to a short biceps femoris. That can be corrected by lengthening the biceps femoris and performing a simple myoskeletal alignment technique. You may choose to refer this client out, as this abnormal end feel can indicate significant damage of the structures of the knee such as torn ligaments, torn meniscus, or cartilage. Do not traction the knee if it is hypermobile. See the section on the meniscus later in this chapter.

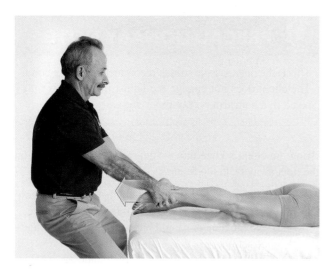

FIGURE 3-18
Traction Knee.

Move to the end of the table and grasp the client's ankle. Lean back and gently traction the leg to decompress the knee, as long as it is not hypermobile (Figure 3-18 ■).

PLANTARIS STRAIN

A muscle strain of the plantaris is one of the most commonly misdiagnosed injuries of the knee. The origin of the plantaris is on the lateral epicondyle of the femur and the insertion is on the calcaneus. Its action is to flex the knee and plantar flex the ankle. The client will typically experience pain behind the knee when moving quickly from a kneeling or seated position to a standing position. Examples would be attempting to stand up after sitting and watching a long movie or a baseball catcher moving quickly from a squat to standing. The best way to identify this problem is with a resisted test. If the client experiences pain during this test and locates it by pointing to the area directly behind the knee, he or she has a plantaris strain.

Step 4: Assess Resisted Range of Motion (RROM)

Goal: to assess if there is a plantaris strain present and exactly where it is located.

If there is a torn muscle or tendon, treat it *last,* after you have balanced out opposing muscle groups and addressed the problems in the muscle belly leading to the muscle tear.

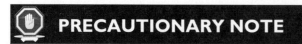

PRECAUTIONARY NOTE

Do not move too fast, or use too much force while performing a resisted test.

- The client is prone with the knee flexed to 90 degrees and the ankle dorsiflexed.
- The client gently attempts to plantar flex the ankle and flexes the knee using 20 percent of his or her strength against your resistance.
- Gently attempt to extend the knee and dorsiflex the ankle to increase the intensity of the test if there is no pain.
- Pain? Ask the client to point to the specific area of pain (Figure 3-19 ■). This indicates a muscle strain and will be worked last. See video clip on www .myhealthprofessionskit.com.

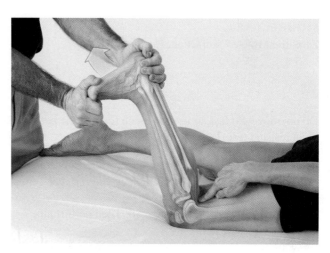

FIGURE 3-19
Resistance Test, Plantaris Strain.

Step 5: Area Preparation

Goal: to prepare the client for myofascial release.

The client is prone, with a bolster under the ankles. Do *not* use ice on the muscle belly unless there is inflammation (heat, redness, or swelling). In that case therapy should not be done until inflammation is resolved. Ice may cause the fascia to become less mobile and restrict movement. This is counterproductive to the mobilizing and healing process, which the therapy work is promoting.

Step 6: Myofascial Release

Goal: to warm up, soften, and mobilize the plantaris.

Perform myofascial spreading directly behind the knee with your finger pads or knuckles, using moderate pressure. This will bring blood flow and oxygen to this ischemic area. Use slow strokes, working proximal to distal on the muscle belly to mobilize and soften the fascia.

Step 7: Cross-Fiber Gliding Strokes/Trigger Point Therapy

CROSS-FIBER GLIDING STROKES

Goal: to tease apart tight plantaris muscle bands.

Perform cross-fiber gliding strokes to tease through and gently spread any tight plantaris muscle bands. This will loosen up tight muscle fibers that often feed and contribute to trigger points, allowing the tissue to move more freely and independently.

TRIGGER POINT THERAPY

Goal: to release trigger points in the plantaris muscle belly, if found.

Palpate for trigger points or tender spots. If there is a specific area of pain that radiates or refers, apply trigger point therapy (Figure 3-20 ■).

- Use direct, moderate pressure for 10 to 12 seconds.
- As the trigger point softens, compress the tissue several times.
- Gently stretch the fascia feeding the ischemic tender area.

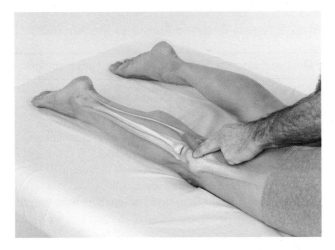

FIGURE 3-20
Cross-Fiber Gliding Stroke and Trigger Point Work, Plantaris.

CORE PRINCIPLE

The vascular structures behind the knee are very deep and it is unlikely that you will harm them using moderate pressure. However, find out if the client has lymphatic problems, and consult with an expert on lymphatic drainage.

Step 11: Stretching (During Therapy)

Goal: to create the normal range of motion of 20 to 30 degrees of dorsiflexion and 0 degrees of knee extension.

Contracting the muscle against resistance to fatigue the muscle prior to the stretch becomes a muscle resistance test and the client may report pain in a specific area, which is a muscle strain. If so, proceed to multidirectional friction (step 8), pain-free movement (step 9), and eccentric scar tissue alignment (step 10) until the client is pain-free.

- The client is prone with the knee bent 90 degrees.
- Ask the client to gently attempt to plantar flex the ankle and flex the knee while you provide resistance at 20 percent force for 5 to 10 seconds.
- He or she relaxes, takes a deep breath, and on exhale dorsiflexes the ankle and fully extends the knee for about 2 seconds as you traction the ankle and assist the stretch.
- At this new position, repeat the contract-relax, contract-antagonist with active assisted stretching two or three times, or until achieving the normal range of motion of 20 to 30 degrees of ankle dorsiflexion and 0 degrees of knee extension.

Then, fully straighten the client's knee, traction the ankle, lean back, and pull the leg into a stretch. Release slowly. This stretch will create additional space in the knee joint, decompressing the forces on the articulating cartilage.

Step 8: Multidirectional Friction

Goal: to soften the collagen matrix by working in multiple directions to prepare for a more functional mobilization of scar tissue fibers.

If there is not a muscle–tendon strain or ligament sprain, multidirectional friction would *not* be part of the treatment.

- Pain? Ask the client to isolate the painful area by pointing to it.
- Perform multidirectional friction on the exact spot for *only* 20 to 30 seconds. Ease up on your pressure or slow down if the client indicates that the area is tender (Figure 3-21 ■).

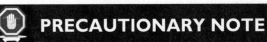
PRECAUTIONARY NOTE

Do not overwork the area and create inflammation.

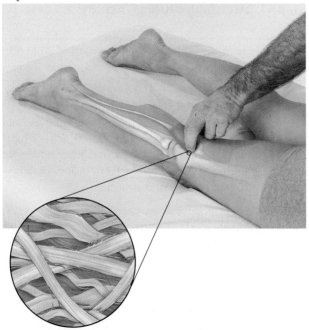

Disorganized scar tissue

FIGURE 3-21
Multidirectional Friction, Plantaris.

Step 9: Pain-Free Movement

Goal: to determine if the client can actively perform knee extension while dorsiflexing the ankle without pain. If so, this gives permission to proceed with pain-free eccentric scar tissue alignment techniques.

- Ask the client to actively flex the knee and plantar flex the ankle followed by extension of the knee and dorsiflexion of the ankle several times. This initiates the alignment of scar tissue fibers.
- Pain-free? Proceed to step 10.
- Pain? Repeat step 8, working slower and deeper, but still pain-free. Repeat step 9 and then proceed to step 10 when there is no pain.

Step 10: Eccentric Scar Tissue Alignment

Goal: to apply pain-free eccentric contraction by lengthening an injured plantaris against mild resistance to realign or redirect the scar tissue.

The greatest error during the eccentric alignment procedure is being too aggressive and not keeping the technique pain-free each time. Too much force in opposing directions can cause a new injury or reinjure the site.

Next, apply eccentric contraction to realign the deeper scar tissue. It must be performed pain-free (Figure 3-22 ■). See video clip on www.myhealthprofessionskit.com

- Ask the client to gently resist knee extension and ankle dorsiflexion.

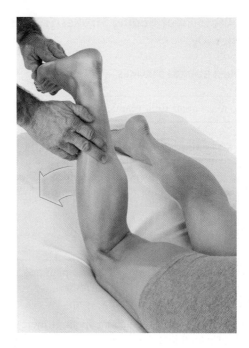

FIGURE 3-22
Plantaris Eccentric Muscle Contraction.

- Tell them to "barely resist, but let me win."
- Start with a pressure of two fingers, and have the client increase resistance only if there is no discomfort.
- Repeat this several times, pain-free.

Step 4: Assess Resisted Range of Motion (RROM)

Goal: to reassess if there is still a plantaris strain present.

Do not move too fast, or use too much force while performing a resisted test. To perform the test:

- The client plantar flexes the foot and gently attempts to flex the knee against your resistance.
- Pain behind the knee? Repeat steps 8 through 10. Then perform the resisted test again.
- Pain-free? Finish with step 11 when there is no longer any pain.

POPLITEUS STRAIN

A muscle strain of the popliteus is very rare and another commonly misdiagnosed injury of the knee. The popliteus origin is the lateral condyle of the femur and the insertion is the posterior, proximal tibial shaft. The action of the popliteus is to initiate knee flexion by medial rotation of the knee. It lies beneath the plantaris and is one of the deepest muscle on the back of the knee.

Medial rotation of the femur or lateral rotation of the tibia will place eccentric stress on this muscle and cause posterior knee pain. This results in myofascial pain and may lead to a muscle strain. The client will complain of pain behind the knee after sitting and then standing up too quickly.

To differentiate between a plantaris or popliteus strain, perform the resistance test for plantaris. If he or she experiences pain directly behind their knee, with resisted ankle dorsiflexion and knee extension, the pain is probably from the plantaris.

Step 4: Assess Resisted Range of Motion (RROM)

Goal: to assess if there is a popliteus strain present and exactly where it is located.

If there is a torn muscle or tendon, treat it *last,* after you have balanced out opposing muscle groups and addressed the problems in the muscle belly leading to the muscle tear. Do not move too fast, or use too much force while performing a resisted test.

- The client is prone with the knee bent 90 degrees, and the femur is in neutral position (not medially or laterally rotated).
- Laterally rotate the tibia about 10 to 20 degrees and have the client gently attempt to medially rotate the tibia using 20 percent strength against your resistance (Figure 3-23 ■).
- You control the intensity of the test.
- Pain? Ask the client to point to the specific spot behind the knee. This indicates a muscle strain and will be worked last.

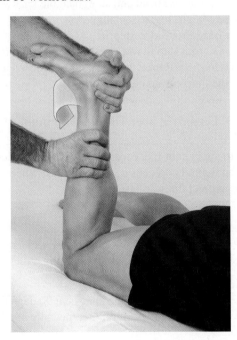

FIGURE 3-23
Popliteus Strain Test.

Step 5: Area Preparation

Goal: to prepare the client for myofascial release.

Do *not* use ice unless there is inflammation (heat, redness, or swelling). Ice may cause the fascia to become less mobile

and may restrict movement. This is counterproductive to the mobilizing and healing process, which the therapy work is promoting.

Treat the cause of pain before the symptoms or specific area of pain by making sure any abnormal rotation patterns in the knee are corrected first. Look especially for the combination of medial femur rotation and lateral tibial rotation. In this case you would first stretch the internal hip rotators and then the lateral hamstrings to treat the primary cause of popliteus stress (Figure 3-24A ■). Perform the internal hip rotator stretch and lateral hamstring stretch at this time if needed to resolve shearing forces of the knee. (Figure 3-24B ■).

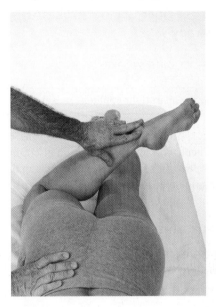

FIGURE 3-24A
Internal Hip Rotator Stretch.

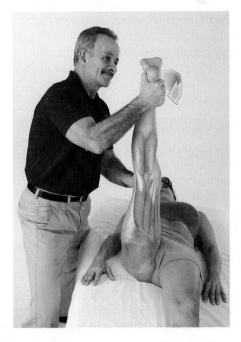

FIGURE 3-24B
Distal Lateral Hamstring Stretch.

Step 6: Myofascial Release

Goal: to warm up, soften, and mobilize the popliteus.

Always perform myofascial release *before* proceeding to deeper, more specific work.

The client is prone with their knee bent 90 degrees. Start by performing myofascial spreading of the area directly behind the knee with your finger pads or knuckles. This will bring blood flow and oxygen to this ischemic area. Use slow strokes, working progressively deeper to mobilize or lengthen the fascia.

Step 7: Cross-Fiber Gliding Strokes/Trigger Point Therapy

CROSS-FIBER GLIDING STROKES

Goal: to tease apart tight popliteus muscle bands.

Perform cross-fiber gliding strokes along the tight bands of the popliteus working from origin to insertion (lateral to medial). Repeat this several times to loosen up tight muscle fibers that often feed and contribute to active trigger points, allowing the tissue to move more freely and independently.

TRIGGER POINT THERAPY

Goal: to release trigger points in the muscle belly, if found.

Palpate for trigger points or tender spots. If there is a specific area of pain that radiates or refers, apply trigger point therapy:

- Use direct, moderate pressure for 10 to 12 seconds.
- As the trigger point softens, compress the tissue several times.
- Gently stretch the fascia the feeds the tender ischemic area.

CORE PRINCIPLE

The vascular structures behind the knee are very deep and it is unlikely you will harm them using moderate pressure. Make sure he or she does not have lymphatic problems.

Step 8: Multidirectional Friction

Goal: to soften the collagen matrix by working in multiple directions to prepare for a more functional mobilization of scar tissue fibers.

If there is not a muscle–tendon strain or ligament sprain, multidirectional friction would *not* be part of the treatment.

- Pain during the stretch or resisted range of motion test? Stop and ask the client to isolate the painful area by pointing to the specific spot. Place your finger on it and then ask if the pain is directly under your finger.
- If so, perform multidirectional friction on the exact spot for *only* 20 to 30 seconds. If you continue for longer than this, you may cause inflammation.

 PRECAUTIONARY NOTE

Do not overwork the area and create inflammation.

Step 9: Pain-Free Movement

Goal: to determine if the client can actively perform knee flexion and extension without pain.

If so, this gives permission to proceed with pain-free eccentric scar tissue alignment techniques.

- Ask the client to bend and straighten the knee several times to begin scar tissue alignment.
- Pain-free? Proceed to step 10.
- Pain? Repeat step 8, working slower and deeper, but still pain-free. Repeat step 9 and then proceed to step 10 when there is no pain.

Step 10: Eccentric Scar Tissue Alignment

Goal: to apply pain-free eccentric contraction by lengthening an injured popliteus against mild resistance to realign or redirect the scar tissue.

The greatest error during the eccentric alignment procedure is being too aggressive and not keeping the technique pain-free each time. Too much force in opposing directions can cause a new injury or reinjure the site.

- The client is prone with the knee bent 90 degrees, with the femur in neutral position (not medially or laterally rotated).
- Hold the back of the heel with one hand. Place the other hand on the foot to stabilize the ankle.
- Ask the client to gently resist medial tibial rotation performed by you. Do not exceed 10 degrees in internal tibial rotation.
- Tell him or her to "barely resist, but let me win."
- If there is no discomfort, the client can increase the resistance.
- Repeat this several times.

This will lengthen the popliteus and help realign the deeper scar tissue.

Step 4: Assess Resisted Range of Motion (RROM)

Goal: to reassess if there is still a popliteus strain present.

 PRECAUTIONARY NOTE

Do not move too fast, or use too much force while performing a resisted test.

Perform a popliteus resisted test.

- The client is prone with the knee bent. Attempt to medially rotate the tibia against his or her resistance.
- Pain behind the knee? Repeat steps 8 through 10. Then perform the resisted test again.

MEDIAL MENISCUS INJURY AND MEDIAL COLLATERAL LIGAMENT (MCL) SPRAIN

As stated earlier, the menisci are "c" shaped fibrous cartilage located in the knee joint between the femur and the tibia. They provide shock absorption and reduce the friction between the contacting bones. They are important for weight distribution and excessive rotational or compressive forces can cause damage to them. Typically, an injury will occur to the medial meniscus, as this is the weaker side of the knee. The medial collateral ligament, which stabilizes the medial knee, is usually involved also. Meniscus tears that we can access and treat are surface tears (Figure 3-25 ■). However we have seen some benefits to deeper meniscus problems when the muscles around the knee are lengthened and balanced to eliminate compressive and shearing forces of the knee. "The two most common causes of a meniscus tear are due to traumatic injury (often seen in athletes) and degenerative processes (seen in older clients who have more brittle cartilage). The most common mechanism of a traumatic meniscus tear occurs when the knee joint is bent and the knee is then twisted."[11]

 PRECAUTIONARY NOTE

Significant or deep disruption of the meniscus, usually associated with trauma, needs surgical repair.[12]

Step 4: Assess Resisted Range of Motion (RROM)

Goal: to assess if there is a surface meniscus tear or MCL sprain present and exactly where it is located.

 PRECAUTIONARY NOTE

Do not perform this test with hypermobile knee joints.

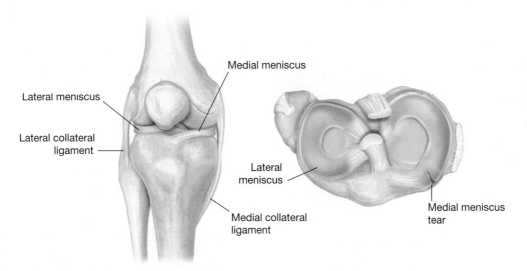

FIGURE 3-25
Internal Knee Structures.

If there is a torn meniscus, or MCL sprain, treat it *last,* after you have balanced out opposing muscle groups around the knee and reduced the compressive and rotational forces on the knee. Do not move too fast, or use too much force while performing these tests. Keep in mind that the Apley compression and Apley distraction tests, performed earlier, are more accurate in differentiating an injured medial meniscus from an injured medial collateral ligament. The author suggests these tests and the Valgus stress test done for an MCL sprain be repeated at this time. The painful or mildly injured structures may no longer test positive once the compressive and rotational forces to the knee are eliminated. Also, it is more common than not to injure both structures when there is a compressive and rotational force, but this is an additional test in preparation to working the MCL and medial meniscus.

Stand or sit at the side of the table. The client is seated or supine with the leg straight.

- Have the client attempt gentle hip adduction, bringing their leg toward the midline as you gently press against the lateral side of the knee with one hand, while gently pulling back toward you just below the knee with your other hand This is almost identical to the Valgus stress test taught earlier in this chapter. (Figure 3-26).
- This will mildly gap the area around the medial meniscus, create joint space, and may relieve the pressure on the meniscus.
- If the client experiences pain on the medial side of the knee, ask him or her to point to the specific spot. The client will usually identify both the MCL and medial meniscus areas along the medial joint line. The following treatment will address both the MCL and the medial meniscus at the same time.
- This is an additional test that helps differentiate a medial meniscus injury and a medial collateral ligament injury, and the injured medial structures should only be

worked after all the compressive forces and rotational forces from the surrounding muscles are released.

Step 5: Area Preparation

Goal: to release all muscles surrounding the knee before treating the superficial meniscus tear.

Treat the cause of pain before the symptoms or specific area of pain. Start with and follow the entire protocol for pelvic stabilization to restore normal muscle resting lengths to the medial and lateral hip rotators, quadriceps, ITB, hamstrings, and also the gastrocnemius, popliteus, and plantaris to decompress the knee and correct abnormal rotation in the knee before you proceed to the next step. All of these muscles *must* be relaxed before working the injured or damaged structures of the knee.

🛑 PRECAUTIONARY NOTE

Never treat a muscle–tendon strain or ligament sprain until those structures are brought back to their normal resting positions. Do not treat a strain in a muscle–tendon unit that is long or short. And do not treat a ligament sprain that is under tension from rotational or misalignment forces at that joint!

Step 8: Multidirectional Friction

Goal: to soften the collagen matrix by working in multiple directions to prepare for a more functional mobilization of scar tissue fibers.

If there is not a surface meniscus tear or MCL sprain, multidirectional friction would *not* be part of the treatment.

- The client is sitting on the table, with the leg straight
- Pain during the resisted test? Ask the client to isolate the painful area by pointing to it.
- Perform multidirectional friction on the medial side of the knee to the specific area of pain for *only* 20 to 30 seconds.
- Use a supported finger to apply pressure without gliding. Use only enough pressure to soften the collagen matrix and make sure you do not overwork the area (Figure 3-27).

🛑 PRECAUTIONARY NOTE

Do not create inflammation.

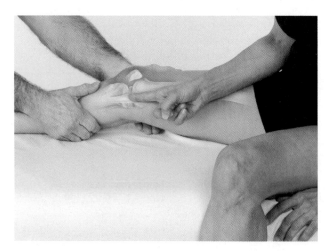

FIGURE 3-26
Valgus Stress/MCL Sprain Test.

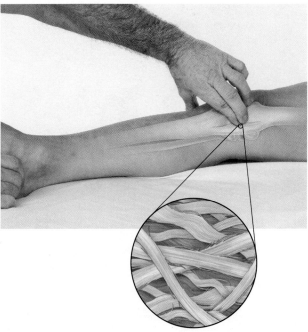

Disorganized scar tissue

FIGURE 3-27
Multidirectional Friction, MCL/Medial Meniscus.

Step 9: Pain-Free Movement

Goal: to determine if the client can actively perform knee flexion and extension without pain. If so, this gives permission to proceed with pain-free eccentric scar tissue alignment techniques.

- The client is sitting on the table. Have him or her flex and extend the knee several times.
- Pain-free? Proceed to step 10.
- Pain? Repeat step 8, working slower and deeper, but still pain-free. Repeat step 9 and then proceed to step 10 when there is no pain.

Step 10: Eccentric Scar Tissue Alignment

Goal: to apply pain-free eccentric stretch by reducing compressive forces surrounding an injured meniscus against mild resistance to realign or redirect the scar tissue.

 PRECAUTIONARY NOTE

After surgery, do not disrupt the proper healing of scar tissue by beginning this protocol too soon. Consult the client's physician before treatment.

The greatest error during the eccentric alignment procedure is being too aggressive and not keeping the technique pain-free each time. Too much force in opposing directions can cause a new injury or reinjure the site.

Apply a mild eccentric stretch to gently realign the deeper layers of scar tissue. It *must* be performed pain-free. Since the MCL and medial meniscus are not contractile structures like a muscle tendon unit, this technique is slightly different.

- The client is supine or sitting on the table with the unaffected leg off the side of the table for stabilization.
- Stand or sit on the side of the table next to the lateral side of the client's leg. Place one hand on the lateral side of the knee, supporting the lateral joint line, and the other hand on the upper medial gastrocnemius.
- With the leg straight, apply gentle pressure on the lateral joint line and a gentle downward traction on the medial gastrocnemius (Figure 3-28 ■).

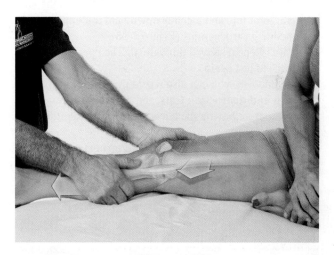

FIGURE 3-28
MCL/Medial Meniscus Eccentric Force.

- This will slightly "gap" the medial knee. The leg does not move. This will help realign multiple layers of collagen and will create space in the area of the injured meniscus. The light stretch on the MCL helps align the collagen and one hypothesis is that as the damaged meniscus is decompressed, the gentle gapping can create a force to realign the disorganized collagen around the surface tear of the meniscus. Keep in mind this is only for minor surface tears. If in doubt, refer out!

It is *imperative* to start with a pressure of only two fingers. Use the whole hand on the outer joint line only if there is zero discomfort. Repeat this several times.

 PRECAUTIONARY NOTE

Pain is *not* okay; the client must let you know if this is uncomfortable. Do not perform this on a client with a hypermobile knee.

Step 4: Assess Resisted Range of Motion (RROM)

Goal: to reassess if there is still a surface medial meniscus tear present.

Do not move too fast, or use too much force while performing a resisted test. To perform the test:

- The client is supine or sitting on the table with the unaffected leg off the side of the table for stabilization.
- Stand or sit on the side of the table next to the lateral side of the client's leg. Place one hand on the lateral side of the knee, supporting the lateral joint line, and the other hand on the upper medial gastrocnemius.
- With the leg straight, apply gentle pressure on the lateral joint line and a gentle downward traction on the medial gastrocnemius (Figure 3-28).
- Pain? Repeat steps 8 through 10. Then perform the resisted test again.
- If you wish, you can also repeat the **Apley compression and distraction tests,** and the Valgus stress test, before having the client stand up for additional evaluations.
- Pain-free? Ask the client to stand up next to the table and gently step side to side, laterally from right to left. If there is no discomfort, have the client gently "hop" on each leg, laterally side to side, increasing the amount of force on the knee.

⚠ PRECAUTIONARY NOTE

It is imperative to tell the client to try to avoid crossing the leg with a medial meniscus injury over the other leg at the knee (lateral hip rotation). This forces the tibia into the medial aspect of the femur and creates too much compression of the medial meniscus (Figure 3-29 ■). If there is a suspected meniscus injury on either side of the knee, do not perform the quadriceps stretch without traction of the tibia away from the femur.

ILIOTIBIAL BAND FRICTION SYNDROME

The iliotibial band (ITB) runs vertically down the lateral thigh over the vastus lateralis and attaches to the tibial tubercle, which is on the lateral side of the tibia. Fibers of the gluteus maximus and tensor fasciae latae (TFL) attach to the proximal end of the ITB and together help stabilize the hip and knee. Excessive stress, or a restricted or contracted condition of the ITB, **iliotibial band friction syndrome,** can cause pain on the lateral side of the knee. The client will report

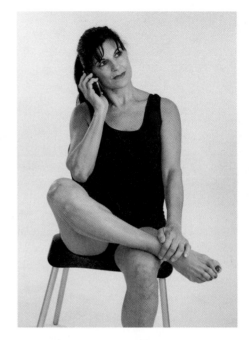

FIGURE 3-29
Poor Posture for Meniscus Problems.

this pain during activity, as it typically diminishes with rest. Going up and down stairs may also create discomfort on the lateral side of the knee. To evaluate for excess tension in the ITB press down on the distal end of the band, just before it passes over the lateral condyle of the femur, and do passive or active flexion and extension of the knee. Usually if the client has iliotibial band friction syndrome pain or discomfort will increase at about 30 degrees of knee flexion (Figure 3-30 ■).

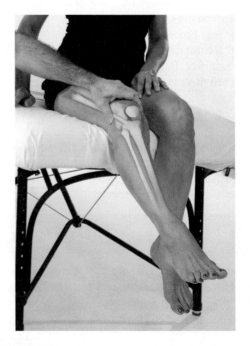

FIGURE 3-30
ITB Friction Test.

Step 4: Assess Resisted Range of Motion (RROM)

Clinical studies indicate that it is best to not friction the distal end of the ITB. The pain on the lateral knee is rarely ever due to scar tissue in the distal end of the band. The tension in the lateral knee is best relieved by creating length in the lateral fibers of gluteus maximus, and the TFL muscle. After lengthening the contractile portion of the band, you can do a myofascial technique to free the band from the underlying vastus lateralis. Then if you correct abnormal external tibia–fibular rotation of the knee, the pain will usually go away. The pain in the lateral knee can be multifaceted and involve the lateral meniscus, lateral collateral ligament, fixated proximal fibular head, and ITB tension. You must identify and treat the correct structures and not look at this as a generic situation like runner's knee.

Step 5: Area Preparation

Goal: to prepare the client before performing myofascial release.

Do *not* use ice unless there is inflammation (heat, redness, or swelling). Ice may cause the fascia to become less mobile and may restrict movement. This is counterproductive to the mobilizing and healing process, which the therapy work is promoting.

You *must* follow the protocol for pelvic stabilization through the anterior quadriceps release before you begin the ITB work.

Step 6: Myofascial Release

Goal: to warm up, soften, and mobilize the ITB, and to move the fascial layers back to normal resting or lengthened position.

Always perform myofascial release *before* proceeding to deeper, more specific work.

After the anterior and medial quadriceps work, work the ITB. Think of it as a tight tendon even though it is a ligamentous structure.

- The client is supine. Bend his or her knee to bring the hip into flexion.
- Start by working into the gluteus maximus and medius with compressions (Figure 3-31 ■).
- Then, over the clothing, perform cross-fiber gliding strokes, and compressions to the TFL (Figure 3-32 ■).
- To locate the TFL, palpate the ASIS and drop laterally off it. Have the client medially rotate the hip and you will feel the TFL move under your fingers. Use your fingers or thumbs and be careful, as this area is likely to be tender.

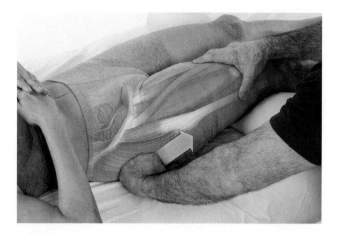

FIGURE 3-31
Gluteus Maximus Compression.

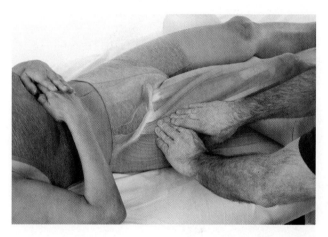

FIGURE 3-32
TFL Myofascial Release.

- Stretch the lateral fibers of gluteus maximus by having the client flex the hip to 90 degrees. Stand on the opposite side of the table. Place one hand on the lateral thigh, supporting the lateral joint line of the knee. The other hand in on the lateral fibers of the gluteus maximus, pressing it down toward the table to stabilize the hip. Assist the stretch as the client actively adducts the leg across the body (Figure 3-33 ■). The hip must stay on the table.
- Then stretch the TFL to help release the ITB tension for better mobilization of the band, as you next free it up from the vastus lateralis. The client is supine with the leg straight. The hip is flexed 30 degrees and laterally rotated. Stand on the opposite side of the table. Place one hand on the ilium with gentle pressure and three fingers on the TFL muscle to stabilize the hip. With your other hand under the thigh also stabilize the lateral joint line of the knee. The client abducts the hip 30 degrees and then actively adducts across the midline as you assist the stretch. Do a pin and stretch

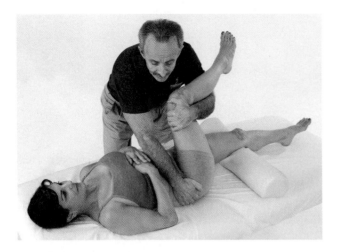

FIGURE 3-33
Gluteus Maximus Lateral Fibers Stretch.

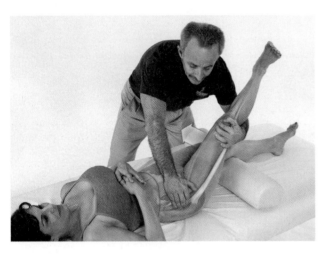

FIGURE 3-34
TFL Stretch.

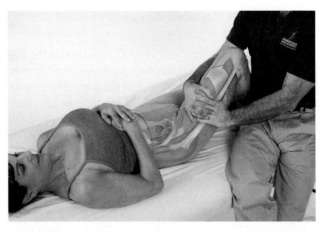

FIGURE 3-35A
ITB Mobilization.

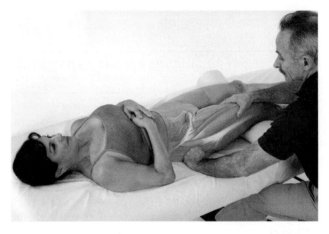

FIGURE 3-35B
Compression Broadening from Gluteus Maximus Distally through Vastus Lateralis (Work from Hip to Knee).

of the TFL. Do not let the hip come up off the table (Figure 3-34 ■).

- Next, using the heel of your hand, hook the inferior angle of the ITB and rotate it from medial to lateral as you draw the skin and band toward the knee. Use your other hand on the other side of the leg to help create a rotational movement (Figure 3-35A ■). Do not slide over the skin. Work from the hip toward the knee to lengthen the band, and thus reduce symptoms over the lateral femoral condyle (work proximal to distal).
- Then perform compressions into the vastus lateralis, working from origin to insertion to create length. If there is lateral tracking of the patella make sure to intentionally lengthen the vastus lateralis. This will help eliminate the lateral patella tracking problem (Figure 3-35B ■).

Pin your elbow into your side and with the palm of your hand and work along the ITB several times (proximal to distal). This will help release adhesions along the ITB. Alternate with compressions. If the vastus lateralis is tender

during the compressions you may not have fully released the ITB. Go back and repeat the rotational movement. Lengthening the vastus lateralis and strengthening the oblique fibers of the vastus medialis can oftentimes eliminate the cause of chondromalacia and patellar tendinosis. Because the cartilage of the patella has minimal or no pain receptors, once you stop the tracking, the underlying damaged cartilage will not cause pain. The pain from lateral patellar tracking is usually due to the nipping of the bursa and fatty sacs of the knee, not the cartilage degeneration under the knee cap.

Step 7: Cross-Fiber Gliding Strokes/Trigger Point Therapy

CROSS-FIBER GLIDING STROKES

Goal: to tease apart tight muscle fibers in muscle groups causing the ITB to be tight.

Remember, the band itself is a relatively nonvascular and noncontractile structure.

Use cross-fiber gliding strokes, working from origin to insertion (proximal to distal) to tease through and gently spread muscle fibers in the gluteus maximus and tensor fasciae latae (TFL).

TRIGGER POINT THERAPY

Goal: to release trigger points in the muscle belly, if found.

If there is a specific area of pain that radiates or refers, apply trigger point therapy.

- Use direct, moderate pressure for 10 to 12 seconds.
- As the trigger point softens, compress the tissue several times.
- Gently stretch the tissue.

Go to the end of the table and lean back and traction the leg. Release very slowly.

Step 11: Stretching (During Therapy)
Refer back to medial gluteus maximus and TFL stretch prior to mobilizing the ITB.

Goal: to create normal range of motion of 30-degree hip adduction.

Contracting the muscle against resistance to fatigue the muscle prior to the stretch becomes a muscle resistance test and the client may report pain in a specific area, which is a muscle strain. If so, proceed to multidirectional friction (step 8), pain-free movement (step 9), and eccentric scar tissue alignment (step 10) until the client is pain-free.

Since the ITB is relatively noncontractile you need to stretch the gluteus maximus and the tensor fasciae latae releasing the forces on the band.

Step 8: Multidirectional Friction

Goal: to soften the collagen matrix by working in multiple directions to prepare for a more functional mobilization of scar tissue fibers.

As mentioned earlier, based on new clinical studies, it is not recommended to friction the distal end of the ITB.

Step 9: Pain-Free Movement

Goal: to determine if the client can actively perform knee flexion and extension without pain. Since the distal band is rarely injured we will skip this step, nor is it required for ITB distal fibers.

- Pain-free? Proceed to step 10.

- Pain? Repeat step 8, working slower and deeper, but still pain-free. Repeat step 9 and then proceed to step 10 when there is no pain.

Step 10: Eccentric Scar Tissue Alignment

Goal: to apply pain-free eccentric contraction by lengthening an injured ITB against mild resistance to realign or redirect the scar tissue (step not required).

 PRECAUTIONARY NOTE

After knee surgery, do not disrupt the proper healing of scar tissue by beginning this protocol too soon. Consult the client's physician before treatment.

The greatest error during the eccentric alignment procedure is being too aggressive and not keeping the technique pain-free each time. Too much force in opposing directions can cause a new injury or reinjure the site.

Step 4: Assess Resisted Range of Motion (RROM)

Goal: to reassess if there is still an ITB strain present (step not required).

- Pain? Repeat steps 8 through 10. Then perform the resisted test again.
- Pain-free? Finish with step 11 when there is no longer any pain.

LATERAL MENISCUS INJURY AND LATERAL COLLATERAL LIGAMENT (LCL) SPRAIN

An injury to the lateral meniscus and the lateral collateral ligament (LCL) occurs less often than an injury to the medial side of the knee. One of the reasons may be because the lateral meniscus has twice the mobility of the medial meniscus.[13] A Varus stress test will result in the client reporting immediate pain on the lateral side of the knee for LCL injuries. The ITB may also be involved and must be released prior to working the lateral side of the knee.

Step 4: Assess Resisted Range of Motion (RROM)

Goal: to assess if there is a surface lateral meniscus tear present and exactly where it is located.

If there is a torn muscle or tendon, treat it *last,* after you have balanced out the surrounding muscle groups and reduced the compressive forces and abnormal rotational forces on the knee. The following test is also performed for an LCL sprain.

PRECAUTIONARY NOTE

Do not move too fast, or use too much force while performing a resisted test.

- The client is supine or seated on the table with one leg straight.
- Varus stress test: Stabilize the medial joint line with one hand and gently press against the medial side of the knee, while gently pulling down on the upper outer gastrocnemius with the other hand.
- This will mildly "gap" the lateral meniscus, creating space and relieving the pressure on the meniscus. If the client points to the lateral joint line it can be an additional positive test for the LCL and the lateral meniscus will be less symptomatic after all the compressive and rotational forces are removed from the knee (Figure 3-36 ■).
- Also refer to the Apley compression and Apley distraction tests performed earlier in this chapter to differentiate lateral meniscus damage from LCL damage (refer to Figure 3-7).

 PRECAUTIONARY NOTE

Do not perform the resisted test on a hypermobile knee or following major trauma.

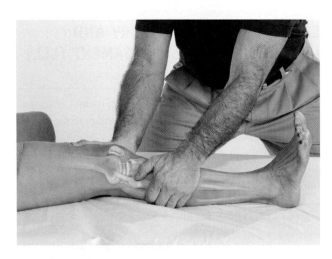

FIGURE 3-36
Varus Stress Test (LCL Sprain Test).

Step 5: Area Preparation

Goal: to release all of the muscles surrounding the knee before treating the superficial lateral meniscus tear.

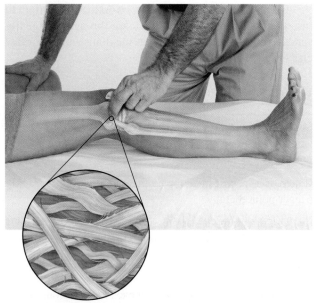

Disorganized scar tissue

FIGURE 3-37
LCL Multidirectional Friction.

You *must* perform the pelvic stabilization protocol through to the ITB work before you proceed with the following lateral knee work.

Step 8: Multidirectional Friction

Goal: to soften the collagen matrix by working in multiple directions to prepare for a more functional mobilization of scar tissue fibers.

If there is not a superficial lateral meniscus tear, multidirectional friction would *not* be part of the treatment.

- Pain during the LCL and meniscus tests? Ask the client to isolate the painful area on the lateral side of the knee by pointing to it.
- Perform multidirectional friction on the specific spot of pain for *only* 20 to 30 seconds. Use a supported finger to apply pressure without gliding (Figure 3-37 ■).
- Use only enough pressure to soften the collagen matrix and make sure you do not overwork the area.

 PRECAUTIONARY NOTE

Do not overwork the area and create inflammation.

Step 9: Pain-Free Movement

Goal: to determine if the client can actively perform knee flexion and extension without pain. If so, this gives permission to proceed with pain-free eccentric scar tissue alignment techniques.

- The client is sitting on the table. Have him or her flex and extend the knee several times. This begins the process of realigning collagen fibers (scar tissue).
- Pain-free? Proceed to step 10.
- Pain? Repeat step 8, working slower and deeper, but still pain-free. Repeat step 9 and then proceed to step 10 when there is no pain.

Step 10: Eccentric Scar Tissue Alignment

Goal: to apply pain-free eccentric stretch by releasing compressive forces surrounding an injured lateral meniscus or injured LCL against mild resistance to realign or redirect the scar tissue.

 PRECAUTIONARY NOTE

After surgery, do not disrupt the proper healing of scar tissue by beginning this protocol too soon. Consult the client's physician before treatment.

The greatest error during the eccentric alignment procedure is being too aggressive and not keeping the technique pain-free each time. Too much force in opposing directions can cause a new injury or reinjure the site.

Next, perform an eccentric force to realign the deeper scar tissue. This *must* be performed pain-free.

- The client is sitting on the table with one leg straight.
- Place one hand on the medial side of the knee and the other on the upper outer gastrocnemius.
- Apply gentle pressure to the medial joint line and mild downward traction to the upper lateral gastrocnemius to slightly gap the knee. The leg does not move. Repeat. (Figure 3-38 ■).
- It is imperative that you start with very light pressure. You can then gently increase pressure on the medial joint line to recruit deeper levels of disorganized collagen, but only if there is zero discomfort.
- Repeat several times, pain-free.

 PRECAUTIONARY NOTE

Make sure you check in with the client to make sure this is not uncomfortable. Pain or extreme discomfort is *not* okay. Do not apply this work to a hypermobile knee.

Step 4: Assess Resisted Range of Motion (RROM)

Goal: to reassess if there is still a lateral meniscus tear or MCL stress present.

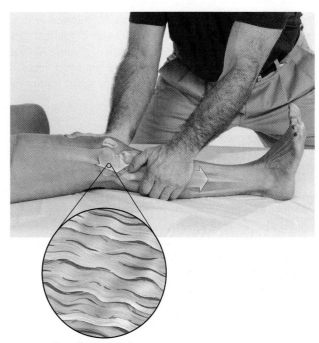
Functional scar tissue

FIGURE 3-38
Eccentric Force LCL (Varus Stress Test).

Perform a lateral meniscus resisted test.

- Have the client gently attempt abduction as you press gently against the medial side of the knee with one hand, while gently pulling distal on the upper fibula with your other hand. (Similar to the Varus stress test.)
- Pain? Repeat steps 8 through 10. Then perform the tests again.
- Pain-free? Ask the client to stand up next to the table and gently step side to side, laterally from right to left. If there is no discomfort, have the client gently hop on each leg, laterally side to side, increasing the amount of force on the knee only if it is pain-free.

Step 11: Stretching (Client Self-Care)

Emphasize client self-care! Client self-care is essential for the client to keep the new normal range of motion that was created during therapy. Clients must learn these techniques and perform them at home to keep the muscle groups balanced and to accustom their minds and bodies to the new pain-free range of motion. Teach the clients active assisted stretching first. Once they understand the stretches and can correctly perform them for you, you can teach them the more advanced PNF stretches. To perform the stretches, the clients need a stretch rope, towel, or long belt.

TECHNIQUES FOR CLIENT SELF-CARE

Goal: for the client to perform stretches demonstrated by you to create normal range of motion in shortened or contracted muscle groups.

In certain states, massage therapists are not allowed to suggest stretches. If you are not competent, or if you feel that suggesting stretches is outside your scope of practice, do *not* follow this step. Be safe, refer out. Wait until you become competent by becoming certified as a personal trainer or certified in active isolated stretching.

✋ PRECAUTIONARY NOTE

Do not have the client stretch beyond normal range of motion, as this could create hypermobile joints and result in injury.

- Tell the client that the stretches will take only a few minutes a day to perform and are necessary for continued results.
- The client should stretch after some movement, moderate exercise, or a hot shower when the fascia and muscles are warm.
- Tell the client to not stretch into pain. He or she needs to differentiate between uncomfortable stretching due to tight muscles and painful stretching that can aggravate a pre-existing clinical condition.
- The client starts the stretches with the tightest side first until normal range of motion and normal muscle resting lengths are achieved. Then he or she can continue to stretch both sides for continued balance and symmetry.
- Suggest only two to four stretches, specific for the condition, each time you see a client. Make sure he or she can perform these correctly before suggesting any additional stretches.
- Print copies of the stretches for your clients to take with them for reference.

PATELLAR TENDINOSIS—QUADRICEPS

1. Have the client perform the following stretch:

   - The client is prone with one knee bent.
   - This stretch *must* be performed with a rolled towel behind the knee, especially if he or she had a meniscus injury to traction the tibia away from the femur. This will help decompress the knee.
   - The client reaches back and grasps the ankle. He or she attempts to extend the knee against his or her own resistance with 20 percent force for 5 to 10 seconds. (The client may use a stretch rope if it is uncomfortable to grab the ankle.)
   - The client relaxes, takes a deep breath, and then on exhale pulls the ankle to the hip for about 2 seconds.
   - This is a passive stretch; the client does not engage the hamstrings, as this may result in a hamstring cramp.
   - The client repeats the stretch 8 to 10 times, then repeats on the other leg, if needed.

2. If the client is not flexible enough to perform the previous stretch, he or she can substitute this one.

   - The client is prone with one knee bent, with a stretch rope looped around the ankle coming up over the back so he or she can hold it.
   - This stretch *must* be performed with a rolled towel behind the knee to traction the tibia away from the femur, to decompress the knee.
   - The client extends the knee against his or her own resistance with 20 percent force for 5 to 10 seconds.
   - He or she relaxes, takes a deep breath, and then on exhale gently pulls on the stretch rope bringing the ankle toward the glutes for about 2 seconds (Figure 3-39 ■).
   - This is a passive stretch; the client does not engage the hamstrings.
   - The client repeats the stretch 8 to 10 times, then repeats on the other leg for balance.

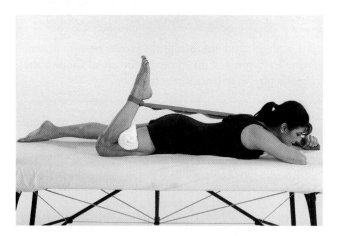

FIGURE 3-39
Quadriceps Stretch.

DISTAL HAMSTRINGS

Oftentimes, especially in the right knee, there will be excessive lateral rotation from the way a person drives a car. This shortens the biceps femoris (lateral hamstring), resulting in problems like posterior fixated fibular head pain. This can mimic or compound pain in other structures such as the ITB, LCL, and lateral meniscus. If this is not corrected, it can create shearing force on the knee, resulting in damage to the ligaments and meniscus of the knee. If lateral rotation of the knee is present, it is critical to stretch the lateral hamstrings to also treat the primary cause of pain in the popliteus. If medial rotation is present in the knee, stretch the distal medial hamstrings to correct rotational problems. Do not stretch the distal lateral or medial hamstrings separately, if there is not rotation in the knee; just stretch all hamstring groups equally.

- The client is supine.
- To stretch the distal hamstrings when there is no rotation at the knee, the client loops the stretch rope around the foot with the strap ending up near the heel.

He or she stabilizes the femur in a neutral position with one hand so it does not rotate, while holding the stretch rope with the other hand, keeping the arm straight (Figure 3-40A ■).
- The client extends the knee, assisting by pulling up on the rope at the lateral side of the leg (Figure 3-40B ■).
- This restores knee extension and takes stress off the structures of the knee.
- The client repeats the stretch on the other leg, if needed.

CORE PRINCIPLE

It is imperative for the client to lift *up* on the stretch rope; otherwise too much pressure is created in the knee. If the gastrocnemius is too tight to allow the leg to straighten, the client should stretch it in addition to this hamstrings stretch. He or she should perform the following plantaris–gastrocnemius stretch separate from this stretch. When stretching the gastrocnemius with the hip flexed and knee extended, it can compress the meniscus and create a secondary injury.

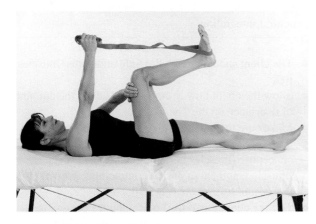

FIGURE 3-40A
Distal Hamstring Stretch—Start.

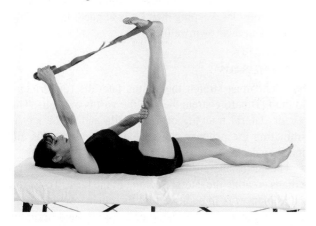

FIGURE 3-40B
Distal Hamstring Stretch—Finish.

PLANTARIS AND GASTROCNEMIUS

- The client is seated with one leg straight with the stretch rope around the ball of that foot.
- He or she brings the ankle to dorsiflexion to lengthen the plantaris and gastrocnemius.
- Then the client plantar flexes the ankle against the resistance of the rope for 5 to 10 seconds at 20 percent force.
- He or she relaxes, inhales, then on exhale actively dorsiflexes the ankle and fully extends the knee while gently pulling back on the rope for about 2 seconds (Figure 3-41 ■).
- At this new position, the client repeats the stretch several times, repeating it on the other leg, if needed.

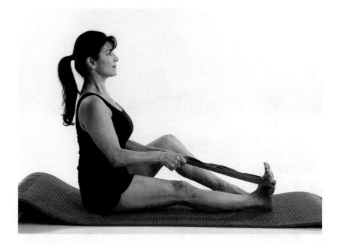

FIGURE 3-41
Gastrocnemius Stretch.

GLUTEUS MAXIMUS LATERAL FIBERS
The client performs this stretch to eliminate ITB pain.

- The client is supine with both the knee and the hip flexed 90 degrees.
- He or she stabilizes the hip of the involved leg with one hand and places the other hand on the lateral side of the knee.
- He or she actively medially rotates the hip.
- The client attempts hip abduction at 20 percent force against his or her own resistance for 5 to 10 seconds (Figure 3-42 ■).
- He or she relaxes, takes a deep breath, and on exhale actively adducts the leg across the body as he or she assists the stretch for about 2 seconds.
- At this new position, the client repeats the stretch two or three times.

TENSOR FASCIAE LATAE
The client performs this stretch to eliminate ITB pain.

- The client is supine.

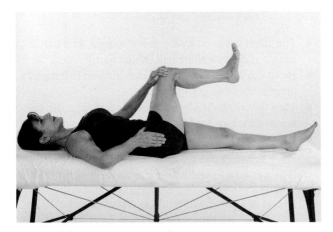

FIGURE 3-42
Gluteus Maximus Lateral Fiber Stretch.

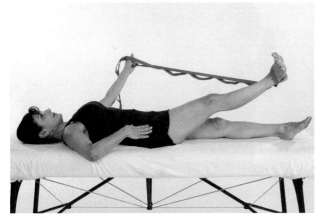

FIGURE 3-43
TFL Stretch.

- He or she places a stretch rope around the ankle of the involved leg, coming around the outside of the ankle and then under that leg.
- The client laterally rotates (turns outward) this leg and places a hand on the hip to stabilize it.
- Then he or she exhales and adducts the leg for about 2 seconds, assisting with the rope while keeping the arm straight out to the side (Figure 3-43 ■).
- He or she repeats the stretch 8 to10 times, then repeats it on the other leg, if needed.

MEDIAL AND LATERAL MENISCUS

There are no self-stretches for the client, as the risk for reinjury is too great. He or she should have someone gently traction the knee to decompress the muscles in that area, and keep the muscle groups around the knee released and balanced.

Step 12: Strengthening (Client Self-Care)

The client must stretch the tight, contracted muscles before strengthening the opposing weak muscles.

 PRECAUTIONARY NOTE

To prevent reinjury after treating a strain, have the client refrain from beginning a strengthening program for 7 to 10 days, or until he or she is pain-free. To facilitate healing, have the client stretch the tight antagonist muscles, taking the tension off the injured muscles.

The final step in the twelve-step approach to pain management is strengthening the weak, inhibited, and sometimes overstretched muscles. These muscles may lack blood flow and oxygen and need to be strengthened to allow complete structural balance throughout the body. Strengthening is essential to a client's continued improvement and recovery, and prevention of injury. Demonstrate the strengthening exercises for the client and then instruct him or her on how to practice the movements at home. The only items needed are a Thera-Band (for resistance) and a towel.

TECHNIQUES FOR STRENGTHENING

Goal: to strengthen weak, inhibited muscle groups around a joint creating muscle balance throughout the body— structural integration.

- The client should stretch the tight antagonist muscles first.
- Show the client how to control and adjust the amount of resistance on the Thera-Band.
- Make sure the client's movements while performing the exercises are slow and controlled during both the concentric (muscle shortening phase) and eccentric (muscle lengthening phase) contractions, *placing more emphasis on the eccentric phase.*
- Tell the client that only 5 to10 minutes per day is needed to perform both stretching and strengthening exercises for any condition.
- Empower clients to take responsibility for reeducating their muscles, keeping their body aligned, and participating in their own wellness.

VASTUS MEDIALIS

The client must stretch the vastus lateralis (quadriceps) and the ITB before strengthening the vastus medialis. This prevents lateral tracking of the patella and is the key to eliminating the primary cause of patellar tendinosis and chondromalacia.

The vastus lateralis is typically stronger than the vastus medialis creating the lateral tracking of the knee. To correct this problem it is imperative that the client strengthen the vastus medialis to return the knee to proper and optimum balance and to prevent injury in the future. See video clip on www.myhealthprofessionskit.com.

CASE STUDY

Fran is a 45-year-old dance instructor that naturally has tight lateral hip rotators and strong quadriceps and hamstrings. She has especially strong calf muscles from being on her toes for many years in ballet.

Fran decides one day to play recreational softball with her team from work. On the first day of practice Fran hits a line drive, and as she begins to round first base and head to second, she feels a painful twisting motion in her knee and grabs her knee in extreme pain. She is evaluated by an orthopedic physician and diagnosed with a medial meniscus tear. Fran is placed in a knee brace and surgery is recommended. Fran is very active, so wearing the knee brace and not being able to dance or participate in sports is unbearable.

Fran's husband is an international lecturer on advanced clinical massage therapy and orthopedic massage, and feels that surgery should be the last option for her condition. After several weeks of ice, pain medications, and wearing a knee brace, Fran is evaluated by her husband. There is no longer inflammation or swelling to the area. When the knee brace is removed, Fran has pain on the medial side of her knee when she walks, and the pain increases when she does a squat, goes up and down steps, or moves side to side in a lateral or medial direction.

Fran's active range of motion evaluation shows the following:

- Medial hip rotation is limited to 15 degrees, indicating tight lateral hip rotators.

- Knee flexion is limited to 90 degrees, indicating tight quadriceps and ITB.

- Dorsiflexion of the ankle is limited to 10 degrees, indicating tight gastrocnemius and soleus.

This is valuable information because the quadriceps, hamstrings, ITB, and gastrocnemius all put tension in the knee joint and contribute to joint tension affecting the articulating cartilage and the scar tissue surrounding the meniscus. Excessive lateral hip rotation compromises the knee situation more by creating torsion in the knee area, especially if it is accompanied by internal tibial rotation.

Passive range of motion end feel for knee flexion indicates the meniscus is being compromised, as Fran has a rather abrupt end feel that seems to be coming both from client splinting to protect the area and from strained or sprained fibers on the inside of the knee. A muscle resistance test indicates a small muscle strain in the medial hamstring insertion of semitendinosus, the Valgus stress test indicates slight sprain in the medial collateral ligament, the Apley compression test is also positive for medial meniscus pain.

Treatment starts by performing pelvic stabilization, with special attention being paid to lengthening the deep six lateral hip rotators to restore 45 degrees of medial hip rotation. Then, the clinical massage therapist massages and lengthens the quadriceps and ITB to bring knee flexion close to 135 degrees. A towel or bolster is placed behind the knee to protect the meniscus when stretching the quadriceps (see Figure 3-39). The therapist then lengthens the hamstrings and gastrocnemius to increase space around the knee. When stretching the gastrocnemius the knee is tractioned in the extended position to protect the meniscus.

In evaluating the hamstrings, Fran points to a muscle strain on the medial side of the knee in the semitendinosus.

- The therapist follows the hamstring protocol and treats that spot last after releasing tension in the muscle belly.

- The therapist then performs multidirectional friction on the medial collateral ligament and the area of the surface tear in the joint surrounding the medial meniscus.

- This is followed by slightly gapping the medial knee joint to create functional scar tissue in the ligament and around the edges of the meniscus.

Fran follows this treatment by walking without the brace. She does not experience pain. She then does a few squats, with no pain. Fran then jumps laterally from side to side, with no pain. The final test is when Fran attempts to jog on the treadmill and is able to do so, with no pain. She is given self-care exercises to stretch the following muscle groups in the following order:

1. Lateral hip rotators (deep six)
2. Quadriceps (must place a towel behind the knee to protect the meniscus)
3. ITB (gluteus maximus lateral fibers and TFL)
4. Medial hamstring (must be done pain-free, allowing enough time for the hamstring strain to heal)
5. Gastrocnemius stretch (performed with caution to protect the meniscus)

These stretches are customized for Fran to maintain muscular balance around the hip and knee, and allow adequate joint space in the knee, so the newly created functional scar tissue in the hamstring, ligament, and meniscus can heal properly.

Fran has been pain-free for five years after only two treatments and feels only occasional discomfort when she neglects doing her self-care.

✋ PRECAUTIONARY NOTE

This treatment is highly successful for surface meniscus tears. It would not be performed for a traumatic injury that creates a deep meniscus tear, ruptured ligament, or extreme ACL hypermobility. *If in doubt, refer out!*

CHAPTER SUMMARY

This chapter was written to offer the clinical massage therapist a variety of tools to evaluate, identify, and properly address the most common clinical conditions of the knee. The author wants to stress the importance of combining the work presented in Chapter 2 on pelvic stabilization, to achieve better results when treating complicated knee conditions. Manual therapists should stop using generic catchall terms like "runners knee" and instead, sort out the multiple possibilities presenting themselves as knee pain.

The intention of this chapter was to ensure that the therapist eliminate any underlying causes of specific clinical conditions of the knee prior to treating the resulting symptoms. It is important to continue looking at the major contributing factors of knee pain as manual therapists balance out the muscle groups of the foot and ankle in Chapter 4 to eliminate ascending syndromes into the knee.

REVIEW QUESTIONS

1. What would you expect to find during a positive test for ACL or PCL instability?
   a. a soft, mushy end feel
   b. a ligamentous end feel
   c. minimal movement
   d. normal range of motion

2. A tight plantaris and popliteus will limit what range of motion?
   a. knee flexion
   b. ankle plantar flexion
   c. knee extension
   d. knee medial rotation

3. If there is pain during the Apley compression test what is most likely injured?
   a. ACL
   b. PCL
   c. meniscus
   d. patellar tendon

4. What is chondromalacia?
   a. ligament degeneration
   b. meniscus injury
   c. patellar tendinosis
   d. degeneration of cartilage under the patella

5. Patellar tendinosis is caused by _____.
   a. tight hamstrings
   b. overuse of rectus femoris, and possibly lack of balance between vastus medialis and vastus lateralis
   c. unresolved tight ITB problems
   d. tight tibialis anterior pulling on the patellar ligament

6. What is the first thing to do before working on a distal hamstrings strain?
   a. stretch the hamstrings and return them to normal muscle resting lengths
   b. work and stretch the quadriceps
   c. strengthen the hamstrings
   d. align eccentric scar tissue

7. How do you test for a popliteus strain?
   a. The client is prone, knee bent 90 degrees. Laterally rotate the tibia and have the client gently attempt to medially rotate the tibia against your resistance.
   b. The client is prone, knee bent 90 degrees. Medially rotate the tibia and have the client gently attempt to laterally rotate the tibia against your resistance.
   c. The client is supine, knee bent 90 degrees. Laterally rotate the tibia and have the client extend the knee.
   d. The client is supine, knee bent 90 degrees. Medially rotate the tibia and have the client extend the knee.

8. The client presents with pain somewhere behind the knee. If you perform the popliteus resisted test and the client does not report a specific spot of pain directly behind the knee, what three other muscles could be strained?
   a. patellar ligament, distal hamstrings, proximal gastrocnemius
   b. plantaris, proximal hamstrings, distal gastrocnemius
   c. plantaris, distal hamstrings, distal gastrocnemius
   d. plantaris, distal hamstrings, proximal gastrocnemius

9. What is the best way to treat iliotibial band friction syndrome?
   a. create length in gluteus maximus and TFL
   b. myofascial release of the band from the vastus lateralis
   c. correct abnormal tibia rotation of the knee
   d. all of the above

10. The client has excessive lateral rotation of the tibia and resultant meniscus pain. Which muscles do you stretch and lengthen?
    a. medial hamstrings
    b. quadriceps
    c. lateral hamstrings
    d. gastrocnemius

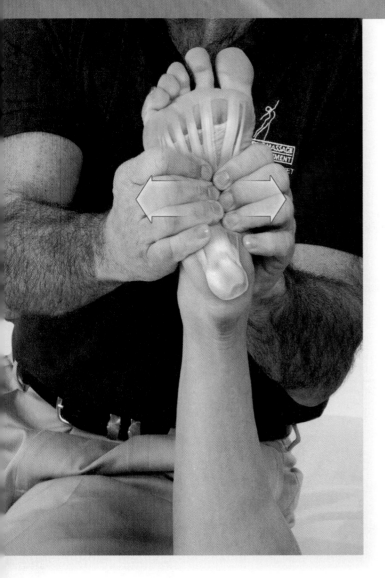

CHAPTER

4 Lower Leg, Ankle, and Foot Conditions

 CHAPTER OUTLINE

Twelve-Step Approach to Lower Leg, Ankle, and Foot Conditions

Achilles Tendinosis

Gastrocnemius Protocol to Address Achilles Tendon Pain

Soleus Protocol

Posteromedial Shin Splints

Flat Feet and Fallen Arches and Hyperpronation

Plantar Fasciitis

Anterior Compartment Syndrome (ACS)

Anterolateral Shin Splints

Inversion Ankle Sprain and Strain

Stress Fracture

LEARNING OBJECTIVES

Upon completing this chapter the reader will be able to:

- Choose the appropriate massage modality or treatment protocol for each specific clinical condition of the lower leg. Based on restoring normal range of motion throughout the body, and normal muscle resting lengths, the focus is to work on the contracted muscle groups typically short and tight—gastrocnemius, soleus, and tibialis posterior—before working the weak, inhibited antagonists—tibialis anterior, extensor digitorum longus, extensor hallucis longus, and peroneals. This will ensure
  - structural integration—balance of the opposing muscle groups
  - that the therapist eliminates the underlying soft-tissue cause of the lower leg conditions before addressing the clinical symptoms
- Restore pain-free ankle joint normal range of motion

- Create ankle stability
- Differentiate between soft-tissue problems caused by
  - myofascial restrictions
  - muscle–tendon tension
  - trigger point tension
  - strained muscle fibers
  - sprained ligaments
  - nerve compression
  - bony fixations
- Teach the client self-care stretching and strengthening exercises (if needed) to perform at home to maintain musculoskeletal balance and pain-free movement following therapy

KEY TERMS

Arthrokinetics   122

Bony fixations 118

Bunion   128

Dorsiflexion   119

Eversion   119

Hammer toe   128

Inversion   119

Neuroma   128

Plantar fascia   129

Plantar flexion   119

Retinaculum   134

Sheathed tendon   135

This chapter addresses a structural approach to treating specific clinical conditions of the lower leg. The goal is to balance the muscle groups of the lower leg, based on normal muscle resting lengths, to restore normal range of motion of the foot and ankle, ensure proper foot strike biomechanics, and create foot and ankle stability. Muscle groups are worked superficial to deep with the focus on the short, contracted muscles *limiting* movement, before working on the weak, inhibited antagonists. This will allow you, as therapist, to treat the cause of lower leg conditions before the symptoms.

PRECAUTIONARY NOTE

Do not work on a client with a recent injury (acute condition), exhibiting inflammation, heat, redness, or swelling. RICE therapy (rest, ice, compression, elevation) would be the appropriate treatment in this situation.

Imbalances in the hips can create distortions that affect the knees and lower legs. Therefore, it is suggested that the clinical massage therapist perform pelvic stabilization along with lower leg work. When assessing active, passive, and resisted ranges of motion of the lower leg this text focuses on the tight, contracted muscle groups *limiting* the movement, not the muscle group creating the movement. Then determine if the problem is myofascial restriction, tight bands, trigger point tension, strained muscle fibers, sprained ligaments, or **bony fixations**. The suggested treatment will be specific to the musculoskeletal imbalances that limit normal pain-free movement.

TWELVE-STEP APPROACH TO LOWER LEG, ANKLE, AND FOOT CONDITIONS

Following are the main conditions that are presented in this chapter:

- Achilles tendinosis
- Posteromedial shin splints
- Flat feet and fallen arches and hyperpronation
- Plantar fasciitis
- Anterior compartment syndrome (ACS)
- Anterolateral shin splints
- Inversion ankle sprain and strain
- Stress fracture

The chapter also covers joint arthritis, bunions, hammer toes, and neuromas.

Step 1: Client History

A thorough client history taken will offer you valuable insights to a client's condition. In addition to the basic information completed on the client history form, ask the client when, where, and how the problem began. Also ask the client to describe the area of pain and what makes it better or worse. This will give you a starting point from which to assess his or her active range of motion.

Step 2: Assess Active Range of Motion (AROM)

The client is prone, knee flexed 90 degrees. Ask him or her to actively perform each of the four primary single-plane

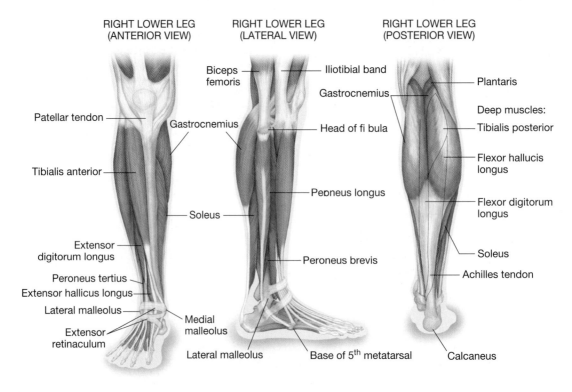

FIGURE 4-1
Lower Leg Muscles.

movements of the ankle joint—**plantar flexion, dorsiflexion, inversion,** and **eversion**—with zero discomfort. Determine if the range of motion is normal. Please understand that the normal degrees for each ankle range of motion will vary with different references. The degrees listed in this text are accurate estimates for clients with healthy ankles. If the ROM is less than average, identify which muscle groups are restricted and therefore preventing normal movement. Dorsiflexion and plantar flexion occur at the talocrural joint. Inversion and eversion occur at the subtalar joint.

Focus on releasing these restricted, antagonist muscle groups (Figures 4-1 ■ through 4-5 ■):

- Plantar flexion occurs when the foot moves away from the anterior surface of the leg. If plantar flexion is less than 30 to 50 degrees, work on releasing the dorsiflexors (antagonists)—extensor digitorum longus, extensor hallucis longus, peroneus tertius, and tibialis anterior—to restore normal muscle resting lengths.
- Dorsiflexion occurs when the dorsal surface of the foot moves toward the anterior surface of the leg. If dorsiflexion is less than 20 to 30 degrees, work on releasing the plantar flexors (antagonists)—gastrocnemius, soleus, tibialis posterior, flexor digitorum longus, flexor hallucis longus, peroneus brevis, peroneus longus, and plantaris—to restore normal muscle resting lengths.
- Inversion occurs as the plantar surface of the foot moves towards the midline of the body. If inversion is less than 30 to 50 degrees, work on releasing the evertors (antagonists)—extensor digitorum longus, peroneus brevis, peroneus longus, and peroneus tertius—to restore normal muscle resting lengths.
- Eversion occurs as the plantar surface of the foot moves away from the midline of the body. If eversion is less than 15 to 20 degrees, work on releasing the invertors (antagonists)—extensor hallucis longus, flexor digitorum longus, flexor hallucis longus, tibialis anterior, and tibialis posterior—to restore normal muscle resting lengths.

ANKLE JOINT SINGLE-PLANE MOVEMENTS—PRIMARY MUSCLES

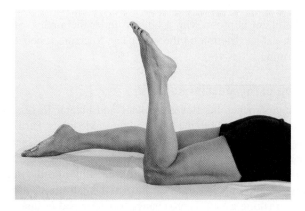

FIGURE 4-2
Ankle Plantar Flexion, 30–50 degrees.

Plantar Flexion, 30 to 50 Degrees

- flexor digitorum longus
- flexor hallucis longus
- gastrocnemius
- peroneus brevis and longus
- plantaris
- soleus
- tibialis posterior

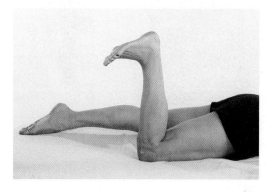

FIGURE 4-3
Ankle Dorsiflexion, 20–30 degrees.

Dorsiflexion, 20 to 30 Degrees

- extensor digitorum longus
- extensor hallucis longus
- peroneus tertius
- tibialis anterior

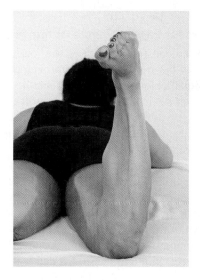

FIGURE 4-4
Ankle Inversion, 30–50 degrees.

Inversion, 50 Degrees

- extensor hallucis longus
- flexor digitorum longus
- flexor hallucis longus
- tibialis anterior
- tibialis posterior

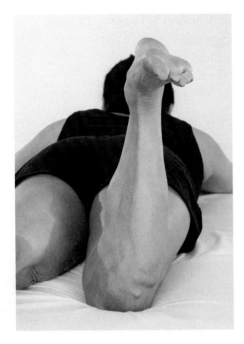

FIGURE 4-5
Ankle Eversion at Subtalar Joint 15–20 Degrees.

Eversion, 15 to 20 Degrees

- extensor digitorum longus
- peroneus brevis
- peroneus longus
- peroneus tertius

Step 3: Assess Passive Range of Motion (PROM)

Determine the end feel of each of the four single-plane movements of the ankle joint by performing passive ROM tests. For dorsiflexion the end feel should be a soft-tissue stretch. Plantar flexion should feel like a soft-tissue stretch and ligamentous, as you are also stretching ligaments. Inversion should also feel like a soft-tissue stretch and ligamentous but more abrupt due to the limitation of the anterior talofibular ligament. Ligaments have less capability to stretch than muscle and tendons. The end feel for eversion is a bone-on-bone or abrupt solid feeling created by contact between the lateral malleolus and the talus. Abnormal passive end feel of the ankle alerts you to certain underlying clinical conditions. For example, if ankle inversion is more than 50 degrees with a tissue stretch end feel that is soft, rather than ligamentous, the client either had a previous ankle sprain or is normally hypermobile. A bone-on-bone end-feel in any direction other than eversion alerts you to a bony fixation or severe ankle arthritis.

Step 4: Assess Resisted Range of Motion (RROM)

The client attempts each of the four single-plane movements of the ankle using 20 percent of his or her strength while you apply resistance. For precaution, start the test with minimal resistance or applied forces, and then slowly increase the reverse resistance to fully recruit the muscle fibers. If the client experiences pain, ask him or her to point to the specific area. This indicates a probable muscle strain to one or more of the muscles being tested and this area will be worked last.

The previous functional assessments may determine if one or more of the following conditions are present in the lower extremity.

ACHILLES TENDINOSIS

Achilles tendinitis is not a typical "-itis," as in many cases it does not produce redness or inflammation. A better term would be *tendinosis,* which is the tearing of tendon fibers in the absence of an inflammatory process.[1] Repetitive motions of running, jumping, and landing on the toes are the primary cause of Achilles tendinosis.[2] The problem usually occurs at the muscle–tendon junction of the gastrocnemius or soleus, or at the periosteal attachment on the calcaneus due to very poor blood supply there.[3]

The client typically feels pain during active or passive dorsiflexion, which will increase with resisted plantar flexion. Make a visual assessment of the foot with the client prone, knee flexed 90 degrees. If the relaxed foot is plantar flexed, then the gastrocnemius, soleus, and Achilles tendon are tight and contracted. The soleus is usually the main cause of Achilles tendinosis, as most clients do not stretch their calves with their knee bent.

GASTROCNEMIUS PROTOCOL TO ADDRESS ACHILLES TENDON PAIN

Step 4: Assess Resisted Range of Motion (RROM)

The client is prone with the leg straight. Have the client dorsiflex the ankle. Ask him or her to attempt plantar flexion while you provide resistance. If the client experiences pain, have him or her point to the specific spot. This indicates a muscle strain and will be worked last.

Step 5: Area Preparation

The client is prone with a bolster under the ankles. Start with palmar friction on the lower leg, to create superficial warming.

Step 6: Myofascial Release

The gastrocnemius flexes the knee and plantar flexes the ankle. It crosses both the knee and the ankle joints. Perform myofascial spreading at a 45-degree angle into the tissue on the gastrocnemius to the Achilles tendon, working proximal to distal. Start with palmar strokes, hooking into the deep investing fascia at 45 degrees, and spreading the tissue laterally, making a "v." Then, change to finger pad or knuckle strokes as you work progressively deeper (Figure 4-6 ■).

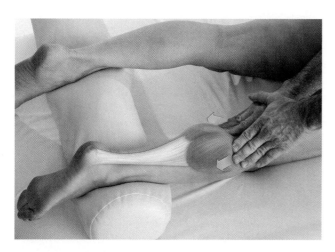

FIGURE 4-6
Myofascial Spreading, Gastrocnemius.

You want to expand the connective tissue that encases the gastrocnemius and surrounds the Achilles tendon. This process will increase blood flow at the capillary level, can move metabolic wastes out of the area, and will mobilize the fascia, allowing it to adapt to a new lengthened position. It also takes the tension off, and unloads, the Achilles tendon.

Alternate the myofascial spreading with slow, gentle, compressive stretches into the muscle belly hooking and moving the tissue back to normal muscle resting lengths. Compression and compressive stretches enhance your myofascial work, so you can work deeper with less effort (Figure 4-7 ■).

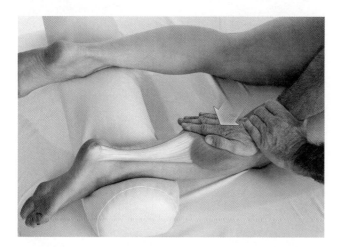

FIGURE 4-7
Compression, Gastrocnemius.

Step 7: Cross-Fiber Gliding Strokes/Trigger Point Therapy

CROSS-FIBER GLIDING STROKES

Tease through and gently spread tight muscle bands with cross-fiber gliding strokes, moving proximal to distal, toward the ankle. Use the pads of your fingers or thumbs to broaden the tissue. This will reduce trigger point activity (Figure 4-8 ■).

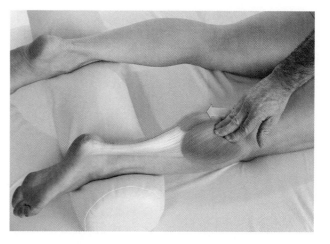

FIGURE 4-8
Cross-Fiber Gliding Strokes and Trigger Point Work, Gastrocnemius.

TRIGGER POINT THERAPY

If there is a muscle belly trigger point—a specific area of pain that radiates or refers—use direct, moderate pressure for 10 to 12 seconds (refer back to Figure 4-8). As the trigger point softens, compress the tissue several times and then gently stretch it. Continue the myofascial work as needed, working slower and deeper, but still pain-free.

ANKLE JOINT PLAY OR ARTHROKINETICS

Gently compress and then traction the ankle several times to decompress the joint. Then grasp the bottom of the foot with one hand and stabilize the ankle with the other hand. Pump the foot gently into the ankle joint with nonsynchronized movements several times to soften any adhesions and distract the client from splinting the area. Follow this with deep traction and dorsiflexion to create joint space. This looks like gentle compressive forces followed by decompression. The sequence is distraction, distraction, traction, and dorsiflexion (Figures 4-9A ■ and 4-9B ■). It also can be called joint play,

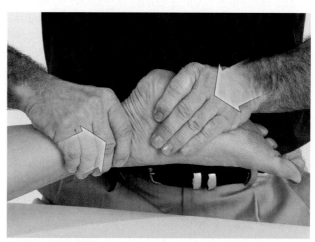

FIGURE 4-9A
Arthrokinetics, Compression.

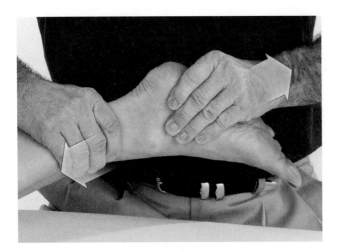

FIGURE 4-9B
Arthrokinetics, Decompression.

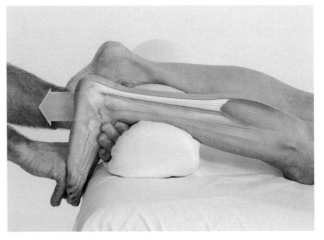

FIGURE 4-10
Gastrocnemius Stretch.

arthrokinetics, or joint mobilization. These non-synchronized, distraction and traction movements may also help decompress the cartilage. Repeat the arthrokinetics and deep traction of the ankle to decompress it, and then repeat the sequence, if needed. When the ankle joint is moving freely, perform the stretch.

Step 11: Stretching (During Therapy)

 PRECAUTIONARY NOTE

Stretching is not suggested for the muscle groups around a hypermobile joint. Strengthening would be more appropriate to stabilize any joint that has excessive movement due to ligamentous laxity.

The client is prone with a bolster under the ankle. This is a pivotal ankle joint opening and decompressive stretch. To protect the joint cartilage of the ankle while stretching the gastrocnemius, place one hand on the front of the ankle and lean back to traction the client's ankle (Figure 4-10 ■).

Ask the client to plantar flex for 5 to 10 seconds at 20 percent force while you provide resistance. He or she relaxes, takes a deep breath, and then on exhale dorsiflexes for about 2 seconds as you traction the ankle and pivot the front of the ankle over your hand and assist the stretch with your other hand. At this new position repeat the contract-relax, contract-antagonist with active assisted stretching two or three times, or until achieving the normal range of motion of 20 to 30 degrees dorsiflexion.

Next, fully straighten the client's leg, traction the ankle, lean back, and pull the leg into a stretch to decompress the hip, knee, and ankle joints. Make sure you perform gentle, sustained ankle traction for about 5 seconds and then release very slowly (Figure 4-11 ■).

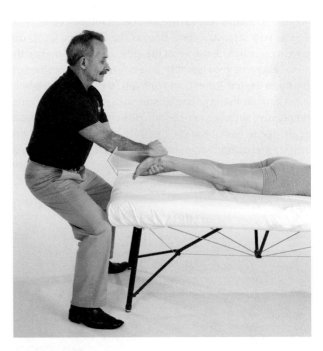

FIGURE 4-11
Ankle Decompression.

Step 8: Multidirectional Friction

If the client experiences discomfort during the previous stretches, stop and ask him or her to point to the specific area. Perform multidirectional friction to the specific area to free up the collagen or scar tissue that is causing the pain. Use a supported finger and work for only 20 to 30 seconds. Ease up on your pressure or slow down if the area is tender.

Step 9: Pain-Free Movement

Ask the client to actively dorsiflex and plantar flex the ankle several times. This begins the process of realigning collagen fibers. If there is no pain, perform the eccentric work. If there is any discomfort, return to the multidirectional friction working a little deeper and slower, but still pain-free.

Step 10: Eccentric Scar Tissue Alignment

Apply eccentric contraction to enhance deeper scar tissue alignment. It must be performed pain-free. Traction the client's ankle. Have the client resist gentle dorsiflexion performed by you. Tell him or her to "barely resist, but let me win." Start with a pressure of only two fingers and then ask the client to increase resistance only if there is zero discomfort. Repeat this several times.

Step 4: Assess Resisted Range of Motion (RROM)

To reassess RROM, repeat the resisted test. If there is still pain, return to the multidirectional friction and then the pain-free movement. Repeat the eccentric work. Finish with the stretch when there is no longer any pain.

SOLEUS PROTOCOL

Step 4: Assess Resisted Range of Motion (RROM)

The client is prone with the knee bent 90 degrees. Have him or her dorsiflex the ankle. Then ask the client to attempt plantar flexion while you provide resistance. If he or she experiences pain, have the client point to the specific spot. This indicates a muscle strain. Work this area last (Figure 4-12 ■).

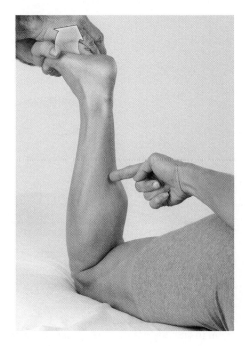

FIGURE 4-12
Muscle Resisted Test, Soleus.

Step 6: Myofascial Release

A shortened and contracted soleus is the number one cause of Achilles tendinosis. The soleus originates on the posterior surfaces of the tibia and fibula and attaches to the Achilles tendon. It is located deep to the gastrocnemius and its medial and lateral fibers are wider than the gastrocnemius. Its action is to plantar flex the ankle.

Sit on the table. Bend the client's knee to 90 degrees to isolate the soleus. The foot can rest on your shoulder, with the ankle plantar flexed. This allows better access to the soleus by shortening and relaxing the gastrocnemius. With finger pad strokes, work proximal to distal to the Achilles tendon at a 45-degree angle, going progressively deeper. Lift and pull up and out through the heads of the gastrocnemius. Curl your fingers in and spread laterally from the middle to affect most of the soleus. Then, move the gastrocnemius medially and laterally out of the way to affect more fibers of the soleus (Figure 4-13 ■).

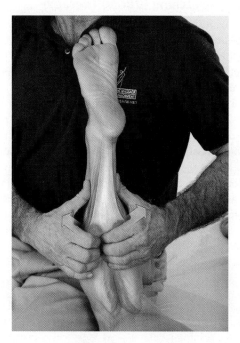

FIGURE 4-13
Myofascial Release of Soleus.

Step 7: Cross-Fiber Gliding Strokes/Trigger Point Therapy

CROSS-FIBER GLIDING STROKES

Next, use gentle cross-fiber gliding strokes through the soleus while pulling the heads of the gastrocnemius in opposing directions from side to side, working distal toward the Achilles. This will lengthen and broaden tight muscle bands, reducing trigger point activity. Do not work the junction of the Achilles tendon as this is the weak link. Instead, release everything that feeds that spot and contributes to the problem. Close your eyes and tune in to find any tender or tight muscle bands, or restrictions, or congestion in the tissue. During your strokes, you can also ask the client for feedback on your pressure or if there is any pain.

TRIGGER POINT THERAPY

Release any muscle belly trigger points, if found, with direct, moderate pressure for 10 to 12 seconds. As it softens, gently compress and stretch the area.

After you have released and lengthened the soleus, stand at the side of the table. The client's knee is bent 90 degrees. Clasp your hands with interlocking fingers around the client's ankle. Gently shake the ankle, to create distraction, for several seconds. Then, while still shaking the ankle, traction the ankle and lift gently, just short of the knee coming off the table. This will create joint space in the ankle. Repeat the shake–distraction–traction sequence several times, as needed to create better joint mobility and decompress the articulating cartilage. (Figure 4-14 ■).

Step 11: Stretching (During Therapy)

Stretching will effectively lengthen the soleus and reduce the tension on the Achilles tendon. With the client's knee flexed 90 degrees, support and gently traction the client's calcaneus with a "c" clamp; using gentle, evenly displaced pressure (Figure 4-15 ■).

Ask the client to plantar flex the ankle for 5 to 10 seconds at 20 percent force while you resist. He or she relaxes, takes a deep breath, and then on exhale dorsiflexes the ankle for about 2 seconds while you gently traction to leverage the ankle and then assist the stretch. From this new position, repeat the contract-relax, contract-antagonist with active assisted stretching until achieving the normal range of motion of 20 to 30 degrees of dorsiflexion.

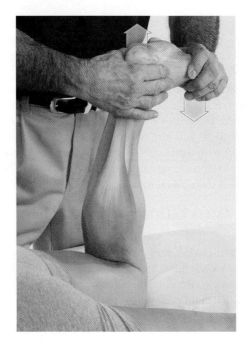

FIGURE 4-15
Soleus Stretch.

Step 8: Multidirectional Friction

If the client experiences pain during the contraction portion of the previous stretch, isolate the exact spot by having the client put a finger directly on it (Figure 4-16A ■). Perform multidirectional friction to the area for only 20 to 30 seconds. If the area is tender, use light pressure. Proceed with the next step (Figure 4-16B ■).

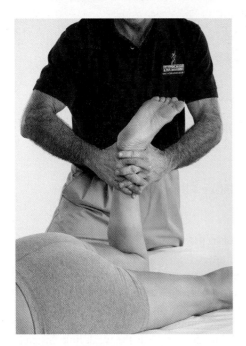

FIGURE 4-14
Ankle Distraction and Traction.

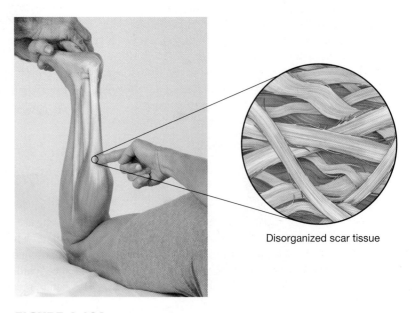

Disorganized scar tissue

FIGURE 4-16A
Muscle Resistance Test, Soleus.

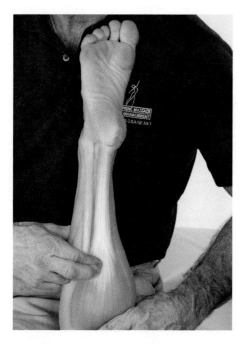

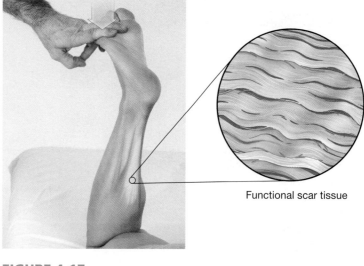

FIGURE 4-17
Eccentric Muscle Contraction, Soleus.

FIGURE 4-16B
Multidirectional Friction, Soleus.

Step 9: Pain-Free Movement

Ask the client to move the ankle through plantar flexion and dorsiflexion several times. This initiates alignment of strained fibers. If there is no pain, continue with the eccentric work. If there is some discomfort, return to the multidirectional friction, working slower and deeper.

Step 10: Eccentric Scar Tissue Alignment

Realign the deeper scar tissue with eccentric contraction, performed pain-free. With the knee flexed, ask the client to gently resist dorsiflexion performed by you. Tell him or her to "barely resist, but let me win." It is critical that pain-free dorsiflexion occur. Use only two fingers for pressure at first. If there is no pain the client can increase the resistance (Figure 4-17 ■). Repeat this several times. If there is still discomfort, return to the multidirectional friction and work slightly deeper and slower, pain-free. Then repeat the pain-free movement and the eccentric contraction. When the pain is gone, perform the stretch.

Step 4: Assess Resisted Range of Motion (RROM)

To reassess RROM, repeat the resisted test. If there is still pain, return to the multidirectional friction and then the pain-free movement. Then repeat the eccentric work. Finish with the stretch when there is no longer any pain.

Step 6: Myofascial Release

Now that you have released the tight cables—gastrocnemius and soleus—attached to the Achilles tendon, you can directly release the fascia surrounding the tendon. Perform a visual assessment.

- If the ankle is inverted use a two-finger gliding stroke and work proximal to distal on the medial side, toward the heel, and distal to proximal, toward the knee, on the lateral side. Perform gentle, deep myofascial spreading, returning the ankle to neutral position. Follow with passive ankle dorsiflexion (Figure 4-18A ■).

- If the ankle is in neutral position, work proximal to distal, toward the heel, on both sides of the Achilles tendon while dorsiflexing the ankle to lengthen the tissue. Hook the fascia and scoop under the tendon like you are lifting it away from the bone, followed by passive dorsiflexion performed by you or active dorsiflexion performed by the client (Figure 4-18B ■).

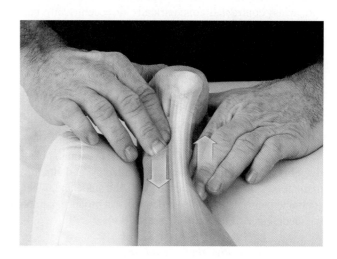

FIGURE 4-18A
Myofascial Release, Right Achilles Tendon.

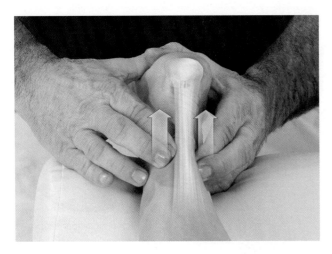

FIGURE 4-18B
Myofascial Release, Right Achilles Tendon.

Lengthening the connective tissue will create myofascial unwinding around the tendon. Seek out any restrictions of the fascia by softening and broadening it. Once you release these adhesions and reduce the tension in the soleus and the gastrocnemius, the pain and discomfort in the Achilles tendon will usually disappear.

POSTEROMEDIAL SHIN SPLINTS

Shin splints is a generic term used interchangeably for pain of the lower leg. It often begins when an athlete trains too fast or too hard, usually early in the season. It is caused by an imbalance of muscles in the lower leg due to overuse, muscle tension, or injury.[4]

Posteromedial shin splints is an overuse condition common among runners. It involves primarily the tibialis posterior muscle. This muscle originates on the proximal posterior tibia, wraps around the medial malleolus, and attaches to the foot. It inverts and plantar flexes the ankle and, when contracted concentrically or eccentrically can produce pain on the medial side of the shin. This can be a challenging condition to work on as this muscle is located deep under the soleus and is almost inaccessible. However, a relaxed soleus can be compressed medially into the muscle fibers and tendon of the tibialis posterior, between the soleus and the medial tibial shaft. Be gentle, since applying direct pressure in this area may cause the client discomfort, along with referred pain down the distal medial third of the tibia.

The tibialis posterior originates on the proximal, posterior tibia, wraps around the medial malleolus, and attaches to the foot. It inverts and plantar flexes the ankle and, when contracted, or eccentrically overloaded, can produce pain on the medial side of the shin (Figure 4-19 ■).

Note: It is imperative that you address this work prior to foot work if the client has limited active eversion or excessive inversion.

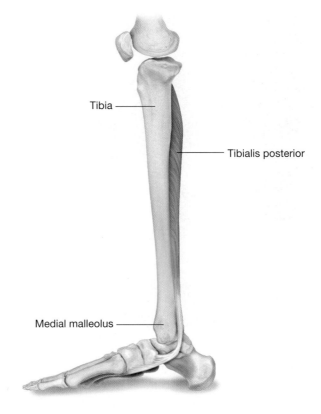

Tibia

Tibialis posterior

Medial malleolus

FIGURE 4-19
Tibialias Posterior Review.

Tibialis Posterior Protocol

The author suggests that manual therapists also evaluate the client in the weight bearing or standing position. In this position, the therapist can evaluate for excessive supination and hyperpronation. Supination is motion around diagonal axis and is a combination of inversion, adduction, and plantar flexion. "Excessive supination is considered a dynamic postural disorder because it involves the foot's movement through the weight bearing phase of locomotion rather than in a static position." Clients that oversupinate are more susceptible to other lower extremity conditions such as ankle sprains and strains. Treatment in this case would focus on lengthening the ankle inverter muscles.[5]

Overpronation or hyperpronation is also a movement dysfunction during the weight bearing phase of gait. "Pronation is an important part of the normal gait pattern and includes abduction, eversion and dorsiflexion. Hyperpronation results when the foot moves either too far or too fast through the phase of pronation, placing more weight on the medial side of the foot during gait. Tibialis posterior weakness is one of the primary factors leading to overpronation."[6] The therapist would have the client strengthen the tibialis posterior, as part of client self-care, to benefit this condition. For detailed information on excessive supination, hyperpronation, and ascending syndromes refer to *Orthopedic Assessment in Massage Therapy* by Whitney Lowe or *Advanced Myoskeletal Techniques* by Dr. Erik Dalton.

Step 5: Area Preparation

With the client prone and the knee flexed 90 degrees, assess the position of the relaxed foot. If it is both inverted and plantar flexed you must first release the tension from the gastrocnemius and the soleus before working on the tibialis posterior. Follow the steps outlined previously under Achilles tendinosis.

Step 4: Assess Resisted Range of Motion (RROM)

The client is prone with the knee flexed 90 degrees. Have him or her evert the ankle. Then ask the client to attempt to invert the ankle while you provide resistance. If he or she experiences pain, have the client point to the specific spot. This indicates a muscle strain and will be worked last (Figure 4-20 ■).

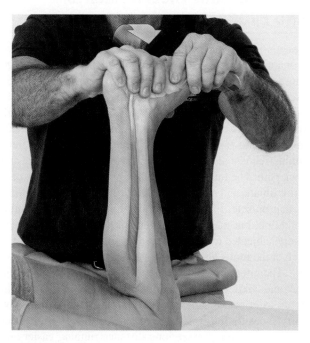

FIGURE 4-20
Muscle Resistance Test, Tibialis Posterior.

Step 6: Myofascial Release

If the client has excessive weight bearing supination or limited active eversion, indicating a tight posterior tibialis, follow the following protocol.

The client is prone with the knee flexed 90 degrees. Start by using palmar friction to warm up the medial side of the lower leg. To release the fascia surrounding the tibialis posterior, work from proximal to distal, from the knee toward the ankle. Place your fingers on the tibia and then move off it medially, sinking slowly into the soleus. Sneak your fingers around the tibia posteriorly, to find the back of it, and displace the soleus into the fibers of the tibialis posterior. Go *very* slowly and curl your fingers into the muscle

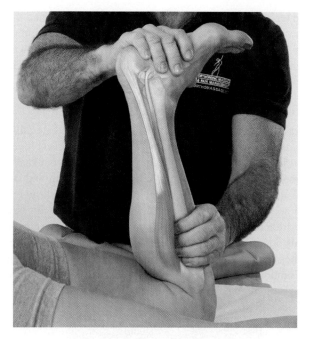

FIGURE 4-21
Myofascial Release, Tibialis Posterior.

using the pads of your fingers. Keeping your fingers here, grasp the client's foot with your other hand (Figure 4-21 ■).

Now fatigue the tibialis posterior. Ask the client to invert the ankle against your resistance for 5 to 10 seconds using only 20 percent of their strength. Then have the client take a deep breath and relax. As the muscle relaxes and you achieve post isometric relaxation, you can slowly sink into the tissue deeper than before. Perform gentle compressions, and cross-fiber gliding strokes moving distally, and move the tissue back and forth and up and down to make sure there are no adhesions. Gently scrub the back of the tibia. Visualize massaging the back of the tibia on the medial side. Move your fingers toward the ankle a few inches and again fatigue the tibialis posterior repeating the above sequence. Continue fatiguing, moving, and releasing the tissue all the way to the medial malleolus.

Next, place your fingers just above the medial malleolus and move the ankle through inversion and eversion, which lengthens and shortens the muscle and tendon. Refer to tendon of posterior tibialis in Figure 4-21. You will feel subtle movement of the tendon under your fingers. If it is not moving, and there are adhesions here, you need to gently friction

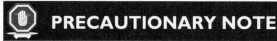

PRECAUTIONARY NOTE

There is an acupressure point approximately four fingers above the medial malleolus and a reflexology point between the malleolus and calcaneus. Avoid direct pressure on these areas on pregnant women.[7]

the tendon and get it to move back and forth. Continue this down and around the medial malleolus to the insertion on the bottom of the foot. Release the tender points there with gentle finger pad compressions and circular friction. The goal is to warm up, soften, and mobilize the tissue.

Step 11: Stretching (During Therapy)

Grasp the client's foot, give it a subtle lift to create ankle traction, and move it to eversion. Then have the client invert for 5 to 10 seconds at 20 percent force against your resistance. He or she relaxes and takes a deep breath and, on exhale you give a subtle lift to the ankle and he or she everts for about 2 seconds while you assist the stretch. At this new position repeat the contract-relax, contract-antagonist, evert plus dorsiflex, with active assisted stretching two or three times. You want to create the normal 15- to 20-degree range of motion of eversion and minimize excessive weight bearing supination (Figure 4-22 ■).

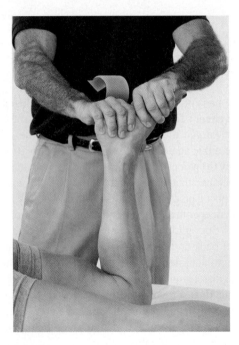

FIGURE 4-22
Posterior Tibialis Stretch.

Step 8: Multidirectional Friction

If the client reports a specific spot of pain during the stretch and during the muscle resistance test, have him or her isolate it by pointing to it. Use multidirectional friction on the exact spot for only 20 to 30 seconds. Working any longer may cause inflammation.

Step 9: Pain-Free Movement

Ask the client to invert and evert the ankle several times to change the proprioception and to encourage neuromuscular reeducation. If there is no pain, perform the eccentric work. Return to the multidirectional friction if the client still has some discomfort in the area of the strain.

Step 10: Eccentric Scar Tissue Alignment

Grasp the client's foot, give it a subtle lift to create ankle traction, and move it to neutral. Then have him or her gently resist eversion performed by you. Tell the client to "barely resist, but let me win." Pain-free eversion needs to occur. Start with a light pressure and have the client increase resistance only if there is zero discomfort. Repeat this several times. This eccentric contraction will help realign the deeper scar tissue.

Step 4: Assess Resisted Range of Motion (RROM)

To reassess RROM, repeat the resisted test. If the client complains that the area is still tender, go back and perform the multidirectional friction, pain-free movement, and then the eccentric work again. When the pain is gone, perform the stretch.

FLAT FEET AND FALLEN ARCHES AND PRONATION

Pes planus is the medical term for flat feet.[8] Excessive pronation causes the foot's arch to collapse, which in turn causes the foot to twist outward. Undiagnosed and untreated excessive pronation may lead to serious foot and lower body injuries. Among the most common associated injuries are flat feet, weak arches, **bunions, hammer toes,** corns, calluses, plantar fasciitis, Achilles tendinosis, **Morton's neuroma,** frequent ankle sprains, shin splints, and knee, hip, and back pain. The fallen arch places constant stress on the posterior tibialis and may actually be the cause of the symptoms in that muscle. Flat feet are most commonly a congenital condition, but may be acquired as a result of being repetitively subjected to hard surfaces, eventually weakening the arch of the foot. Other causes can be obesity and pregnancy.[9]

The client needs to keep the muscles that stabilize the foot and ankle balanced and the bones in proper alignment to act as effective shock absorbers. Many shoe stores now carry shoes for hyperpronated feet. "The shoes designed for hyperpronated feet make long distance running easier and less tiring as they correct for the positional abnormality."[10]

The client should see a podiatrist to determine if a custom-made orthotic can stabilize the foot and ankle. Special insoles can provide biomechanical support for the feet to function more efficiently and better align bones of the foot and ankle. A number of health care practitioners believe that many lower body conditions benefit by proper stabilization of the foot and ankle and may eliminate the cause of other symptoms or conditions throughout the body. Conditions that start in the foot and move up to affect the rest of the body are called *ascending syndromes,* according to Dr. Erik Dalton.[11]

In addition to soft-tissue balance and proper orthotics, a visit to a good chiropractor is highly recommended. It is also a good idea to see an expert on posturology to evaluate for a short leg, and possibly get a full custom lift built into the client's shoes to eliminate a "true" short leg problem, confirmed by reliable x-ray methods.

PLANTAR FASCIITIS

Plantar fasciitis is an overuse condition of the foot causing disorganization and irritation of the **plantar fascia** (Figure 4-23 ■). It results from improper forces to the foot. Fallen arches can be a critical factor. The most common cause is tight gastrocnemius and soleus muscles. These muscles can create excessive plantar flexion, placing the client on his or her toes, which stresses the longitudinal muscles of the foot. This can occur from participating in sports, wearing high heels, trauma, weight gain, and pregnancy.[12]

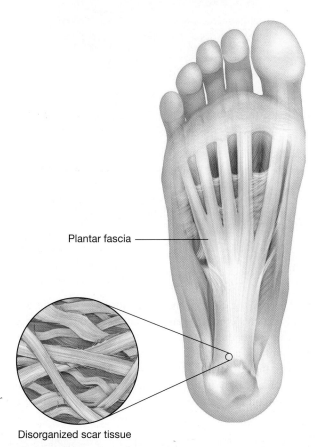

Plantar fascia

Disorganized scar tissue

FIGURE 4-23
Plantar Fasciitis.

Another muscle that can lead to plantar fasciitis is the tibialis posterior. When it is tight and contracted it causes the client to walk or run on the outside of the foot, which stresses the plantar fascia in a diagonal direction. When it is stressed eccentrically by flat feet or hyperpronation, it also plays a role in plantar fascial pain.

The primary role of the plantar fascia is to absorb shock from the weight of the body by maintaining the longitudinal arch of the foot. Pain is most commonly felt in the heel at the attachment of the plantar fascia to the calcaneus, but can also be found anywhere along the bottom surface of the foot. The pain is usually worse after rest, especially when getting out of bed in the morning.[13] As the client moves around, the gastrocnemius and soleus warm up becoming more pliable and the pain temporarily subsides.

Note: To help prevent a postural contribution to plantar fasciitis, have the client sleep without a blanket covering the feet while supine, or sleep with the feet off the edge of the bed while prone to avoid prolonged plantar flexion.

Step 4: Assess Resisted Range of Motion (RROM)

The client is prone with the knee bent 90 degrees. Have him or her dorsiflex the ankle. Then ask the client to attempt to flex the toes or simply curl the toes in, without moving the ankle, while you provide resistance. If he or she experiences pain, have the client point to the specific spot. Work this area last (Figure 4-24 ■).

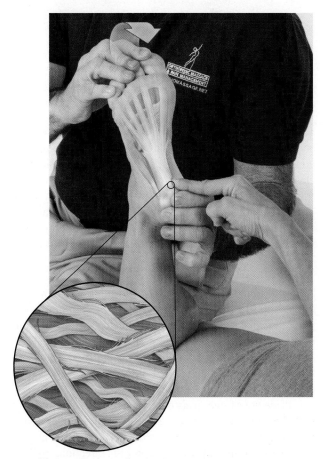

Disorganized scar tissue

FIGURE 4-24
Muscle Resistance Test for Plantar Fascial Strain.

Step 5: Area Preparation

This is a continuation of the previous steps since you must first release the gastrocnemius, soleus, and Achilles tendon, as part of treating this condition. If the client's ankle is excessively inverted, you must also address the posterior tibialis before proceeding. This treats the cause before the symptoms.

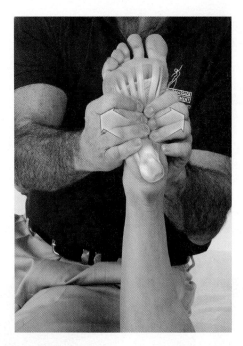

FIGURE 4-25
Compression and Myofascial Spreading, Foot Muscles.

The client is prone with the knee flexed 90 degrees. Perform compressions into the bottom of the foot, using the pads of your fingers, to bring blood and oxygen to the intrinsic muscles of the foot. Support the foot in your palms and use the pad of the fingers of both hands to work longitudinally along the bottom of the foot. Remember, the intent is to warm up and release the entire area *first,* before you work the painful area, or the disorganized collagen fibers (Figure 4-25 ■).

Step 6: Myofascial Release

You want to mobilize the fascia by spreading across the bottom of the foot with the pads of the fingers of both hands, pulling medial to lateral. This will create space in the connective tissue that crosses the bottom of the foot. Repeat this several times. Next, perform compressions, which broaden the muscle belly, for increased blood and oxygen flow to enhance the myofascial spreading.

Place your finger pads on the plantar aspect of the foot and place the pads of your thumbs on the other side. Then push and pull firmly on the long bones of the foot, moving the metatarsals up and down, in opposing directions, to their end feel. This will begin to create space and softening in the deep interosseous membranes, allowing the bones to perform the deepest level of internal myofascial release for you. Work proximal to distal, gliding through the foot. Traction and elongate the foot as you push and pull to decompress each joint articulation. Then, use the pads of your fingers to gently spread the bones and the tissue surrounding them laterally away from each other (Figure 4-26 ■).

Step 7: Cross-Fiber Gliding Strokes

Next, perform cross-fiber gliding strokes longitudinally moving from the heel to the base of the toes. Work between

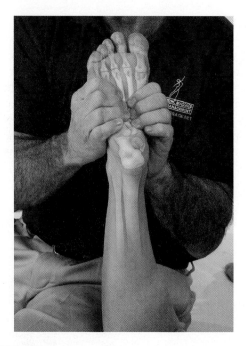

FIGURE 4-26
Massage Intereoseus Membrane Using Long Bones of Foot.

each metatarsal. This will create movement and separation between the bones, pulling the connective tissue away from the nerves, which can reduce certain forms of nerve pain in the foot.

TOE JOINT PLAY OR ARTHROKINETICS

Next, stretch the muscles and plantar fascia that flex the toes. Tight muscles compress and deviate the joints of the toes and can create degeneration, joint fixations, joint arthritis, hammer toes, and bunions. Use your fingers and take all of the toes into extension (Figure 4-27 ■). Perform arthrokinetics on any tight joints.Use nonsynchronized gentle joint compression and then subtle traction movements to soften

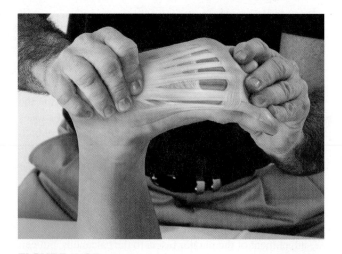

FIGURE 4-27
Stretch Muscles and Plantar Fascia of the Foot by Extending the Toes.

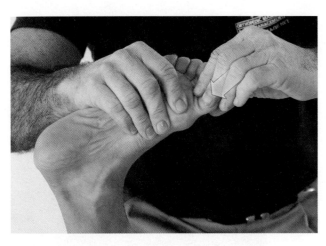

FIGURE 4-28A
Arthrokinetics, Gentle Compression.

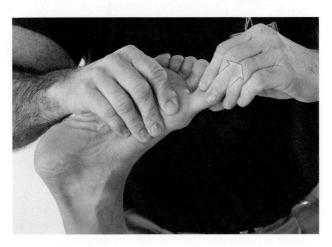

FIGURE 4-28B
Arthrokinetics, Traction.

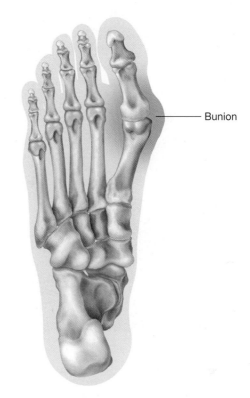

— Bunion

FIGURE 4-29
Bunion.

any adhesions and create joint space. This looks like a gentle pumping motion using compressive forces followed by decompression (Figures 4-28A ■ and 4-28B ■).

Perform arthrokinetics and traction and stretch each individual toe into extension or neutral alignment, as needed. Use a supported thumb as a lever underneath it. Next, perform arthrokinetics followed by gentle lateral flexion of any restricted joint. Then perform arthrokinetics followed by gentle rotation of that joint. This can help reduce calcification or bone spurs. Bone spurs (osteophytes) are bony projections that develop along the edges of bones. The bone spurs themselves are not painful, but they can rub against nearby nerves and bones, causing pain.[14] Generally, abnormal motion of a joint over time can cause a bone spur to form. Spurring of bone can also occur as a result of excessive tension on a bone from a tendon where it attaches to the bone.[15]

"A bunion is a bony bump on the joint at the base of the big toe. As the bump gets bigger, it causes the big toe to turn in toward the second toe."[16] For bunions, use arthrokinetics

to warm up the big toe joint. Then, gently traction and stretch the big toe laterally away from the other toes to create space and realignment. By decompressing and aligning the joints of the toes you can start to reverse the effects of bunions and also hammer toes (Figure 4-29 ■).

Overall, you basically want to get everything moving and released on the bottom of the foot that would connect into the specific area of plantar fascia pain. If the client has developed calluses on the ball of the foot, due to extra pressure there, spend a little extra time working those areas. Now that you have treated the cause, proceed next to the most important steps to eliminate the symptoms of plantar fasciitis.

Step 11: Stretching (During Therapy)

The client is prone with the knee bent 90 degrees. Traction the client's ankle with a "c" clamp with one hand. With the other hand traction the toes with a "c" clamp, bringing them into extension, to lengthen the entire bottom of the foot.

At this position, have the client attempt to flex or "curl" the toes against your resistance for 5 to 10 seconds at 20 percent force. He or she relaxes, takes a deep breath, and on exhale extends the toes and dorsiflexes the ankle down toward the table for about 2 seconds while you traction the ankle and assist the stretch. At this new position, repeat the contract-relax, contract-antagonist with active assisted stretching two or three times (Figure 4-30 ■).

Note: This also stretches the muscles of the foot and the soleus.

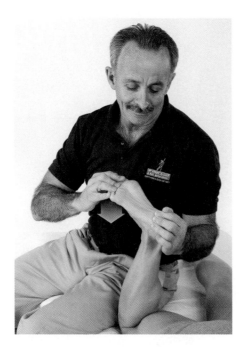

FIGURE 4-30
Stretch Muscles of Foot.

Step 8: Multidirectional Friction

If the client complains of a specific area of pain during the stretch, especially if that pain increases in a specific area as he or she contracts against your resistance, have the client point to it (Figure 4-31 ■).

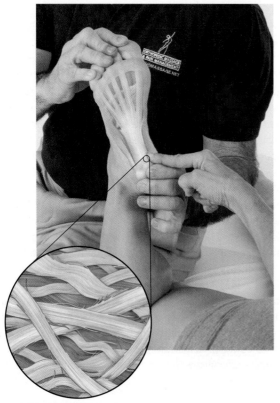

Disorganized scar tissue

FIGURE 4-31
Resisted Test, Plantar Fascia Strain.

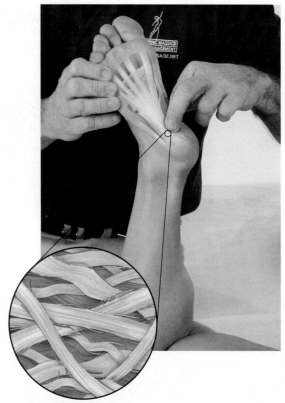

Disorganized scar tissue

FIGURE 4-32
Multidirectional Friction, Plantar Fascia Strain.

Perform pain-free multidirectional friction using a supported finger or fingers to the specific area of tenderness. Go in at different directions to mobilize the collagen fibers, for about 20 to 30 seconds. Make sure you do not overwork the area and use only enough pressure to soften the collagen matrix (Figure 4-32 ■).

Step 9: Pain-Free Movement

Stabilize the ankle so that it does not move. Ask the client to alternately flex and extend the toes without moving the ankle. Repeat this several times. If there is pain, return to the multidirectional friction, working a little slower and deeper. If not, perform the eccentric work.

Step 10: Eccentric Scar Tissue Alignment

This is the eccentric load that begins the process of realigning the deeper scar tissue. Ask the client to flex or curl the toes and hold this position while you apply an eccentric stretch along the base of the foot. The ankle does not move.

Pull your hands away from each other and extend the toes into the stretch to elongate the plantar fascia and help realign the collagen fibers. Ask the client to "barely resist, but let me win" (Figure 4-33 ■). Pain-free toe extension must occur. Repeat this several times if needed using deeper friction on the point of tenderness for approximately 20 to 30 seconds between each set of eccentric stretches.

Note: Stay focused, as the potential to create inflammation increases if the friction is performed longer.

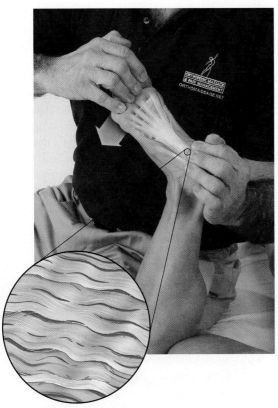

Functional scar tissue

FIGURE 4-33
Eccentric Muscle Contraction, Plantar Fascia Strain.

Step 4: Assess Resisted Range of Motion (RROM)

To reassess RROM, repeat the resisted test, gently going deeper into the stretch. If there is still a tender area when they contract against resistance, return to the multidirectional friction, working a little slower and deeper. Then repeat the pain-free movement and the eccentric work.

 PRECAUTIONARY NOTE

When you take a client's ankle out of inversion and plantar flexion, this may lower the arch and change the foot strike. For clients who wear hard orthotics in their shoes, this can create increased pressure on the plantar fascia. Make sure they are aware of this and consult their podiatrist.

ANTERIOR COMPARTMENT SYNDROME (ACS)

Anterior compartment syndrome (ACS) is a condition of the anterolateral compartment of the lower leg involving the tibialis anterior, extensor digitorum longus, and extensor hallucis longus muscles along with the deep peroneal nerve and anterior tibial artery and vein. These muscles, nerve, and vascular structures are typically under eccentric forces due to tight antagonist muscles—gastrocnemius, soleus, and posterior tibialis (Figure 4-34 ■).

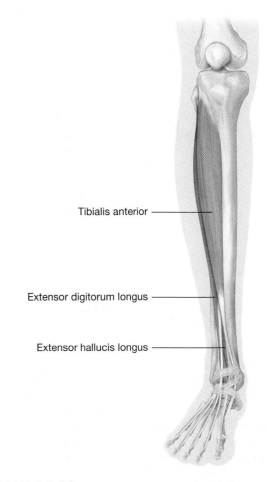

Tibialis anterior

Extensor digitorum longus

Extensor hallucis longus

FIGURE 4-34
Anterior Compartment Muscles.

ACS usually occurs as a result of overuse, which can create swelling in the anterolateral compartment of the lower leg. Causes can include suddenly changing an exercise routine, or running mostly uphill, downhill, or on uneven surfaces. The fascia that wraps around the anterior lower leg muscles is so tough and inelastic that fluid can build up, becoming trapped within the fascial sheath and causing pressure and pain. Symptoms typically are relieved by balancing out opposing muscle groups and rest but may return with activity.[17] The condition can be very severe, which can mean that muscle swelling may compress other structures within the compartment causing neurovascular impairment. This advanced stage of anterior compartment syndrome is rare.

 PRECAUTIONARY NOTE?

If excessive swelling is present, or if in doubt, refer out!

Step 4: Assess Resisted Range of Motion (RROM)

To differentiate between ACS and a muscle strain, have the client dorsiflex the ankle against your resistance. If the pain is described as general or diffuse, it is likely he or she has ACS. The client has a muscle strain if the pain is specific and

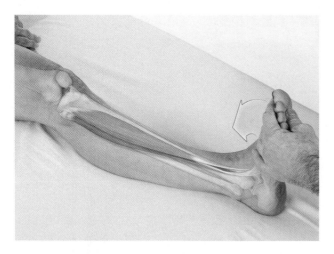

FIGURE 4-35
Muscle Resistance Test on Anterior Compartment Muscles.

he or she can point directly to it during the muscle resistance test (Figure 4-35 ■).

Step 5: Area Preparation

The client is supine. Use palmar friction to warm up the connective tissue of the anterolateral side of the lower leg.

Step 6: Myofascial Release

The angle, direction, and speed of movement are important when performing this release. Start at the **retinaculum** and hook and spread the fascia medial to lateral over the retinaculum to expand it. Repeat this several times (Figure 4-36 ■).

Then go to the lateral side of the tibia just above the ankle using fists, thumbs, index finger pads, or knuckles. Hook the fascia and work at a 45-degree angle into the

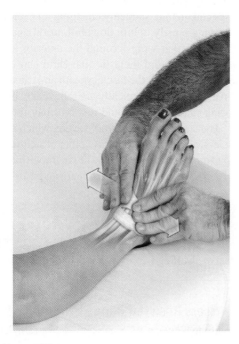

FIGURE 4-36
Retinaculum Release.

tissue. The direction is medial to lateral and distal to proximal, toward the knee and working across the tibialis anterior, extensor digitorum longus, and extensor hallucis longus muscles. Your goal is to move the muscles back to normal muscle resting lengths. The speed is slow to start and then becomes even slower as you work progressively deeper and more specific through the layers of fascia. Move the tissue away from the tibia to increase myofascial space which makes the muscle fibers more pliable. Repeat these strokes up the leg, several times, going even deeper each time. This takes the tissue out of a weak, inhibited, or overstretched position and releases the eccentric tension (Figure 4-37 ■).

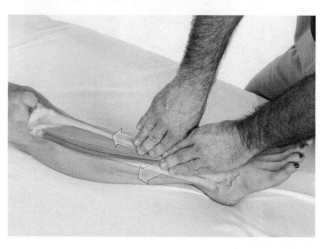

FIGURE 4-37
Myofascial Release, Anterior Compartment

Alternate with gentle compressive broadening to expand the compartment and to increase blood flow to the area. Compressive broadening pumps blood and oxygen deep into the capillary level of the muscle, allowing you to go deeper without discomfort. Compress into the muscles at a 45 degree angle and work insertion to origin to relax these muscles. Pay attention to areas of congestion and be cognizant of the client's comfort level as you work through these tender areas (Figure 4-38 ■).

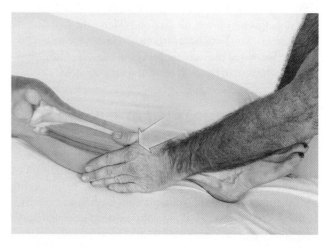

FIGURE 4-38
Compression Broadening.

You can also grasp or hook the tibialis anterior between your thumb and fingers and gently move it back and forth, away from the bone, like moving a big rubber band. Use the muscle belly to soften the surrounding fascial layers and intermuscular septums, creating deep displacement and release of the tissue. Push and pull the muscle groups in the anterior compartment to soften the deep investing fascia and mobilize the muscles. Do not let the tibia move, anchor the bone down, and move only the soft tissue (Figure 4-39 ■).

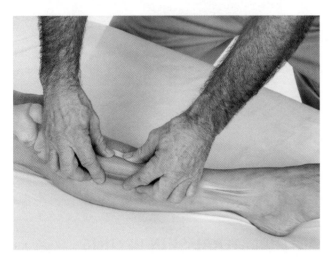

FIGURE 4-39
Release Intermuscular Septums.

You may find adhesions here where the tibialis anterior is literally "stuck" to the tibia. Place your finger pads at a 45-degree angle on the lateral side of the tibia. You need to slowly push the tibialis anterior away from the bone to increase intercompartmental space. This will also reduce the pressure in the anterolateral compartment. Do not glide over the muscle. Start below the knee and work toward the ankle. As you approach the ankle, either slow down your strokes or lighten up on your pressure, as it is likely to be tender (Figure 4-40 ■).

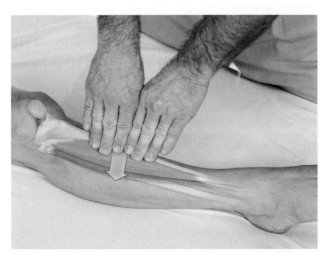

FIGURE 4-40
Release Deep Fascial Adhesions in Anterior Compartment.

Step 7: Cross-Fiber Gliding Strokes/Trigger Point Therapy

CROSS-FIBER GLIDING STROKES

If the tibialis anterior is still tight, you can also perform cross-fiber gliding strokes to further mobilize the tissue. Work distal to proximal to return this typically eccentrically contracted muscle back to its normal muscle resting length.

TRIGGER POINT THERAPY

As you are moving through the tissue, request feedback from the client. Ask if the tender areas refer pain, as direct pressure is applied, which indicates a trigger point. If so, use direct, moderate pressure for 10 to 12 seconds. As the tissue softens, gently compress and continue to relax the surrounding area.

Once you have released the tibialis anterior muscle belly, release the tendons. The retinaculum lies across the top of the ankle and secures the tendons to the ankle. You can soften that again. First, you need to warm up the **sheathed tendons** of the ankle with palmar friction. Then, place your finger pads on the front of the ankle with your thumbs on the bottom of the foot. Push down on the front of the ankle while moving the ankle passively through plantar flexion and dorsiflexion to further warm up the retinaculum. Perform myofascial spreading laterally on the retinaculum (Figure 4-41 ■).

To mobilize the ankle tendons, start with fingertip circular or multidirectional friction and move the tendons back and forth with your finger pads or thumbs to make sure there are no adhesions and to create freely moving tendons. You can also strip through the individual tendons. Slow down

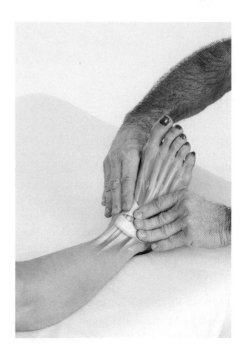

FIGURE 4-41
Retinaculum and Tendon Release Work.

your strokes and check in with the client as this area can be tender. If there are crunchy areas, such as fibrotic tissue, spend a little more time moving and gliding slowly between the tendons that are stuck to the bones. Do not overwork the area and use only enough pressure to release the collagen fibers and fascial adhesions that are gluing the tendons to the underlying bones and ligaments.

For ankle decompression, bring the foot and ankle to neutral. Grasp the ankle with your thumb on the plantar surface of the foot and your fingers over the retinaculum. Perform myofascial gliding strokes across the retinaculum and on the bottom of the foot, as your other hand moves the ankle into neutral with a lot of traction. The thumb is performing cross-fiber gliding work on the bottom of the foot, moving medial to lateral, while the fingers glide across the retinaculum, warming it up. Lean back and use your body weight during these strokes to decompress the ankle. There may be spontaneous alignment of bones during the traction. Repeat this sequence several times (Figure 4-42A ■).

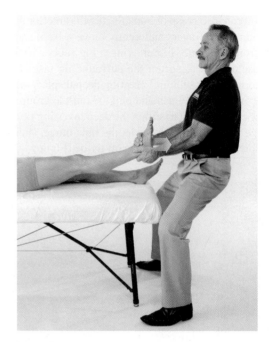

FIGURE 4-42B
Traction Hip, Knee, and Ankle.

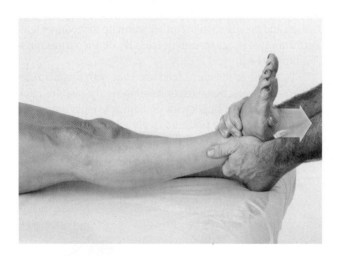

FIGURE 4-42A
Ankle Decompression.

Finally, grasp the client's ankle, lean back, and hold 3 to 5 seconds giving a gentle stretch and traction to the ankle (Figure 4-42B ■). The intent is to decompress the ankle, creating more joint space and reducing the forces that can cause arthritis in the ankle. There will be less wearing down of the cartilage in the joint and every single plane of movement may have less degeneration.

Step 4: Assess Resisted Range of Motion (RROM)

To reassess RROM, have the client dorsiflex the ankle against your resistance. If he or she still reports pain that is described as general or diffuse, return to the myofascial release, working slower and deeper until the pain is gone.

ANTEROLATERAL SHIN SPLINTS

Running or walking downhill can cause excessive plantar flexion, which places eccentric strain on the dorsiflexors of the lower leg: tibialis anterior, extensor digitorum longus, and extensor hallucis longus.

Muscle resistance testing will often isolate the exact problem area if it is a muscle strain. The symptoms and treatment differ from ACS. Be aware of this and apply good functional assessment.

Step 5: Area Preparation

Follow the steps for ACS through the myofascial release.

Step 4: Assess Resisted Range of Motion (RROM)

Determine where the muscle strain is by performing a resisted test. Have the client attempt to dorsiflex the ankle against your resistance. Then ask the client to point to the exact area of pain or tenderness (Figure 4-43 ■). Proceed with the next step.

Step 8: Multidirectional Friction

Perform multidirectional friction directly where the client indicated, on the collagen fibers. Use a supported finger to apply deep pressure (pain-free) with no gliding over the surface. Go in different directions to mobilize the fibers for about 20 to 30 seconds. Use only enough pressure to soften the matrix of fibers. Do not overwork the area.

Step 9: Pain-Free Movement

Have the client dorsiflex and plantar flex the ankle several times to begin aligning the scar tissue. If there is no discomfort, perform the eccentric work. If there is some discomfort, return to the multidirectional friction.

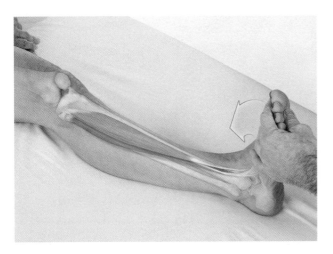

FIGURE 4-43
Muscle Resistance Test.

Step 10: Eccentric Scar Tissue Alignment

Support and traction the client's ankle. Have the client actively dorsiflex the ankle. Then have the client gently resist plantar flexion performed by you. Ask him or her to "barely resist, but let me win." Start with a pressure of only two fingers. The client can increase resistance only if there is zero discomfort. Repeat the eccentric lengthening several times and then proceed with relaxing these tissues. If the client still reports pain, return to all of the previous steps until the pain is gone.

Step 4: Assess Resisted Range of Motion (RROM)

To reassess RROM, repeat the resisted test. If the client reports pain, repeat the multidirectional friction and the eccentric release to alleviate the muscle–tendon strain problem.

Note: Do not stretch the dorsiflexors—tibialis anterior, extensor digitorum longus, and extensor hallucis longus muscles—as they are already weak, inhibited, and overstretched. Instead, stretch the antagonist muscles—gastrocnemius, soleus, and posterior tibialis—to bring the ankle to neutral and then strengthen the dorsiflexors.

INVERSION ANKLE SPRAIN AND STRAIN

This is the most common ankle sprain, usually involving a motion of excess inversion and plantar flexion.[18] The end feel of the ankle during a passive range of motion test of plantar flexion or inversion may be a soft-tissue stretch, not ligamentous, due to muscle, tendon, or ligament tears. Many clients' ankles, are inverted which causes them to walk on the outside of their foot. When they encounter an uneven surface, the integrity of the ankle is compromised due to the weak, inhibited, or overstretched peroneal muscles. The ankle rolls inward creating an inversion ligament sprain or muscle–tendon strain. This can result in tears and injury to the ligaments, muscles, tendons, retinaculum.

The anterior talofibular ligament connects the front part of the fibula to the talus bone on the front-outer part of the ankle joint and is the most commonly injured ligament.[19] However, the calcaneofibular ligament can also be injured during severe inversion sprains (Figure 4-44 ■). Swelling in the area of the lateral malleolus usually occurs along with strain or compensatory spasm of the peroneal muscles.

After the ankle has been evaluated and a fracture has been ruled out, you need to be concerned about inflammation, collagen formation, and fascial restrictions. Begin with RICE therapy (rest, ice, compression, and elevation), with an emphasis on moving the joint pain-free as soon as possible.[20] This will promote proper formation of collagen. One way to achieve this is to have the client "write the alphabet" with the foot. Have the client start with minimal movement and increase the movement only if it is pain-free and it does not increase inflammation.

PRECAUTIONARY NOTE

Do *not* perform massage to the area during the acute stage.

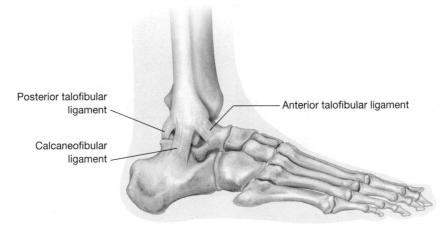

Posterior talofibular ligament

Calcaneofibular ligament

Anterior talofibular ligament

FIGURE 4-44
Ankle Ligaments.

Step 4: Assess Resisted Range of Motion (RROM)

Have the client evert the ankle and point to the specific point of pain. This is usually where the tendons pass behind the lateral malleolus (Figure 4-45 ■).

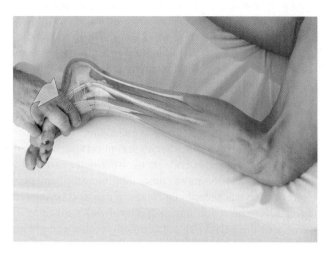

FIGURE 4-45
Muscle Resistance Test, Ankle Strain.

Step 6: Myofascial Release

The client is side lying with a bolster under the knee and ankle. Make sure the ankle is fully supported, in a neutral position, and not inverted. On the lateral side of the leg, perform myofascial spreading at a 45-degree angle into the tissue, on both sides of the fibula, using your closed fists, knuckles, or finger pads. Start just inferior to the lateral malleolus and work from the ankle to the knee, distal to proximal, hooking and taking the connective tissue back to where it belongs (Figure 4-46 ■).

Start superficial and work progressively deeper through the layers of tissue. Myofascial release creates space to allow blood flow to the ischemic muscles and helps decompress the underlying nerves and blood vessels.

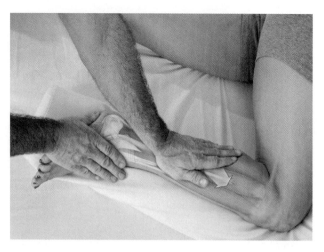

FIGURE 4-47
Compression Broadening, Lateral Lower Leg.

Alternate the myofascial work with gentle compressions for increased blood flow. Compress and hook the fascia upward toward the knee. Your intention is to bring the muscles back to normal muscle resting length, restoring muscle balance (Figure 4-47 ■).

Step 11: Stretching (During Therapy)

Do not stretch the muscles around the lateral ankle. They will be strengthened in client self-care. You can stretch the antagonists to allow the muscles around the lateral ankle to go back to their resting lengths. Support, lift, and traction the client's ankle. Move the ankle to eversion. Fatigue the tibialis posterior by having the client invert the ankle for 5 to 10 seconds at 20 percent force while you provide resistance. He or she relaxes and inhales while you give a subtle lift to the ankle to create traction. As the client exhales he or she everts the ankle for about 2 seconds while you assist the stretch. At this new position, repeat this contract-relax, contract-antagonist with active assisted stretching two or three times until you create the normal 20- to 30-degree range of motion (Figure 4-48 ■).

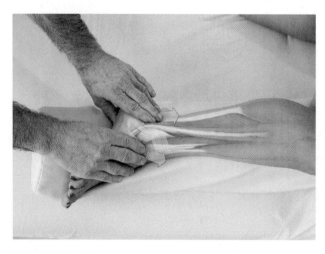

FIGURE 4-46
Myofascial Release, Lateral Lower Leg.

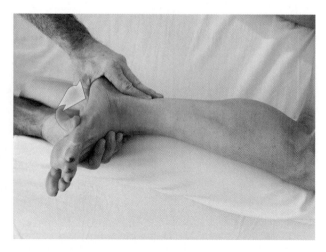

FIGURE 4-48
Stretch Posterior Tibialis.

Step 8: Multidirectional Friction

Have the client evert the foot against your resistance (Figure 4-49 ■). If he or she complains of pain during the muscle resistance test, have the client point to it. Perform multidirectional friction—pain-free, slow, and specific—for 20 to 30 seconds. You may feel adhesions or restrictions here. Adhesions can be tears or tender areas of disorganized collagen known as scar tissue, or fascial adhesions causing tendons, muscles, and ligaments to get stuck together. Whatever is adhesive or restricted needs therapy, especially around the lateral malleolus. You want to soften any abnormal adhesions of the muscles or ligaments with multidirectional friction for 20 to 30 seconds. (Figure 4-50 ■).

Note: Never work on the lateral tendons of the ankle if the client's ankle is still inverted.

Step 9: Pain-Free Movement

Ask the client to invert and evert the ankle several times. If there is no pain, perform the eccentric work. Return to the multidirectional friction if the client reports pain with this movement.

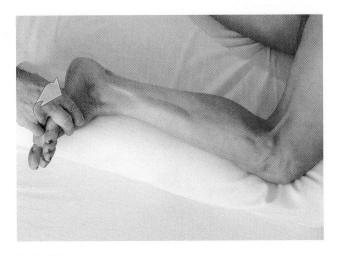

FIGURE 4-49
Muscle Resistance Test, Ankle Strain.

Step 10: Eccentric Scar Tissue Alignment

Apply eccentric contraction to realign the scar tissue of the muscle–tendon strain. Support and traction the client's ankle and bring it into slight eversion. Have the client gently resist inversion performed by you, bringing the ankle back to neutral. Tell him or her to "barely resist, but let me win." Start with a pressure of only two fingers and have the client increase resistance only if there is no discomfort. Repeat the eccentric work several times (Figure 4-51 ■).

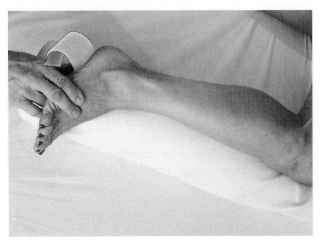

FIGURE 4-51
Eccentric Muscle Contraction.

Step 4: Assess Resisted Range of Motion (RROM)

To reassess RROM, have the client evert the ankle. If there is still a point of pain, return to the multidirectional friction and the pain-free movement. Repeat the eccentric contraction and reevaluate until the client is pain-free.

LIGAMENT SPRAIN

If the client has a ligament sprain, soften the scar tissue around the ligament first using multidirectional friction. Then support the ankle and move it into slight eversion. Next, pin down the origin of the involved ligament(s) while performing a *passive* stretch of the ankle back to the neutral position.

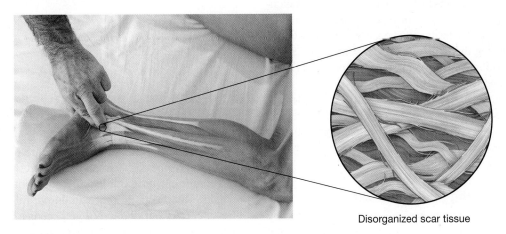

Disorganized scar tissue

FIGURE 4-50
Multidirectional Friction.

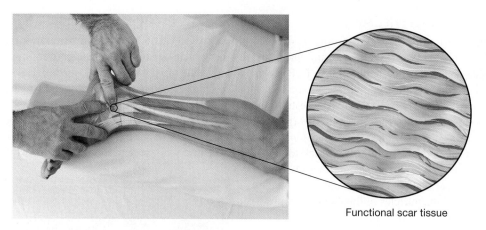

Functional scar tissue

FIGURE 4-52
Eccentric Ligament Technique.

Perform this pin and passive stretch several times to begin to realign the scar tissue in any of the stabilizing ligaments. Limit the amount of inversion during this technique as you do not want to stretch damaged lateral ligaments (Figure 4-52 ■).

Note: Do not stretch the peroneals as they are already overstretched in this situation. However, it is imperative that the client strengthens the peroneal muscles to increase the integrity of the lateral aspect of the ankle and to prevent reinjury in the future. See the strengthening exercises at the end of the chapter. You must also treat the tight inverters and plantar flexors that may have caused the problem. Follow the steps outlined under posteromedial shin splints (Figure 4-53 ■).

STRESS FRACTURE

A stress fracture is often incorrectly assessed as a shin splint. It is an overuse injury that occurs as a result of repetitive stress loading on the weight-bearing tibia—although it can also occur on the fibula. It is usually due to the fact that the surrounding muscles have become inflexible and no longer act as adequate shock absorbers.

This condition is usually seen early in the season when the athlete attempts too much, too soon. The client will complain of a small specific area of pain that doesn't change with muscle resistance testing. Since x-rays are often unreliable in diagnosing this problem, the client should be given a magnetic resonance imaging (MRI) or bone scan if the condition is doubtful or doesn't improve.[21]

A nondisplaced stress fracture will heal faster by increasing blood flow to the immediate area. Therefore, general massage techniques, performed pain-free, such as myofascial release and very gentle compressions are essential for recovery.

Step 11: Stretching (Client Self-Care)

The goal is for the client to perform stretches suggested by you to create normal muscle resting lengths in shortened or contracted muscle groups, and restore normal range of motion to the joint.

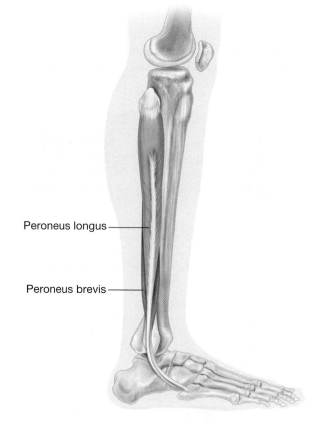

Peroneus longus

Peroneus brevis

FIGURE 4-53
Lateral Leg Muscles.

 PRECAUTIONARY NOTE

In certain states, massage therapists are not allowed to suggest stretches or strengthening exercises. If you are not competent, or if you feel that suggesting stretches is outside your scope of practice, do *not* follow this step. Be safe, refer out. Wait until you become competent by becoming certified as a personal trainer or certified in active isolated stretching.

CORE PRINCIPLE

Suggest only two to four stretches or strengthening exercises, specific to the condition, each time you see a client. Make sure he or she can perform these correctly before suggesting any additional exercises.

- Tell the client that the stretches will take only a few minutes a day to perform and are necessary for continued results.
- The client should stretch after joint movement, exercise, or a hot shower when the fascia and muscles are warm.

PRECAUTIONARY NOTE

Do not have the client stretch beyond normal range of motion, as this could create hypermobile joints and result in injury. Do *not* suggest stretches for weak, inhibited, or overstretched muscle groups. These muscles need to be tonified and strengthened to maintain structural balance. This is based on restoring normal muscle resting lengths of opposing muscle groups, and normal range of motion at that joint.

- Tell the client to not stretch into pain. The client needs to differentiate between uncomfortable stretching due to tight muscles and painful stretching that can aggravate a pre-existing clinical condition.
- The client starts the stretches with the tightest side first until normal range of motion is achieved. Then he or she continues to stretch both sides for continued balance and symmetry.
- Print copies of the stretches for your clients to take with them for reference.

GASTROCNEMIUS

- The client is seated on the floor.
- The affected leg is straight with the stretch rope around the ball of that foot.
- He or she brings the ankle to dorsiflexion to lengthen the gastrocnemius.
- Then the client plantar flexes the ankle against the resistance of the stretch rope for 5 to 10 seconds at 20 percent force.
- He or she relaxes, inhales, and then on exhale actively dorsiflexes the ankle while gently assisting (pulling back) on the stretch rope for about 2 seconds.
- At this new position, the client repeats the stretch several times to lengthen the gastrocnemius and then repeats it on the other leg, if needed (Figure 4-54 ■).

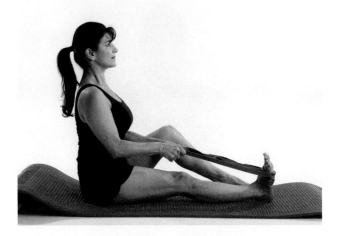

FIGURE 4-54
Gastrocnemius Stretch.

SOLEUS

- The client is seated with one knee bent 90 degrees and with the hands on the ball of that foot.
- The knee *must* be bent to 90 degrees to isolate the soleus.
- The client plantar flexes the ankle against the resistance of the hands for 5 to 10 seconds at 20 percent force.
- He or she relaxes, inhales, and then on exhale actively dorsiflexes the ankle while gently assisting (pulling back) with the hands for about 2 seconds.
- At this new position, the client then relaxes, takes a breath, and on exhale repeats the stretch several times. He or she repeats the stretch on the other leg to prevent compensation and secondary injury, and to balance out the body (Figure 4-55 ■).

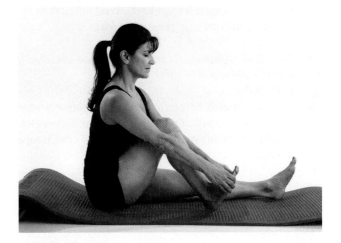

FIGURE 4-55
Soleus Stretch.

TIBIALIS POSTERIOR

If the client has excessive weight bearing supination or is inverted and cannot evert the foot 20 degrees when prone or not weight bearing, suggest this stretch. If he or she is hyperpronated, strengthen the tibialis posterior instead.

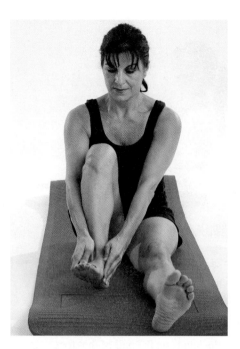

FIGURE 4-56
Posterior Tibialis Stretch.

- The client seated with one knee bent 90 degrees (the knee must not move).
- Using the hands around the ball of the foot, the client inverts the ankle against the resistance of the hands at 20 percent force for 5 to 10 seconds.
- He or she relaxes, inhales, and on exhale actively everts the ankle for about 2 seconds while assisting with the hands.
- At this new position, the client then relaxes, takes a breath, and on exhale repeats the assisted stretch.
- The client repeats this sequence several times, then repeats on the other leg (Figure 4-56 ■).

Note: The tibialis posterior is strengthened, not stretched if the client hyperpronates.

This stretch can also be performed using a stretch rope wrapped around the ball of the foot. The client follows the same directions for this stretch, substituting the stretch rope for the hands.

Step 12: Strengthening (Client Self-Care)
TECHNIQUES FOR STRENGTHENING

Goal: to strengthen weak, inhibited muscle groups around a joint creating muscle balance throughout the body—structural integration.

The client must stretch the tight, contracted antagonist muscles before strengthening the opposing weak, inhibited, and overstretched muscles.

PRECAUTIONARY NOTE

To prevent reinjury after treating a strain, have the client refrain from beginning a strengthening program for 7 to 10 days, or until he or she is pain-free. To facilitate healing, have the client stretch the tight antagonist muscles, taking the tension off the injured muscles until pain-free strengthening can begin.

These exercises are performed on the weak, inhibited muscles. All the client needs is a Thera-Band. The Thera-Band is inexpensive and you could provide it for them. Show the client how he or she can control and adjust the amount of resistance by holding the band.

Make sure the client understands that the movements are slow and controlled during both the concentric contractions (muscle shortening phase) and eccentric contractions (muscle lengthening phase), *spending more time on the eccentric phase.* Suggest roughly 2 seconds in the concentric phase and 4 seconds in the eccentric or lengthening phase. It is imperative that the client strengthens these muscles that are weak and usually overstretched to return the body to proper and optimum balance and to prevent injury in the future.

PERONEALS

CORE PRINCIPLE

This muscle group *must* be strengthened by clients with lateral ankle sprains and damage to the ligaments of the lateral ankle for prevention of reinjury!

- The client is seated with both legs straight.
- The Thera-Band is looped individually around each foot, finishing on the outside of the ankles and held in the client's hands.
- The client everts the ankles while pulling on the Thera-Band to create tension. Adjusting the distance between the feet can control the amount of tension on the tubing.
- If the client doesn't feel a "burn" during the exercise, he or she needs to move the feet further apart.
- The key is to perform the exercise slowly. Since eccentric contraction is more beneficial than concentric contraction, the client everts the ankle for 2 seconds (concentric) and then returns to neutral (eccentric) taking about 4 seconds.
- The client performs one to three sets of 8 to 10 repetitions (Figure 4-57 ■).

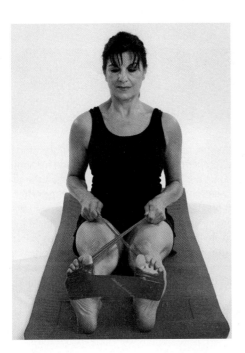

FIGURE 4-57
Strengthen Peroneals.

TIBIALIS POSTERIOR

There are clients who present with a weak tibialis posterior, and possibly tight peroneals, creating hyperpronation of the weight bearing ankle. To balance the ankle, they need to strengthen their tibialis posterior after stretching the peroneals. Have these clients perform the following exercise.

 PRECAUTIONARY NOTE

If this position creates discomfort in the client's knee, do not have him or her perform it.

- The client is seated with both knees flexed, one hip externally rotated.
- The Thera-Band is looped individually around each foot, finishing on the inside of the ankles and held in the client's hands.
- The client inverts the ankles while pulling on the tubing to create tension. Adjusting the distance between the feet can control the amount of tension on the tubing.
- If the client does not feel a "burn" during the exercise, he or she needs to increase the resistance in the band.
- The key here is to perform the exercise slowly. Since eccentric contraction is more beneficial than concentric contraction, he or she inverts the ankle for 2 seconds (concentric) and then returns slower to neutral (eccentric) taking about 4 seconds.
- The client performs one to three sets of 8 to 10 repetitions (Figure 4-58 ■).

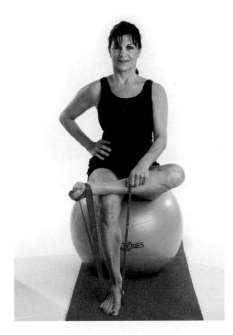

FIGURE 4-58
Strengthen Posterior Tibialis.

ANTERIOR COMPARTMENT SYNDROME

This exercise strengthens the weak, inhibited ankle dorsiflexors to help prevent anterior compartment syndrome.

- The client is seated with the Thera-Band looped around the exercising foot and secured under the other foot.
- The client dorsiflexes the ankle for 1 to 2 seconds (concentric) and then returns to neutral (eccentric) taking about 4 seconds.
- He or she performs one to three sets of 8 to 10 repetitions (Figure 4-59 ■).

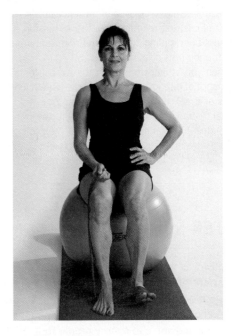

FIGURE 4-59
Strengthen Tibialis Anterior.

CASE STUDY

John is a 30-year-old marathon runner who has been running about 50 miles each week to prepare for a local marathon. He has been feeling pain in his Achilles tendon for about three weeks and pain in the front of his tibia which is what brought him in to your office. His running partner is a doctor and he told John that he has what seems like Achilles tendonitis, and may be developing shin splints.

John states in the client history that this particular pain gets progressively worse about 10 minutes into his run, and diminishes slightly with decreased activity. This indicates the possibility of a myofascial pain syndrome and you suspect anterolateral compartment syndrome. John's doctor friend confirms that evaluation.

Upon initial evaluation, during active range of motion you note that John can dorsiflex his ankle only 10 degrees, indicating tight gastrocnemius and soleus. He also has limited eversion of just 5 degrees, indicating a tight posterior tibialis. You do not see any excessive pronation observing his foot strike. Passive range of motion evaluation finds normal end feel in all directions. When you assess resisted range of motion for the soleus, John points with one finger to a spot at the muscle–tendon junction of the Achilles tendon. There is no redness, swelling, or inflammation, thus indicating Achilles tendinosis—a muscle strain without inflammation. When you perform a muscle resistance test for the muscles that dorsiflex the ankle, John cannot isolate a specific painful area, but points to the entire anterolateral compartment of the lower leg and describes the pain in this area as general and diffuse. Since your evaluation indicates tight gastrocnemius, soleus, and posterior tibialis you treat the gastrocnemius first releasing myofascial tension, tight bands with cross-fiber gliding strokes, and then a few active trigger points found in the soleus.

When you attempt to stretch the soleus, John points to a specific spot of discomfort at the muscle–tendon junction of the Achilles at the Achilles tendon junction. You perform multidirectional friction for 30 seconds, and then pain-free movement that creates 20 degrees of dorsiflexion. You follow that with pain-free eccentric muscle contraction. Then you apply a deep stretch and when John contracts against resistance, he says it

feels much better, but isolates a small spot of discomfort in that same area. You perform multidirectional friction for another 30 seconds, working a little deeper and slower than the previous time, and then John moves the ankle through pain-free dorsiflexion and plantar flexion. You follow that with an eccentric muscle contraction to the soleus and John cannot find the point of pain. You are then able to fully stretch the soleus to its normal resting length, creating 30 degrees of dorsiflexion. You then release the posterior tibialis and restore full pain-free eversion.

Stretching the gastrocnemius, soleus, and posterior tibialis brings the muscle groups of the anterior compartment to a neutral resting position. You then perform myofascial work to the anterior and lateral compartment, working from distal to proximal (insertion to origin), to help relax the muscle groups that are weak and inhibited because of their tight and overpowering antagonists. This increases myofascial space and the pain in the anterolateral compartments diminishes.

Based on your evaluation and treatment to create lower leg muscular balance, with normal muscle resting lengths, you give John the following self-care suggestions. John is given a stretch rope and shown how to stretch the tight muscles from superficial to deep:

- gastrocnemius
- soleus
- posterior tibialis

He is then given a Thera-Band and shown how to strengthen the weak antagonists:

- tibialis anterior
- peroneals

John returns the next week and shows you the self-care he is performing, and reports that he is not only running pain-free, but he has also taken 30 seconds off his 10K time. He is committed to the self-care for injury prevention and performance enhancement benefits, and before leaving your office, gives you the names of three clients whom he wants you to start seeing.

CHAPTER SUMMARY

This chapter was written to offer the clinical massage therapist a variety of tools to evaluate, identify, and properly address the most common clinical conditions of the lower extremity. The author wants to stress the importance of stabilizing the foot and ankle to restore proper foot strike. Excessive supination or hyperpronation will create compensatory

pain in the rest of the body, called ascending syndromes. Manual therapists should stop using generic catchall terms like "shin splints" and instead, sort out the multiple possibilities presenting themselves as pain in the lower extremity.

The intention of this chapter was to ensure that the clinical massage therapist eliminate any underlying causes of specific conditions of the lower extremity prior to treating the resulting clinical symptoms. It is important to look closely at the major contributing factors of lower extremity pain by first balancing out the muscle groups of the foot and ankle. In doing that preparation work, what seem like complicated clinical conditions of the lower extremity can be resolved in just a few sessions. By restoring proper foot strike and performing pelvic stabilization, many of the clinical symptoms of the knee will simply disappear. This will allow your clients to live pain-free and your athletes to achieve peak performance.

REVIEW QUESTIONS

1. Normal range of motion for dorsiflexion is

   _____.

   a. 15 to 20 degrees
   b. 20 to 30 degrees
   c. 10 degrees
   d. 30 to 50 degrees

2. A tight soleus is the number one cause of what condition?
   a. compartment syndrome
   b. bunions
   c. Achilles tendon pain
   d. sprained ankle

3. Pain that is felt in the heel of the foot, which is usually worse in the morning and then feels better as the gastrocnemius and soleus warms up, is called

   _____.

   a. Morton's neuroma
   b. plantar fasciitis
   c. bunion
   d. hammer toe

4. The posterior tibialis performs what two actions?
   a. dorsiflexion and inversion
   b. dorsiflexion and eversion
   c. plantar flexion and eversion
   d. plantar flexion and inversion

5. If the client has sustained an inversion ankle sprain, what muscle or muscles need to be strengthened?
   a. peroneals
   b. posterior tibialis
   c. gastrocnemius
   d. soleus

6. The normal end feel for ankle plantar flexion is

   _____.

   a. ligamentous and abrupt
   b. bone-on-bone

   c. soft and leathery
   d. not limited

7. What two muscles should you stretch to prevent plantar fasciitis?
   a. gastrocnemius and Achilles tendon
   b. gastrocnemius and plantar fascia
   c. gastrocnemius and soleus
   d. gastrocnemius and anterior tibialis

8. If the posterior tibialis is tight, what range of motion is restricted?
   a. eversion
   b. inversion
   c. plantar flexion
   d. knee flexion

9. What test do you use to differentiate between anterior compartment syndrome and a strain in the tibialis anterior?
   a. the client dorsiflexes against therapist resistance
   b. the client inverts the ankle against therapist resistance
   c. the client plantar flexes against therapist resistance
   d. the therapist passively moves the client's ankle through plantar flexion and dorsiflexion

10. Pes planus or fallen arches are described as

    _____.

    a. excessive pronation that causes the foot's arch to collapse
    b. having associated injuries such as bunions, hammer toes, and plantar fasciitis
    c. placing constant stress on the posterior tibialis
    d. all of the above

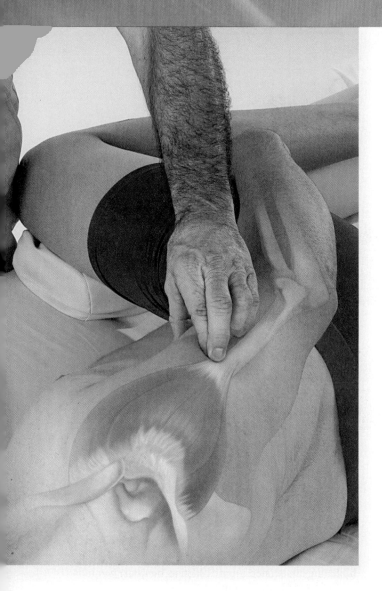

CHAPTER 5

Shoulder Conditions

 CHAPTER OUTLINE

Twelve-Step Approach to Shoulder Conditions

Specific Muscle Resistance Tests

General Shoulder Protocol

Pectoralis Major

Pectoralis Minor

Subclavius

Biceps and Coracobrachialis

Upper Trapezius and Middle Deltoid

Subscapularis

Rhomboids

Triceps and Posterior Deltoid

Scapula Reposition

Supraspinatus and Upper Trapezius

Infraspinatus and Teres Minor

Common Conditions

LEARNING OBJECTIVES

Upon completing this chapter the reader will be able to:

- Choose the appropriate massage modality or treatment protocol for each specific clinical condition of the shoulder
- Work on the short, contracted muscle groups such as pectoralis major, pectoralis minor, subclavius, and subscapularis before working the weak, inhibited antagonists such as rhomboids, middle trapezius, lower trapezius, infraspinatus, and teres minor. This will ensure
  - structural integration—balance of the muscle groups
  - that the therapist eliminates the underlying cause of the shoulder problems before addressing the clinical symptoms
- Restore pain-free shoulder normal joint range of motion
- Restore normal muscle resting lengths in the muscle groups of the shoulder

- Create shoulder stability
- Differentiate between soft-tissue problems caused by
  - myofascial restrictions
  - muscle–tendon tension
  - myoskeletal alignment problems
  - trigger point tension
  - joint capsule adhesions
  - strained muscle fibers
  - scar tissue
- Teach the client self-care stretches and strengthening exercises to perform at home to maintain shoulder structural balance and pain-free movement following therapy

KEY TERMS

Adhesive capsulitis 148

Brachial plexus 190

Bursa 194

Bursitis 192

Coracoid process 153

Deltoid tuberosity 170

Hyperemia 159

Kyphosis 177

Migraine headaches 159

Rotator cuff 192

Subacromial bursa 194

Thoracic outlet syndrome 190

Upper crossed syndrome 195

Vascular headaches 159

The majority of clients' shoulders are forward and medially rotated due to poor postural patterns, repetitive motions, or trauma. The muscles in the front of the shoulder such as pectoralis major, pectoralis minor, subclavius, and subscapularis become tight and contracted, while the opposing muscles such as rhomboids, middle trapezius, infraspinatus, and teres minor become weak, inhibited, and eccentrically contracted or overstretched.

This imbalance around the joint may enhance a neuromuscular response, attempting to restore balance, which also creates tension in the joint. This may lead to joint degeneration or arthritis, as the cartilage wears down from being placed in a tight or imbalanced position during shoulder movement. The resultant discomfort also limits range of motion, possibly contributing to a formation of fascial adhesions inside the joint capsule.

The fascia and osseous membrane surrounding the articulating cartilage acts as "superglue" and essentially glues the humerus to the scapula contributing to a condition called **adhesive capsulitis.**

Adhesive capsulitis usually begins innocently enough. Your shoulder is bothering you, so you don't use it. There is something to be said for resting an overused joint after a weekend softball tournament. But if you've injured your shoulder, or are suffering from chronic shoulder pain, and you don't use your shoulder for a long time, your joint will stiffen up. From there, it becomes a vicious cycle. Your shoulder gets more and more stiff and eventually the lining of the joint gets stiff and you cannot use your shoulder. Although adhesive capsulitis and frozen shoulder are often used to describe the same clinical condition, they are quite different. An early onset fascial adhesion inside the joint capsule is the pathology that limits active and passive shoulder movement in early onset adhesive capsulitis. The pathologies that may be involved in a true frozen shoulder include not only adhesive capsulitis, but also subacromial bursitis, calcific tendonitis, rotator cuff pathology, and other conditions such as shoulder impingement, that all contribute to limited shoulder motion.

In general, frozen shoulder can come on after an injury to your shoulder or a bout with another musculoskeletal condition such as tendinitis or bursitis.[1] It can also develop after a stroke. Quite often its cause cannot be pinpointed. Any condition that causes you to refrain from moving your arm and using your shoulder can put you at risk for developing frozen shoulder. Diabetes is also a risk factor for frozen shoulder. The medical community is still researching why, but one theory involves collagen, one of the building blocks of ligaments and tendons. Collagen is a major part of the ligaments that hold the bones together in a joint. Glucose (sugar) molecules attach to collagen. In people with diabetes, the theory goes, this can contribute to abnormal deposits of collagen in the cartilage and tendons of the shoulder. The buildup then causes the affected shoulder to stiffen up.[2]

Women are more likely to develop frozen shoulder than men, and frozen shoulder occurs most frequently in people between the ages of 40 and 70.[3]

TWELVE-STEP APPROACH TO SHOULDER CONDITIONS

The good news, from the results in treating hundreds of patients in various stages of adhesive capsulitis and complicated frozen shoulder conditions, is there is a protocol to specifically address each specific clinical condition. The inner fascial and capsular work must be performed pain-free, in conjunction with balancing out the muscle groups of the shoulder while systematically treating associated sprains or strains. The deep fascial adhesions inside the joint capsule can be softened and mobilized with precise joint capsule techniques. Pain-free movements, using the head of the humerus to create pressure, movement, and slow velocity stretch to the deepest investing fascia inside the joint capsule, can facilitate myofascial release within the shoulder joint. The head of the humerus can be used as a massage tool to release and reposition the fascia or adhesions in the joint capsule. This is achieved by performing very gentle pain-free movements using the articulating cartilage of the humerus to massage the articulating cartilage, fascia, and osseous membrane of the shoulder within the joint capsule at the exact areas that you find a bone-on-bone-like end feel in the shoulder.

An added plunging technique, by gently compressing and decompressing the scapula with the head of the humerus, seems to even organize the disorganized collagen in the joint capsule itself. The author's hypothesis is that when you gently, but deeply compress the humerus into the scapula, it is a form of strain–counterstrain allowing the fibrin formation in the joint capsule to relax. When you gently traction or decompress the capsule with the humerus, the adhesions or fibrin formations create an eccentric force through resistance to your decompression. Thus, he believes that is what may better organize or realign the fibrin formation or disorganized collagen. The goal is to align with research experts to do clinical studies that will validate this result-driven hypothesis.

This can often release the frozen shoulder in literally one session, especially in early onset adhesive capsulitis. This is a unique technique that is one of the author's trademarks. Although some people in the health care industry are skeptical about the feasibility of releasing long-term frozen shoulders, orthopedic massage practitioners using this technique have witnessed the release of frozen shoulders in many cases where the participants had previously been diagnosed with adhesive capsulitis and true forzen shoulders, by their physicians. (Watch the shoulder joint capsule release video clip at www.myhealthprofessionskit.com). *This shoulder capsule work is one of the most revolutionary techniques you will learn in this book.*

The shoulder protocol involves moving between

- Soft-tissue restrictions: muscle–tendon, fascia, scar tissue
- Bone-on-bone-like end feel: joint capsule
- Client emotions: guarding, fear of pain

This is called "the dance," as the protocol may be different for each client. You will learn how to assess restrictions creating an individualized treatment for each client. The following conditions are covered in this chapter:

- Thoracic outlet syndrome
- Adhesive capsulitis and frozen shoulder
- Rotator cuff tear
- Supraspinatus tendinosis and supraspinatus impingement
- Infraspinatus tendinosis and teres minor tendinosis
- Subscapularis tendinosis versus bicipital and coracobrachialis tendinosis
- Subacromial bursitis
- Upper crossed syndrome

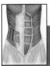

CORE PRINCIPLE

Imbalances in the hips can create distortions that affect the shoulders. It is highly recommended to perform pelvic stabilization before working on the shoulder.

PRECAUTIONARY NOTE

Do not work on a client with a recent injury (acute condition), exhibiting inflammation, heat, redness, or swelling. RICE therapy (rest, ice, compression, elevation) would be the appropriate treatment in this situation. This work cannot be performed on clients with severe shoulder conditions like a complete rupture of a muscle, complicated labrum tears, and fractures.

Step 1: Client History

Goal: to obtain a thorough medical history including precautions and contraindications for treatment of the client's shoulder condition.

As mentioned in Chapter 1, taking a thorough client history will offer you valuable insights into a client's condition. In addition to the basic information completed on the client history form, ask the client when, where, and how the problem began. Also ask the client to describe the area of pain and what makes it better or worse. This will give you a starting point from which to assess the client's active range of motion.

Step 2: Assess Active Range of Motion (AROM)

Goal: to assess range of motion of single-plane movements, performed solely by the client, to identify tight or restricted shoulder muscle groups.

Assess the client's active ROM for the primary single-plane shoulder movements—flexion, extension, abduction, adduction, medial rotation, lateral rotation, horizontal abduction, and horizontal adduction—with zero discomfort. Determine if the range of motion is normal. Please understand that the normal degrees for each shoulder range of motion will vary with different references. The degrees listed in this text are accurate estimates for clients with healthy shoulders. (see the single-plane movement Figures 5-1 ■ through 5-8 ■). If the range of motion is less than average, identify which muscle groups are restricted and therefore preventing normal movement. Focus on releasing these restricted, antagonist muscle groups:

- If flexion is less than 160 to 180 degrees, work on releasing the extensors (antagonists)—latissimus dorsi, pectoralis major (lower fibers), posterior deltoid, teres major, and triceps (long head)—to restore normal muscle resting lengths.
- If extension is less than 50 to 60 degrees, work on releasing the flexors (antagonists)—anterior deltoid, biceps brachii, coracobrachialis, and pectoralis major (clavicular portion)—to restore normal muscle resting lengths.
- If abduction is less than 180 degrees, work on releasing the adductors (antagonists)—latissimus dorsi, pectoralis major, and teres major—to restore normal muscle resting lengths.
- If adduction is less than 30 to 45 degrees, work on releasing the abductors (antagonists)—deltoid (middle), and supraspinatus—to restore normal muscle resting lengths.
- If medial/internal is less than 90 degrees, work on releasing the lateral rotators (antagonists)—infraspinatus, posterior deltoid, and teres minor—to restore normal muscle resting lengths.
- If lateral/external is less than 80 to 90 degrees, work on releasing the medial rotators (antagonists)—anterior deltoid, latissimus dorsi, pectoralis major, subscapularis, and teres major—to restore normal muscle resting lengths.
- If horizontal adduction is less than 135 degrees, work on releasing the horizontal abductors (antagonists)—infraspinatus, posterior deltoid, teres major, and teres minor—to restore normal muscle resting lengths.
- If horizontal abduction is less than 30 to 45 degrees, work on releasing the horizontal adductors (antagonists)—anterior deltoid and pectoralis major—to restore normal muscle resting lengths.

SHOULDER JOINT SINGLE-PLANE MOVEMENTS—PRIMARY MUSCLES

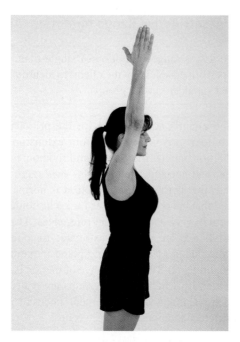

FIGURE 5-1

Shoulder Flexion, 160–180 degrees.

Flexion, 160 to 180 Degrees

- Anterior deltoid
- Coracobrachialis
- Biceps brachii
- Pectoralis major (clavicular portion)

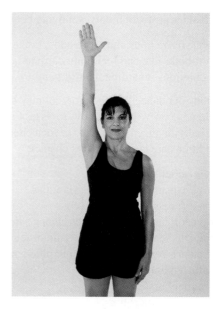

FIGURE 5-3

Shoulder Abduction, 180 degrees.

Abduction, 180 Degrees

- Deltoid (middle portion)
- Supraspinatus

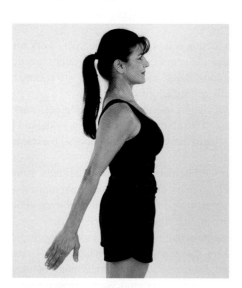

FIGURE 5-2

Shoulder Extension, 50–60 degrees.

Extension, 50 to 60 Degrees

- Latissimus dorsi
- Teres major
- Pectoralis major (lower fibers)
- Teres minor
- Posterior deltoid
- Triceps (long head)

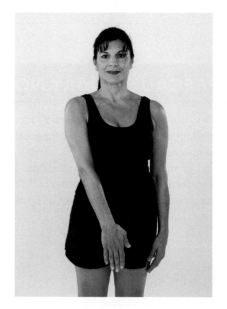

FIGURE 5-4

Shoulder Adduction, 30–45 degrees.

Adduction, 30 to 45 Degrees

- Latissimus dorsi
- Pectoralis major
- Teres major
- Teres minor coracobrachialis

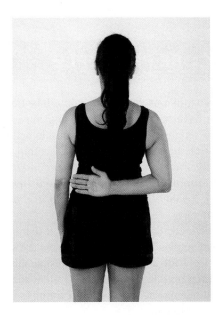

FIGURE 5-5
Shoulder Medial/Internal Rotation, 90–100 degrees.

Medial/Internal Rotation, 90 to 100 Degrees

- Anterior deltoid
- Latissimus dorsi
- Pectoralis major
- Subscapularis
- Teres major

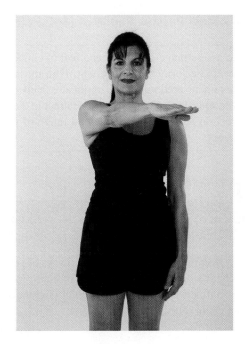

FIGURE 5-7
Shoulder Horizontal Adduction, 135 degrees.

Horizontal Adduction, 135 Degrees

- Anterior deltoid
- Pectoralis major

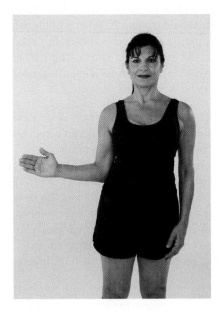

FIGURE 5-6
Shoulder Lateral/External Rotation, 80–90 degrees.

Lateral/External Rotation, 80 to 90 Degrees

- Infraspinatus
- Posterior deltoid
- Teres minor

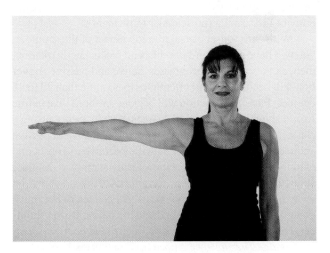

FIGURE 5-8
Shoulder Horizontal Abduction, 30–45 degrees.

Horizontal Abduction, 30 to 45 Degrees

- Infraspinatus
- Posterior deltoid
- Teres major
- Teres minor

Step 3: Assess Passive Range of Motion (PROM)

Goal: to assess range of motion end feel of single-plane movements performed on the client. Pain during passive movement predominately implicates inert tissues. However, muscles and tendons that contract in the opposite direction are stretched at the end range of passive movement.

CORE PRINCIPLE

When performing PROM, you should always be sensitive to the client's breathing and patterns of guarding. Your overall confidence, combined with a calming voice, can help the client relax.

To assess passive range of motion (PROM), gently perform each of the eight shoulder single plane movements on the client, pain-free. The purpose is to determine the end feel of the physiological barrier at the end of the shoulder joint's range of motion.[4] Flexion, extension, abduction, lateral rotation, and horizontal abduction will have a tissue stretch or leathery end feel. Medial rotation, adduction, and horizontal adduction will also have a tissue stretch end feel, but may be associated with a tissue-on-tissue end feel in certain individuals. Make sure the client keeps the head, neck, and shoulders square and that the humerus is moving independently of the scapula (no scapular movement).

With early-onset capsular involvement of the shoulder, you will have a bone-on-bone-like end feel in lateral rotation, then, as the condition progresses, active and passive abduction will become limited oftentimes to no more than 30 to 45 degrees. Passive abduction will be bone-on-bone-like in true frozen shoulders at about 30 degrees of abduction, causing a classical body compensation pattern during active or passive abduction of the shoulder. You will observe early onset and extreme upward scapular rotation during attempted shoulder abduction. The client will also compensate by side bending away from the shoulder being passively abducted. For much greater detail on evaluating and understanding frozen shoulders, refer to Whitney Lowe's book *Orthopedic Assessment in Massage Therapy* (see Appendix C in this textbook) or go to www.orthomassage.net and get our DVD on Orthopedic Massage for Complicated Shoulder Conditions.

Step 4: Assess Resisted Range of Motion (RROM)

Goal: to assess if there is a muscle–tendon strain present and, if so, exactly where it is located.

CORE PRINCIPLE

If there is a torn muscle or tendon, it will be treated *last,* after you have balanced out opposing muscle groups and addressed the problems in the muscle belly leading to the muscle tear. This book will stress this statement continually: *Never treat a muscle–tendon strain, or a ligament sprain, unless the injured muscle–tendon unit, or injured ligament, is brought back to its normal resting position.*

It is believed that too many manual therapists treat strains and sprains while those structures are still under stress or mechanical load. The therapist should balance out opposing muscle groups to bring them back to their normal muscle resting lengths before trying to soften and mobilize scar tissue.

 PRECAUTIONARY NOTE

Do not move too fast, or use too much force while performing a resisted test.

The client attempts each of the eight single-plane movements of the shoulder using 20 percent of his or her strength while you apply gentle reverse resistance. You control the test. If the client experiences pain, ask him or her to point to the specific area. This indicates a muscle–tendon strain and this area will be worked last.

- If the client's pain is in the front of the shoulder, test the following muscles: biceps and coracobrachialis, subscapularis, and pectoralis minor.
- If the client's pain is on top of the shoulder, test the supraspinatus and middle deltoid.
- If the client's pain is in the back of the shoulder, test the infraspinatus, teres minor, and rhomboids.
- The muscle groups we suggested testing are the more common injuries of the shoulder. However, there can be other muscle groups or structures involved.

For precaution, start the test with minimal resistance and then slowly increase the resistance to fully recruit the deeper muscle fibers.

SPECIFIC MUSCLE RESISTANCE TESTS

Keep in mind that testing a muscle, by having the client contract the muscle against the therapists resistance, is done to determine whether or not that particular muscle–tendon unit has a strain. (A = action, O = origin, I = insertion.)

CORE PRINCIPLE

If the client reports pain after you finish the resisted test, this is *not* a positive test and the problem may be in the surrounding or stabilizing muscles. *The pain must be in the muscle you are testing during the test.*

Biceps (Long Head) and Coracobrachialis

A = Biceps: elbow flexion, forearm supination

Coracobrachialis: shoulder adduction, shoulder flexion

O = Biceps: supraglenoid tubercle of scapula

Coracobrachialis: **coracoid process** of scapula

I = Biceps: tuberosity of radius and bicipital aponeurosis

Coracobrachialis: medial surface of midhumeral shaft

Resisted Test: The client is standing, with the shoulder flexed to 90 degrees, palm up (supinated). Place your hands above and below the client's elbow. The client flexes the shoulder, using 20 percent force against your resistance, and may feel pain in the bicipital groove if the long head of the biceps is injured. You control the test. If the client reports pain at the coracoid process there is a muscle–tendon strain in the upper biceps short head or coracobrachialis. Have the client point to the exact area (Figure 5-9 ■).

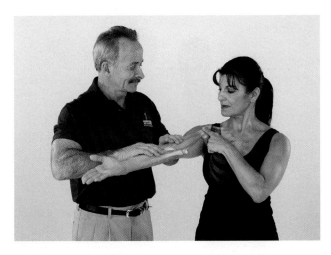

FIGURE 5-9
Muscle Resistance Test, Biceps and Coracobrachialis.

Subscapularis

A = Shoulder medial rotation; stabilizes the head of the humerus

O = Subscapular fossa of scapula

I = Lesser tubercle of humerus

Resisted Test: The client is standing, arm bent 90 degrees, with the elbow tucked in at the side. Pin the client's elbow at the side with one hand and keep the client's wrist straight and supported with your other hand. The client medially rotates the shoulder using 20 percent force against your resistance. You control the test. That means you can increase the intensity of the test, if he or she is unsure about a minor muscle–tendon strain, by moving the shoulder into the opposite direction of the client's gentle contraction. Ask the client to point to the specific spot of pain. This particular injury is rare because the subscapularis tendon is very thick, deep, and well protected by more superficial muscles that are more likely to get injured (Figure 5-10 ■).

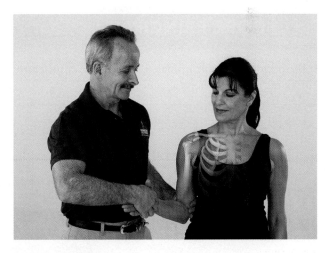

FIGURE 5-10
Muscle Resistance Test, Subscapularis.

Pectoralis Minor

A = Depresses the scapula; downward rotation of the scapula

O = Third, fourth, and fifth ribs

I = Coracoid process of scapula

Resisted Test: The client is standing, with the arm being tested at 135 degrees of shoulder abduction, and the palm facing forward. Stand in front of the client with one hand on the shoulder to stabilize it, and with one hand on the distal end of the humerus. The client attempts to bring the arm across his or her body toward the opposite hip using 20 percent force against your resistance. You control the test. If there is a muscle–tendon strain, the pain is usually at the coracoid process (Figure 5-11 ■).

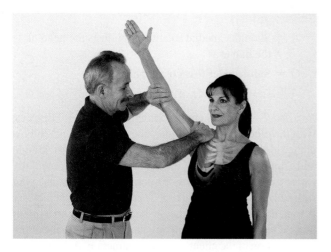

FIGURE 5-11
Muscle Resistance Test, Pectoralis Minor.

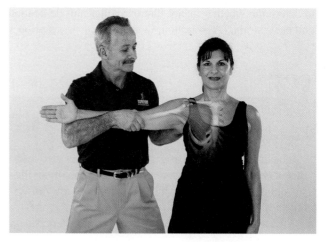

FIGURE 5-12
Muscle Resistance Test, Pectoralis Major.

CORE PRINCIPLE

The pectoralis minor, if injured, can be one of the contributing causes of thoracic outlet syndrome.

Pectoralis Major

CORE PRINCIPLE

This muscle is rarely injured, so this test is seldom performed.

A = Both origins adduct and medially rotate the shoulder. The clavicular origin flexes the shoulder and the sternal origin extends the shoulder.

O = Medial half of clavicle, sternum, cartilage of ribs one to six.

I = Crest of greater tubercle of humerus.

Resisted Test: The client is standing, arm at the side at 90-degree abduction, with the palm facing forward. Place one hand on the client's elbow, the other on the shoulder to stabilize it. The client moves the shoulder to horizontal adduction using 20 percent force against your resistance. You control the test. Ask the client to point to the specific area of discomfort (Figure 5-12 ■).

Supraspinatus

A = Shoulder abduction; stabilizes the head of the humerus

O = Supraspinous fossa of scapula

I = Greater tubercle of humerus

Resisted Test: The client is standing, arm at the side abducted 20 to 30 degrees, with the palm facing backward (pronated, thumb facing toward the body). Place one hand above the client's elbow, the other on the client's hip to stabilize it. The client resists shoulder adduction with you controlling the amount of pressure applied for the test. Have him or her point to the painful area This test will usually only be positive if there is a significant strain in the supraspinatus. The injury will usually be at the muscle–tendon junction under the acromion (Figure 5-13 ■).

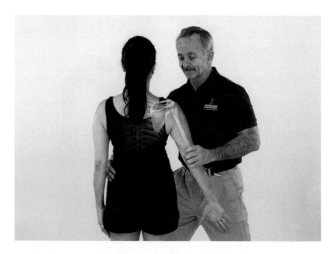

FIGURE 5-13
Muscle Resistance Test, Supraspinatus.

Infraspinatus

A = Shoulder lateral rotation, shoulder abduction; stabilizes the head of the humerus

O = Infraspinous fossa of scapula

I = Greater tubercle of humerus

Resisted Test: The client is standing, elbow bent 90 degrees, with the *arm* 10 degrees abducted away from the side. He or she laterally rotates the shoulder using 20 percent force against your resistance. You control the test. Make sure to stabilize the client's elbow at the side with one hand and also keep his or her wrist straight and supported with your other hand. If there is discomfort, have the client pinpoint the exact area, by pointing to it (Figure 5-14 ■).

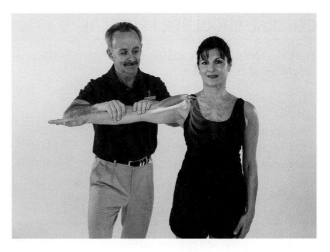

FIGURE 5-15
Muscle Resistance Test, Middle Deltoid.

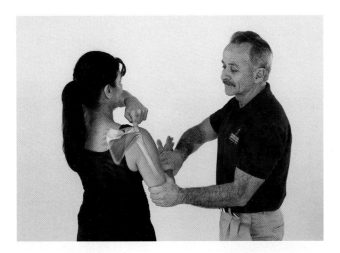

FIGURE 5-14
Muscle Resistance Test, Infraspinatus, and Teres Minor.

Teres Minor

A = Shoulder lateral rotation, shoulder adduction; stabilizes the head of the humerus

O = Superior half of lateral border of scapula

I = Greater tubercle of humerus

Resisted Test: Use the same test as for the infraspinatus (Figure 5-14).

Middle Deltoid

A = Shoulder abduction

O = Lateral border of acromion process

I = Deltoid tuberosity

Resisted Test: The client's arm is abducted 90 degrees at the side of the body, with the palm facing down. The therapist places his or her hands above and below the clients elbow. The client abducts the shoulder using 20 percent force against your resistance. You control the test. If

there is pain, have the client point to it with one finger (Figure 5-15 ■).

Rhomboid Major and Minor

A = Scapula adduction, elevation, and downward rotation

O = Major: spinous processes T2 to T5; minor: spinous processes C7, T1

I = Medial border of scapula between spine of scapula and inferior angle

Resisted Test: The client's arms are crossed in front of the body at 90-degree abduction. The therapist places his or her hands on the client's elbows. The client pulls the elbows back, and tries to pull the scapulas together using 20 percent force against your resistance. You control the test. Have him or her point to the specific spot of pain (Figure 5-16 ■).

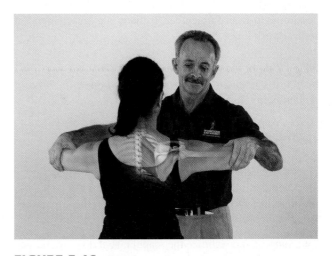

FIGURE 5-16
Muscle Resistance Test, Rhomboid Major and Minor.

GENERAL SHOULDER PROTOCOL

There is a specific order for releasing and balancing the muscle groups of the shoulder:

1. Pectoralis major
2. Pectoralis minor
3. Subclavius
4. Biceps and coracobrachialis
5. Upper trapezius and middle deltoid
6. Subscapularis
7. Rhomboids
8. Triceps brachii and posterior deltoid
9. Scapular reposition
10. Supraspinatus and upper trapezius
11. Infraspinatus and teres minor

The protocol may change, however, depending on the problems found during the initial range of motion assessments. The goal is to bring muscle groups of the shoulder back to their normal resting states, creating structural balance, normal range of motion, and joint capsule release for pain-free movement.

Work superficial to deep, one muscle at a time. Start with the client supine to release the tight anterior muscles first. This takes the tension off the weak, inhibited, or overstretched posterior muscles, which are typically full of tender points. These tender points are myofascial pain patterns that cannot be effectively treated like muscle belly trigger points. Once the opposing muscle groups of the shoulder are balanced, the tender points often will disappear.

As you balance and release all of the muscle groups surrounding the shoulder, be aware of the difference between soft-tissue restrictions, muscle strains, emotional guarding, and joint capsule adhesions. If at anytime you find a bone-on-bone-like end feel, stop the protocol and go to the joint capsule work. (See video clip at www.myhealthprofessionskit.com) If you feel as if you are chasing the client's pain, because the location keeps changing, it is most likely caused by myofascial restrictions. Stay attuned to the client and keep the session pain-free. Remember, if there is a muscle–tendon injury, work it last.

Note: If there isn't a muscle–tendon injury, do not apply deep cross-fiber or multidirectional friction to the area of tendon pain.

Joint Capsule Work

As previously stated, this unique technique is one of the author's trademark techniques. It will be used whenever any shoulder range of motion end feel appears to be bone-on-bone-like. With the client supine, abduct the arm to the first bone-on-bone-like restriction.

- Support and stabilize the scapula, so it does not move, from either on top of or under the client's shoulder with one hand, using evenly displaced pressure.

PRECAUTIONARY NOTE

If the client tested positive for a muscle–tendon strain, it is highly recommended that you bring that muscle back to resting length, and treat the strain prior to attempting joint capsule work. If the client is guarded due to shoulder discomfort during the capsule work, you will not be able to access and release the deep fascial adhesions inside the shoulder capsule.

- Use your other hand to hold the arm just proximal to the elbow.
- Perform a gentle plunging technique using the head of the humerus as a massage tool. This mimics a mortar and pestle effect. Gently and slowly compress the humerus into the joint capsule simulating your hands coming together (Figure 5-17A ■).

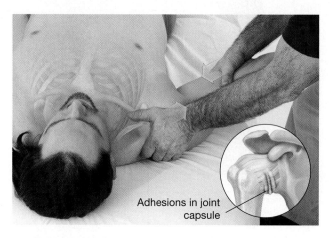

Adhesions in joint capsule

FIGURE 5-17A
Joint Capsule Release, Compression.

- Ask the client if this is uncomfortable. It usually isn't, as you are actually shortening the fascial adhesions and taking the pressure off the joint capsule. Have the client relax and visualize the capsule softening and letting go.
- Make contact in the joint capsule, using the cartilage of the humerus to massage the fascia gluing it against the cartilage of the scapula.
- Rotate the arm gently, and then pull back out. Contract the scapula, rotate the humerus, and then decompress the scapula. Continually repeating this sequence allows the head of the humerus to soften and mobilize the fascia deep inside the joint capsule, because what can create myofascial release is heat, pressure, movement, and gentle, slow-velocity fascial stretching.
- Make your plunges nonsynchronized and then slowly stretch the inner fascia and surrounding joint capsule

when the client least expects it, to prevent him or her from guarding or helping during this work.

● Rotate the arm externally to the restriction and repeat the plunging technique several times. Then perform a deep fascial and capsular stretch externally. Back off the stretch, return to neutral position, and then pull back out of the joint capsule (Figure 5-17B ■). See video clip at www.myhealthprofessionskit.com

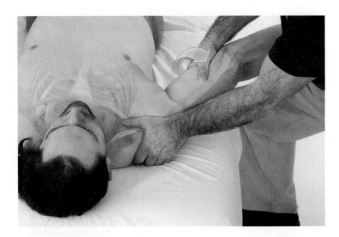

FIGURE 5-17B
Joint Capsule Release, External Rotation.

● Next, rotate the arm internally to the restriction and repeat the plunging technique several times, ending with a deep fascial and capsular stretch internally. Back off the stretch, return to neutral, and then pull back out. Repeat the sequence again, if needed (Figure 5-17C ■).
● Decompress the joint capsule (Figure 5-17D ■).
● For hand placement doing the same technique to the left shoulder, refer to Figure 5-18 ■.

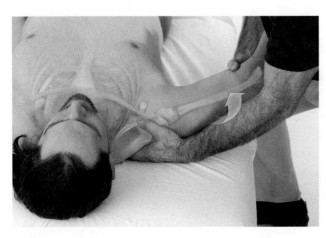

FIGURE 5-17C
Joint Capsule Release, Internal Rotation.

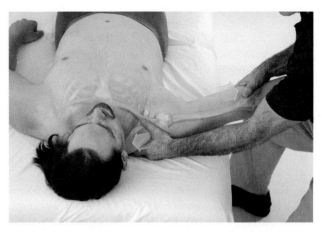

FIGURE 5-17D
Joint Capsule Release, Decompression.

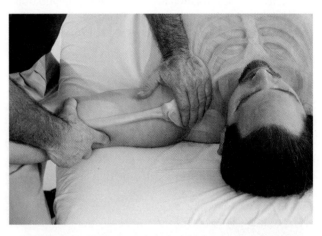

FIGURE 5-18
Joint Capsule Work, Different Hand Position for Left Arm.

You must rotate the arm to the left and to the right because there could be multiple adhesions in different directions and also at different degrees of abduction. Most people have more lateral rotation restriction due to tight medial shoulder rotators, therefore more restrictions will usually be found as you move toward lateral rotation and progress into further abduction. With a large client you can rest the arm on your hip and initiate the plunging action from your hip. You may feel some popping and releasing of the fascia as you create more freedom in the joint capsule. It is critical to perform this work *totally pain-free,* as even minor guarding prevents effective joint capsule work.

CORE PRINCIPLE

You must change the protocol and perform the joint capsule work anytime during the session if you find a bone-on-bone-like end feel.

"Velvet Glove" Technique

George Kousaleos's "velvet glove" technique is a myofascial release technique performed on the upper trapezius and cervical muscles to warm and stretch the connective tissue to be able to affect the deeper muscles. This also helps move the fascia back toward the spine, where it belongs, to allow a more neutral neck posture. Before beginning the velvet glove technique, here are some basics:

- The client is supine.
- Sit at the head of the table.
- The client slowly rotates his or her head, only to where it is comfortable, away from the side you are working on during all four strokes. Tell him or her to keep the neck straight and do not allow lateral flexion to occur. The hair should be heard rolling across the table. Active cervical rotation activates reciprocal inhibition, which may enhance the release. Place one hand on the client's forehead to control the speed of rotation.

- Use the back of your other hand in a loose fist, leading with your fingers, to perform the velvet glove myofascial release technique.
- The first three strokes will overlap as you work distal to proximal up the cervical spine.
- Use slow, smooth, progressively deeper strokes. See video clip at www.myhealthprofessionskit.com

To use the velvet glove technique, perform the four strokes as follows:

1. Start just above (superior to) the clavicle and move the back of your hand down over the upper trapezius, hooking the tissue and bringing it toward the table and the spine (Figure 5-19A ■).
2. The next stroke is over the curve of the neck, again hooking the tissue while moving the back of your fist toward the table (Figure 5-19B ■).
3. The third stroke goes over the entire cervical spine. Hook or catch the SCM (sternocleidomastoid)

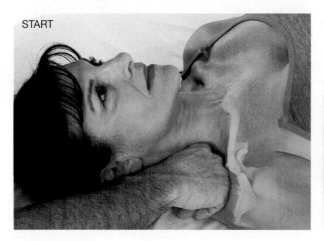
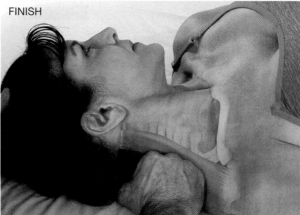

FIGURE 5-19A
Myofascial Release, Upper Trapezius (Ends at Spinous Processes).

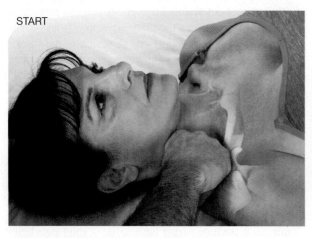
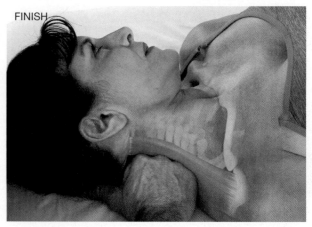

FIGURE 5-19B
Myofascial Release, Upper Trapezius/Curve of Neck (Overlaps Previous Stroke by About 50 percent).

START

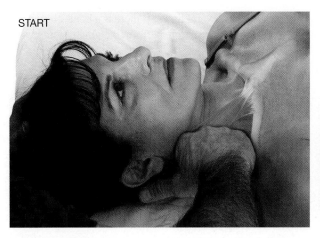

FINISH

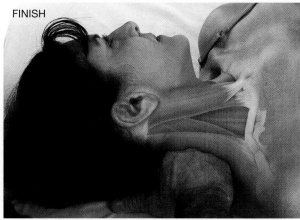

FIGURE 5-19C
Myofascial Release, SCM and Trapezius.

START

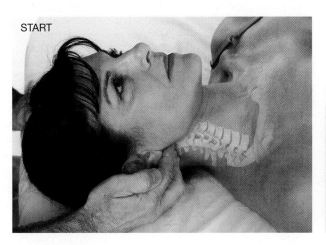

FINISH

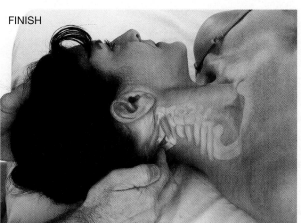

FIGURE 5-19D
Myofascial Release, Suboccipital Attachments.

and the scalenes to bring them into the myofascial release. This will effectively start to increase blood flow to the area of the SCM and scalene muscles. Stay off the carotid artery. If you feel a pulse, don't apply any pressure, and reposition your hand. (Figure 5-19C ■).

4. Use your fingerpads and work the suboccipitals under the base of the skull, moving lateral to medial. Tight suboccipital muscles can create ischemic **vascular headaches,** C1 and C2 immobilization, and pain. For clients who experience **migraine headaches**, repeat this stroke multiple times (Figure 5-19D ■).

Repeat the entire velvet glove sequence, strokes 1 to 4, several times. The neck may look like it is sunburned when you are through, as this technique brings increased blood flow **(hyperemia)** to the area.

PECTORALIS MAJOR

The pectoralis major is a powerful, superficial chest muscle; it is worked and stretched first so that you can access the deeper pectoralis minor and subclavius fibers. It originates on the medial half of the clavicle, the sternum, and cartilage of ribs one to six. It inserts on the crest of greater tubercle of humerus. Both origins adduct and medially rotate the shoulder. The clavicular origin flexes the shoulder and the sternal origin extends the shoulder.

Step 5: Area Preparation

Goal: apply only two drops of a light lubricant with palmer friction to help warm and mobilize the superficial fascia of the pectoralis major. This will help you restore normal muscle resting length to the pectoralis major before beginning deeper and more specific work.

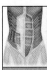

CORE PRINCIPLE

Treat the cause of pain before the symptoms or specific area of pain.

The client is supine on the table. If you are working on a female, you can have her place her opposite hand on her breast tissue and push it down and lateral to hold it in place out of your way.

Step 6: Myofascial Release

Goal: to warm up, soften, and mobilize the fascia and to move the fascial layers back to normal, neutral position.

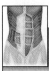

CORE PRINCIPLE

Always perform myofascial release *before* proceeding to deeper, more specific work.

- Stand at the side of the table. Start at the sternal insertion of the pectoralis major to affect the inferior fibers of the muscle.
- Work diagonally up toward the top of the shoulder with a myofascial stroke using the palm of your hand.
- Use your other hand to hold the client's wrist and gently rock the arm, with their elbow bent at 90 degrees, to help relax and distract the client.
- As you finish the stroke near the top of the shoulder, laterally rotate the humerus to effectively stretch the pectoralis major (Figure 5-20A ■).

- Repeat this several times. If there is a bone-on-bone-like end feel on this stretch, perform the joint capsule work.

Next, start at the sternalclavicular location and using the heel and palm. Of your hand follow the medial fibers of the pectoralis major outward along the inferior angle of the clavicle onto the arm, as you continue to rock the arm and draw the humerus laterally, with the shoulder abducted 90 degrees. Repeat this stroke several times, working progressively deeper. Avoid pressing on any bony landmarks during both strokes.(Figure 5-20B ■).

Step 7: Cross-Fiber Gliding Strokes/Trigger Point Therapy

CROSS-FIBER GLIDING STROKES

Goal: to tease apart tight pectoralis major muscle bands (contracted, shortened muscle group).

Use cross-fiber gliding strokes to tease through and gently spread any tight muscle bands. This will loosen up tight muscle fibers that often feed and contribute to trigger points, allowing the tissue to move more freely and independently. Tight muscles, with pain located directly under your pressure? This requires cross-fiber gliding strokes working from origin to insertion on the pectoralis major. Start at the sternal insertion of the pectoralis major to affect the inferior fibers of the muscle and work diagonally up toward the top of the shoulder. Continue to work the entire muscle belly from origin to insertion to restore normal muscle resting length.

TRIGGER POINT THERAPY

Goal: to release trigger points in the muscle belly, if found.

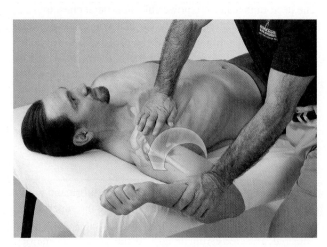

FIGURE 5-20A
Myofascial Release, Inferior Fibers Pectoralis Major.

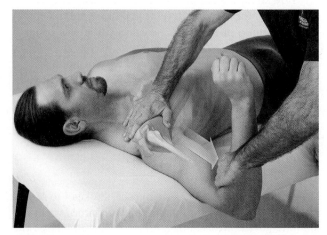

FIGURE 5-20B
Myofacial Release, Superior Fibers Pectoralis Major.

CORE PRINCIPLE

You should first perform trigger point work on the contracted, tight muscles, before addressing weak, inhibited muscle groups.

If there is a specific area of pain that radiates or refers when direct pressure is applied, and this referral pain pattern can be predicted and mapped out as described by Dr. Janet Travell, apply sustained direct pressure for 10 to 12 seconds.

- As the trigger point softens, compress the tissue several times.
- Gently stretch through the tissue.

PECTORALIS MINOR

The pectoralis minor lies deep to the pectoralis major. It originates on the third, fourth, and fifth ribs and inserts on the coracoid process. It abducts the scapula and draws it anteriorly and downward. It also raises the ribs in forced inhalation (if the scapula is stabilized). It is imperative to work the pectoralis minor, as it is one of the multifaceted causes of thoracic outlet syndrome.

Step 5: Area Preparation

Goal: to prepare the pectoralis minor for best access before starting myofascial release.

The client is supine on the table. If you are working on a female, you can have her place her hand on her breast tissue and push it down and lateral to hold it in place out of your way. This will give the therapist better access to treat the pectoralis minor.

Step 7: Cross-Fiber Gliding Strokes/Trigger Point Therapy

CROSS-FIBER GLIDING STROKES

Goal: to tease apart tight pectoralis minor muscle bands (contracted, shortened muscle).

- Stand or sit at the head of the table.
- The client's arm is at the side, shoulder medially rotated with the hand across the body. This position relaxes the pectoralis major.
- Work the pectoralis minor with a cross-fiber gliding stroke, using the knuckles or two to three fingers, from the third, fourth, and fifth ribs to just before the attachment on the coracoid process (origin to insertion). Be careful to not apply pressure to the coracoid process at the end of the stroke. Be attuned to the client when you work the inferior fibers, as they may be tender. You can slow down the stroke or lighten your pressure if the stroke is not comfortable, but try to stay deep.
- Repeat the strokes several times (Figure 5-21 ■).

You can also access the pectoralis minor via the armpit. Stand at the client's side. Lift up and go under the lateral edge of the pectoralis major. Use your thumbs and strum the fibers of the pectoralis minor to tease the tight muscle fibers apart. If you want to make sure you are on the pectoralis minor, have the client depress the shoulder (Figure 5-22 ■).

TRIGGER POINT THERAPY

Goal: to release trigger points in the muscle belly if found.

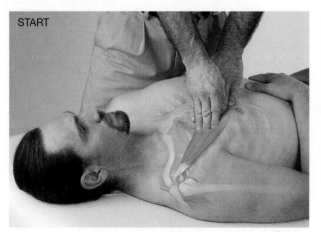
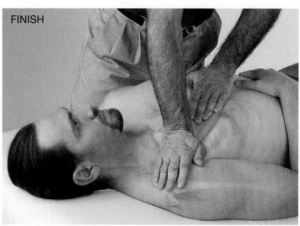

FIGURE 5-21
Cross-Fiber Gliding Strokes and Compressive Stretch, Pectoralis Minor.

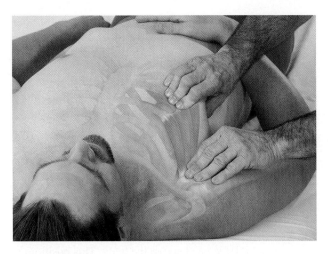

FIGURE 5-22
Work Pectoralis Minor using Thumbs under Pectoralis Major.

CORE PRINCIPLE

You should primarily perform trigger point work on the contracted, tight muscles groups prior to treating the weak, inhibited muscle groups.

If there is a specific area of pain that radiates or refers, when moderate direct pressure is applied, use trigger point therapy.

- Apply sustained direct, moderate pressure for 10 to 12 seconds.
- As the trigger point softens, compress the tissue several times.
- Gently stretch through the tissue.

Step 11: Stretching (During Therapy)

Goal: to restore normal muscle resting lengths.

PRECAUTIONARY NOTE

Stretching is not suggested for the muscle groups around a hypermobile joint. Strengthening would be more appropriate to stabilize any joint that has excessive movement due to ligamentous laxity.

CORE PRINCIPLE

Contracting the muscle against resistance to fatigue the muscle prior to the stretch becomes a muscle resistance test and the client may report pain in a specific area, which is a muscle strain. If so, proceed to multidirectional friction (step 8), pain-free movement (step 9), and eccentric scar tissue alignment (step 10) until the client is pain-free.

- Reposition the client so that the shoulder closest to you is on the edge of the table.
- The client's arm is straight and the shoulder abducted 135 degrees.
- Stabilize the uninvolved shoulder.
- Ask the client to take the arm across the body toward the opposite hip at 20 percent force for 5 to 10 seconds while you provide resistance.
- Have the client relax, inhale, and then on exhale have the client engages the antagonist muscles by moving the arm and shoulder toward the table and floor while you assist the stretch for about 2 seconds (Figure 5-23 ■).

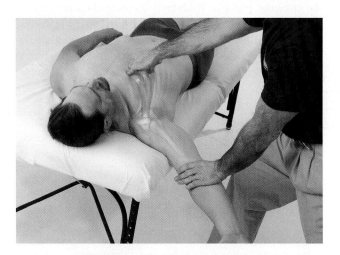

FIGURE 5-23
Pectoralis Minor Hand Placement for Stretch.

- At this new position, repeat the contract-relax, contract-antagonist with active assisted stretching two or three times or just until you stretch the muscle back to it's normal resting length.

To enhance this stretch, place three fingers close to the origin of the pectoralis minor and pin the attachments of that muscle down while performing the stretch (Figure 5-24 ■). While you are stretching this muscle the client may complain of pain in the back of the shoulder. As you release the anterior shoulder muscles, the overstretched posterior muscles may have no space to move into. If that is the case,

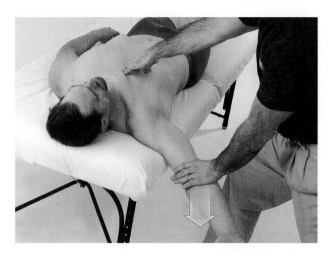

FIGURE 5-24
Hand Placement and Direction of Pectoralis Minor Stretch.

change the protocol. Have the client turn over and perform myofascial spreading to the posterior shoulder to create space for movement into the back of the shoulder. See the infraspinatus and teres minor myofascial release section; then return to this section and continue the protocol.

Note: Myofascial release can be done to the back of the shoulder, for just a minute or two, prior to starting the entire anterior shoulder protocol, to avoid this last step from being needed. However, do not do specific work to weak inhibited muscles in the back of the shoulder prior to releasing the short, tight anterior shoulder muscles.

If you feel a bone-on-bone-like end feel during this stretch, you may need to perform joint capsule work again and then return to the stretch.

 CORE PRINCIPLE

Sometimes during this stretch the client can experience parasthesia (pins and needles sensation), tingling or numbness into the arm, hand, and fingers. Don't be alarmed, as this is the probably the result of the shortened pectoralis minor and subclavius *temporarily* pressing on the brachial plexus of nerves. After the muscle is lengthened, and the shoulder relaxed, the increased temporary sensations should quickly disappear.

Step 8: Multidirectional Friction

Goal: to soften the collagen matrix by working in multiple directions to prepare for a more functional mobilization of scar tissue fibers.

 **CORE PRINCIPLE**

If there is not a muscle–tendon strain or ligament sprain, multidirectional friction would *not* be part of the treatment.

- Pain during the contraction against resistance or the stretch? Ask the client to isolate the painful area by pointing to it (Figure 5-25 ■).
- Put your finger on the spot and ask if the pain is directly under your finger. If so, this is a muscle strain, which will most likely be at the muscle–tendon junction.
- Perform multidirectional friction to the specific area to free up the scar tissue that is causing the pain (Figure 5-26 ■).
- Use a supported finger and work for only 20 to 30 seconds each time.

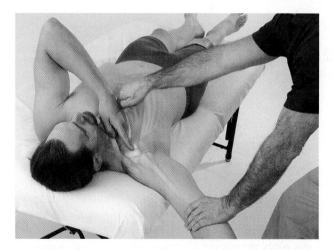

FIGURE 5-25
Muscle Resistance Test For Pectoralis Minor Strain.

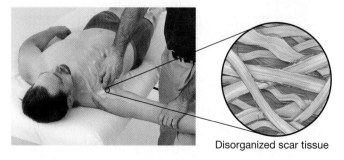

Disorganized scar tissue

FIGURE 5-26
Pectoralis Minor Multidirectional Friction.

PRECAUTIONARY NOTE

Do not overwork the area and create inflammation.

Step 9: Pain-Free Movement

Goal: to determine if the client can actively move the arm from 135-degree abduction to the opposite hip and back without pain. If so, this gives permission to proceed with pain-free eccentric scar tissue alignment techniques.

This begins the process of realigning the scar tissue. Ask the client to move the arm from the position of 135-degree shoulder abduction to the opposite hip and then back. Have him or her repeat this several times to begin to redirect or align the injured fibers.

- Pain-free? Proceed to step 10.
- Pain? Repeat step 8, working slower and deeper, but still pain-free. Repeat step 9 and then proceed to step 10 when there is no pain.

Step 10: Eccentric Scar Tissue Alignment

Goal: to apply pain-free eccentric contraction by lengthening an injured pectoralis minor against mild resistance to realign or redirect the scar tissue.

PRECAUTIONARY NOTE

After surgery, do not disrupt the proper healing of scar tissue by beginning this protocol too soon. Consult the client's physician before treatment. Do not proceed with the eccentric muscle contraction if the previous movement is not pain-free.

CORE PRINCIPLE

The greatest error during the eccentric alignment procedure is being too aggressive and not keeping the technique pain-free each time. Too much force in opposing directions can cause a new injury or reinjure the site.

Apply eccentric contraction to realign the deeper scar tissue. It must be performed pain-free.

- Have the client abduct the shoulder to 135 degrees. He or she begins to bring the arm across the body toward the other hip.
- Have the client resist gentle abduction performed by you.
- Tell him or her to "barely resist, but let me win." Use a two-finger pressure to start and have the client increase resistance only if there is zero discomfort (Figure 5-27 ■).
- You can use your other hand to stabilize the origin of the pectoralis minor.
- Repeat this several times, pain-free.
- This work promotes functional or aligned scar tissue.

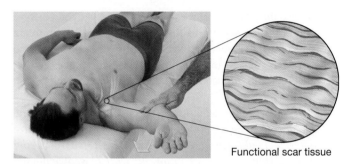

Functional scar tissue

FIGURE 5-27
Eccentric Muscle Contraction for Scar Tissue Alignment.

Step 4: Assess Resisted Range of Motion (RROM)

Goal: to reassess if there is still a pectoralis minor muscle strain present and exactly where it is located.

Perform the pectoralis minor resisted test.

- The client is supine with the arm at 135-degree of shoulder abduction, with the palm facing forward.
- Stand in front of the client with one hand on the shoulder to stabilize it, and with one hand on the distal end of the humerus.
- The client gently attempts to bring the arm across the body using only 20 percent of their strength toward the opposite hip against your resistance.
- You control the force of the test by applying a counter force if needed to recruit the deepest fibers.
- Pain? Repeat steps 8 through 10. Then perform the resisted test again.
- Pain-free? Finish with step 11 when there is no longer any pain.

PRECAUTIONARY NOTE

Do not move too fast, or use too much force while performing a resisted test.

SUBCLAVIUS

The subclavius is located deep to the pectoralis major, underneath the clavicle. Its action is to elevate the first rib and move the clavicle anteriorly and inferiorly. It also stabilizes the sternoclavicular joint.

Step 7: Cross-Fiber Gliding Strokes/Trigger Point Therapy

CROSS-FIBER GLIDING STROKES

Goal: to tease apart tight subclavius muscle bands (contracted, shortened muscle).

- Stand at the side of the table.
- Relax the client's shoulder and hook or scoop under the clavicle near the sternoclavicular joint with two fingers.
- Keep your fingers closest to the midline curled under, so they are not on the client's throat, as this could trigger an emotional response.
- Use a cross-fiber gliding stroke and work from the sternum outward, medial to lateral (Figure 5-28 ■).
- Tease through tight muscle fibers with cross-fiber gliding strokes to release the subclavius.
- This will also slightly affect the anterior scalene muscle. Clearing out this inferior clavicular region may help eliminate a contributing factor in thoracic outlet

syndrome. This book will take a much closer look at the critical role that the anterior and posterior scalenes play in causing thoracic outlet problems in the cervical chapter.
- You must communicate with the client. If the area is tender, you are probably working the correct muscles, since the subclavius can be very hypertonic and ischemic. If it hurts or is extremely uncomfortable, you are working too fast or too deep.

TRIGGER POINT THERAPY

Goal: to release trigger points in the subclavius muscle belly, if found.

CORE PRINCIPLE

You should primarily perform trigger point work on the contracted, tight muscles, prior to addressing weak, inhibited muscle groups.

If there is a specific area of pain that radiates or refers when direct pressure is applied, apply trigger point therapy.

- Use direct, moderate pressure for 10 to 12 seconds.
- As the trigger point softens, compress the tissue several times.
- Gently stretch through the tissue.

Step 11: Stretching (During Therapy)

Goal: to restore normal muscle resting lengths.

CORE PRINCIPLE

Contracting the muscle against resistance to fatigue the muscle prior to the stretch becomes a muscle resistance test and the client may report pain in a specific area, which is a muscle strain. If so, proceed to multidirectional friction (step 8), pain-free movement (step 9), and eccentric scar tissue alignment (step 10) until the client is pain-free.

- Gently grasp the client's elbow with the arm abducted 90 degrees and move the shoulder and arm laterally.
- Pin down the front of the client's shoulder and ask him or her to lift up into your hand with 20 percent force for 5 to 10 seconds. Make sure you shape your

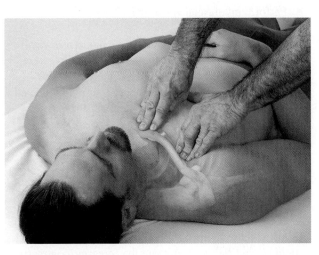

FIGURE 5-28
Subclavius Myofascial Release.

hand to stay off the coracoid process and any other bony prominence.

- Have the client relax, inhale, and then on exhale you draw the shoulder laterally and the client actively brings it posteriorly toward the table with your assistance for about 2 seconds (Figure 5-29 ■).
- At this new position repeat the contract-relax, contract-antagonist with active assisted stretching two or three times if needed to restore normal muscle resting length.

CORE PRINCIPLE

During this stretch the client may experience parasthesia, numbness, or tingling into the arm, hand, or fingers. Don't be alarmed, as this is probably the result of a shortened subclavius and pectoralis minor *temporarily* pressing on the brachial plexus of nerves. This will diminish when you relax the tissue, after the stretch.

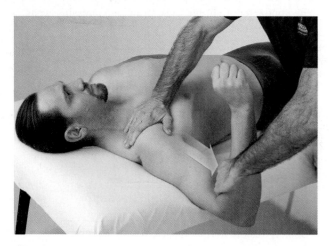

FIGURE 5-29
Subclavius Stretch.

BICEPS AND CORACOBRACHIALIS

The biceps is a superficial muscle on the anterior arm. It has a long and a short head which merge to form the belly of the muscle. It flexes the elbow and the shoulder and supinates the forearm. Typically, an injury will occur to the tendon of the long head of the biceps.

The coracobrachialis flexes and adducts the shoulder. It originates at the coracoid process and this is where an injury usually occurs.

Step 5: Area Preparation

Goal: to prepare the biceps or coracobrachialis for myofascial release.

The client is supine with the arm supinated and supported on the massage table.

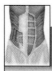

CORE PRINCIPLE

Do *not* use ice on the muscle belly unless there is inflammation (heat, redness, or swelling). Ice may cause the fascia to become less mobile and restricts movement. This is counterproductive to the mobilizing and healing process, which the therapy work is promoting.

CORE PRINCIPLE

Treat the cause of pain before the symptoms or specific area of pain.

Step 6: Myofascial Release

Goal: to warm up, soften, and mobilize the biceps or coracobrachialis fascia.

CORE PRINCIPLE

Always perform myofascial release *before* proceeding to deeper, more specific work.

- Perform myofascial spreading 45 degrees into the tissue.
- Work proximal to distal, down the humerus away from the tendon attachments. This will help restore normal muscle resting lengths. (Figure 5-30A ■).
- Alternate with light compressions to bring blood and oxygen to the muscle belly (Figure 5-30B ■).

Step 7: Cross-Fiber Gliding Strokes/Trigger Point Therapy

CROSS-FIBER GLIDING STROKES

Goal: to tease apart tight muscle groups that flex the shoulder and flex and supinate the forearm (contracted, shortened muscles).

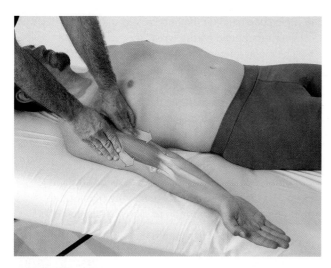

FIGURE 5-30A
Biceps Myofascial Release.

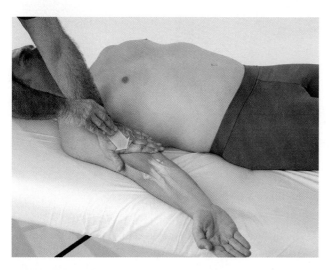

FIGURE 5-30B
Compression Stretch, Biceps.

Use cross-fiber gliding strokes to tease through and gently spread any tight muscle bands. This will loosen up tight muscle fibers that often feed and contribute to active trigger points, allowing the tissue to move more freely and independently.

- Tight muscles, with pain located directly under your pressure?
- This requires cross-fiber gliding strokes working from origin to insertion (proximal to distal) on muscles such as the biceps and coracobrachialis.

TRIGGER POINT THERAPY

Goal: to release trigger points in the biceps or coracobrachialis muscle belly, if found.

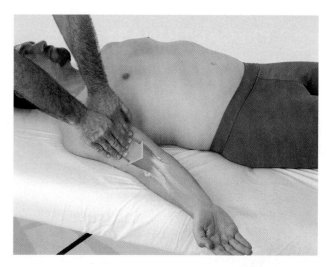

FIGURE 5-30C
Cross-Fiber Gliding Strokes/Trigger Point Work.

CORE PRINCIPLE

You should perform trigger point work on the contracted, tight muscles, before addressing the weak, inhibited muscle groups.

If there is a specific area of pain that radiates or refers when direct pressure is applied, apply trigger point therapy.

- Use direct, moderate pressure for 10 to 12 seconds.
- As the trigger point softens, compress the tissue several times (Figure 5-30C ■).
- Gently stretch through the tissue.

Step 11: Stretching (During Therapy)

Goal: to create the normal 50- to 60-degree range of motion of shoulder extension.

CORE PRINCIPLE

Contracting the muscle against resistance to fatigue the muscle prior to the stretch becomes a muscle resistance test and the client may report pain in a specific area, which is a muscle strain. If so, proceed to multidirectional friction (step 8), pain-free movement (step 9), and eccentric scar tissue alignment (step 10) until the client is pain-free.

✋ PRECAUTIONARY NOTE

Do not stretch beyond normal range of motion, as this could create hypermobile joints and result in injury.

To stretch the proximal biceps and coracobrachialis:

- To stretch the upper fibers of the biceps, have the client move so that the shoulder is still supported on the table, but the arm is off the table.
- The client's arm is straight at the side, palm facing up, and supinated.
- Place your hands above and below the client's elbow.
- The client flexes the shoulder against your resistance with 20 percent force for 5 to 10 seconds.
- He or she relaxes, takes a deep breath, and on exhale extends the arm toward the floor with your assistance for about 2 seconds (Figure 5-31 ▪).
- At this new position, repeat the contract-relax, contract-antagonist with active assisted stretching two or three times or until achieving the normal 50- to 60-degree range of motion of shoulder extension.

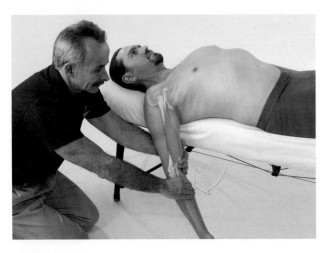

FIGURE 5-31
Contract-Relax Stretch, Upper Biceps.

Step 11: Stretching (During Therapy)

Goal: to create the normal 0-degree range of motion of elbow extension.

To stretch the distal biceps:

- To stretch the lower fibers of the biceps, have the client move so that the shoulder and humerus are still supported on the table, but the forearm is off the table.
- The client's arm is straight at the side, palm facing up, supinated.

- Place one hand on the humerus to stabilize it. Place your other hand on the wrist.
- The client attempts to flex the elbow and supinate the forearm against your resistance with 20 percent force for 5 to 10 seconds.
- He or she relaxes, takes a deep breath, and on exhale the client fully extends the elbow and pronates the forearm with your assistance for about 2 seconds (Figure 5-32 ▪).
- At this new position, repeat the contract-relax, contract-antagonist with active assisted stretching two or three times or until achieving the normal 0-degree range of motion of elbow extension.

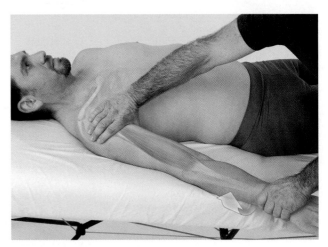

FIGURE 5-32
Distal Bicep Stretch.

This may prevent bicipital tendon aponeurosis strain. Tendinosis to the distal biceps aponeurosis on the proximal head of the ulna can scar down the median nerve and create symptoms similar to medial epicondylitis and carpal tunnel syndrome.

Note: The test for bicipital aponeurosis tendinosis will be shown in Chapter 7, with elbow, forearm, wrist, and hand conditions. This is one of the contributing muscles creating pain in the area of the medial epicondyle. It is often generically called medial epicondylitis, even though the biceps tendon and biceps apeneurosis attaches below the medial epicondyle. Make sure to restore normal muscle resting length to the biceps using this part of the shoulder protocol prior to treating that strain if the test for bicipital aponeurosis tendinosis is positive.

Step 8: Multidirectional Friction

A proximal biceps strain to the long head of the biceps in the bicipital groove or a strain to the coracobrachialis and short head of the biceps at the attachment on the coracoid process is much more common than a distal biceps strain involving the bicipital aponeurosis just below the elbow. The muscle

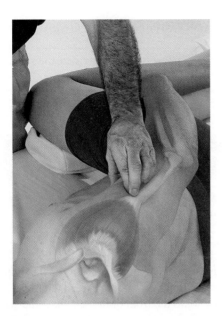

FIGURE 5-38B
Multidirectional Friction, Middle Deltoid.

PRECAUTIONARY NOTE

Do not overwork the area and create inflammation.

Step 9: Pain-Free Movement

Goal: to determine if the client can actively perform shoulder abduction and adduction without pain. If so, this gives permission to proceed with pain-free eccentric scar tissue alignment techniques.

Ask the client to move the shoulder through abduction and adduction several times to initiate the process of realigning the strained fibers.

- Pain-free? Proceed to step 10.
- Pain? Repeat step 8, working slower and deeper, but still pain-free. Repeat step 9 and then proceed to step 10 when there is no pain.

Step 10: Eccentric Scar Tissue Alignment

Goal: to apply pain-free eccentric contraction by lengthening an injured middle deltoid against mild resistance to realign or redirect the scar tissue.

PRECAUTIONARY NOTE

After surgery, do not disrupt the proper healing of scar tissue by beginning this protocol too soon. Consult the client's physician before treatment.

CORE PRINCIPLE

The greatest error during the eccentric alignment procedure is being too aggressive and not keeping the technique pain-free each time. Too much force in opposing directions can cause a new injury or reinjure the site.

Apply eccentric contraction to realign the deeper scar tissue. This must be performed pain-free.

- Have the client abduct the straight arm to 90 degrees with the palm facing down.
- Have him or her resist gentle adduction performed by you from 90 degrees of abduction down to 30 degrees.
- Tell the client to "barely resist, but let me win."
- Start with a pressure of only two fingers and then have the client increase resistance only if he or she has no discomfort (Figure 5-39 ■).
- Repeat this several times.

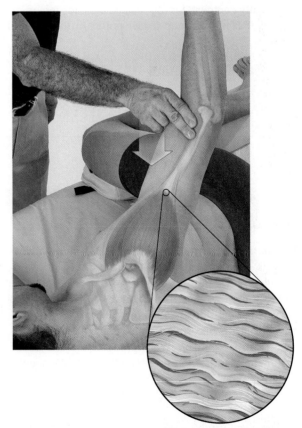

Functional scar tissue

FIGURE 5-39
Eccentric Muscle Contraction, Middle Deltoid.

Step 4: Assess Resisted Range of Motion (RROM)

To reassess RROM, repeat the middle deltoid resisted test. If there is still a specific area of pain, return to multidirectional friction working even slower and deeper, but pain-free and then repeat the eccentric work. Reassess and repeat any or all of the previous steps until the client is pain-free.

The middle deltoid work can also be performed with the client prone or supine.

SUBSCAPULARIS

The deep subscapularis is one of the four rotator cuff muscles, and it is the only one that rotates the shoulder medially. It is located on the anterior surface of the scapula and has a broad, flat, wide tendon where it inserts on the humerus, so it is rarely injured.

When the subscapularis and the pectoralis minor are tight and contracted, the medially rotated position of the shoulder can create an impingement of the fibers of the supraspinatus that will be painful and restrict abduction, but will not show up as a tear. This can lead to supraspinatus tendinosis and possibly contribute to a resultant frozen shoulder. Therefore, it is imperative to release these two muscle groups before working the supraspinatus. Also, a contracted subscapularis creates weak and inhibited or eccentrically contracted infraspinatus and teres minor, creating myofascial pain and tender points in these muscle groups.

Step 5: Area Preparation

Goal: to prepare the subscapularis before performing myofascial release.

CORE PRINCIPLE

Do *not* use ice during myofascial mobilization, unless there is minor inflammation (heat, redness, or swelling). Ice may cause the fascia to become less mobile and restrict movement. If the pain receptors need to be calmed, apply Biofreeze. Otherwise use a warming ointment that has a viscosity to minimize glide, such as Prossage Heat. Ice may be counterproductive to the fascial mobilizing and healing process, which the therapeutic work is promoting.

The client can be worked on side lying, at the edge of the table nearest you, with support under the neck and a bolster under the top bent leg.

Step 6: Myofascial Release

Goal: to warm up, soften, and mobilize the subscapularis fascia.

CORE PRINCIPLE

Always perform myofascial release *before* proceeding to deeper, more specific work.

- The client is side lying.
- Lift up the client's arm toward the ceiling, and place your hand into the armpit between the ribcage and the scapula, onto the front of the scapula—the subscapular fossa.
- Perform gentle, rocking movements to distract and relax the client.
- Then lift the arm toward the opposite side of the table and fold it or "drape" the scapula over your hand. Stabilize the shoulder with your other hand (Figure 5-40A ■).
- Perform gentle compressions using the pads of your fingers into the subscapularis to maximize blood flow.
- Then have the client exhale as you sink a little deeper onto the subscapularis. Perform gentle, slow myofascial strokes with your fingerpads, alternating with compressions.

On the side-lying client perform the above steps and then:

- Gently sink in with your finger pads and engage the inferior and lateral fibers of the subscapularis. Hook the fascia up against the scapula.

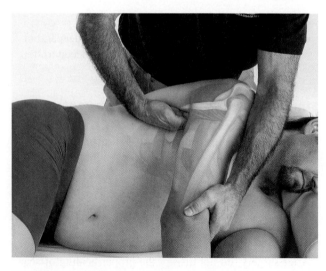
FIGURE 5-40A
Subscapularis Myofascial Release.

- Start to slowly drag and hook the tissue as you depress the shoulder and pull and rotate the inferior scapula back toward the midline several times. This will also stretch the upper trapezius and middle deltoid. Make sure you drag the tissue with a myofascial pull first using the hand under the scapula, and then move the scapula posterior and inferior, rotating it back to where it is supposed to be (Figure 5-40B ■).

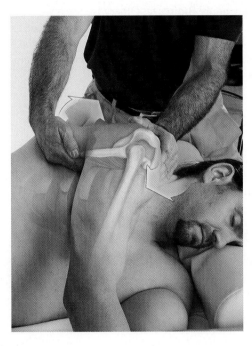

FIGURE 5-40B
Downward Scapular Rotation.

Step 7: Cross-Fiber Gliding Strokes/Trigger Point Therapy

CROSS-FIBER GLIDING STROKES

Goal: to tease apart tight muscle bands in the subscapularis (tight, contracted muscle).

Perform gentle cross-fiber gliding strokes to further soften the tissue. Mobilize the deeper investing fascia with your fingerpads and downward rotate the scapula again, if necessary.

TRIGGER POINT THERAPY

Goal: to release trigger points in the subscapularis muscle belly, if found.

Palpate for trigger points and tender spots which will most likely be at the inferior, lateral border of the scapula. If there is a specific area of pain that radiates or refers when moderate direct pressure is applied, do trigger point therapy.

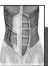
CORE PRINCIPLE

You should primarily perform trigger point work on the contracted, tight muscles, prior to working the weak, inhibited antagonists.

- Use direct, moderate pressure for 10 to 12 seconds.
- As the trigger point softens, compress the tissue several times.
- Gently stretch though the tissue.

Step 11: Stretching (During Therapy)

Goal: to create the normal 80- to 90-degrees range of motion of shoulder lateral rotation.

CORE PRINCIPLE

Contracting the muscle against resistance to fatigue the muscle prior to the stretch becomes a muscle resistance test and the client may report pain in a specific area, which is a muscle strain. If so, proceed to multidirectional friction (step 8), pain-free movement (step 9), and eccentric scar tissue alignment (step 10) until the client is pain-free.

PRECAUTIONARY NOTE

Do not stretch beyond normal range of motion, as this could create hypermobile joints and result in injury.

Side-lying client:

- The client is still side lying, with the elbow bent 90 degrees and tucked in at the side.
- Place one hand on the humerus above the elbow, the other on the forearm and wrist. Rotate the humerus laterally to the restriction, to lengthen the subscapularis muscle.
- Have the client attempt medial rotation of the humerus against your resistance for 5 to 10 seconds with only 20 percent force.
- He or she relaxes, takes a deep breath, and on exhale engages the antagonist muscles and laterally rotates the arm for about 2 seconds.

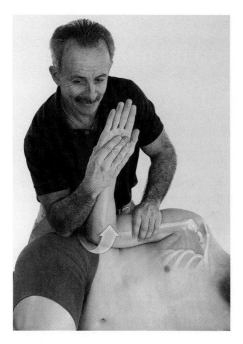

FIGURE 5-41
Subscapularis Stretch.

- You assist by laterally rotating the humerus (Figure 5-41 ■).
- At this new position, the client repeats the contract-relax, contract-antagonist with active assisted stretching two or three times or until achieving the normal 80- to 90-degrees range of motion of shoulder lateral rotation.

RHOMBOIDS

The rhomboids consist of the rhomboid major and rhomboid minor. Their muscle fibers run at an oblique angle between the spinal column and the scapula. They are located deep to the trapezius and superficial to the erector spinae. They are typically weak, inhibited muscles, allowing the scapula to fall away from the spine further contributing to forward shoulder posture.

Step 5: Area Preparation

Goal: to prepare the rhomboids with heating ointments to facilitate myofascial release.

This muscle group will now be in a relaxed and neutral position due to the previous anterior shoulder and upper trapezius work. Move to the head of the table. The client is prone with the arms at 90-degree shoulder abduction, off the side of the table. Start with several myofascial strokes using minimal lubrication. Work through the rhomboids from the upper traps to T12, to warm up the tissue.

CORE PRINCIPLE

Do *not* use ice during myofascial mobilization, unless there is minor inflammation (heat, redness, or swelling). Ice may cause the fascia to become less mobile and restrict movement. If the pain receptors need to be calmed, apply Biofreeze. Otherwise use a warming ointment that has a viscosity to minimize glide, such as Prossage Heat. Ice may be counterproductive to the fascial mobilizing and healing process, which the therapeutic work is promoting.

Step 6: Myofascial Release

Goal: to warm up, soften, and mobilize the rhomboid fascia and to move the fascial layers back to their normal resting position.

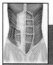

CORE PRINCIPLE

Always perform myofascial release *before* proceeding to deeper, more specific work.

- Perform myofascial strokes, using the back of your fists with your thumbs as a guide, in the lamina groove (Figure 5-42 ■).
- Keep your wrists straight, with your fingers curled in. Hook and lift the upper traps with your knuckles, as you lean forward sinking into the tissue, and perform a short gliding stroke.
- Continue working down the back through the lamina groove and the belly of the rhomboids, finishing the strokes at the inferior rhomboids.

If the client has a forward thoracic curve without vertebral rotation (smooth lamina grooves):

- Ask him or her to arch the back into neutral and slowly extend the thorax with zero discomfort, as you perform the short gliding stroke (Figure 5-43 ■).
- Then ask the client to lower his or her head toward the face cradle as you gently hold and press down, pinning the tissue, to allow an additional myofascial stretch.
- Only if it is 100 percent pain-free, have the client continually repeat this sequence as you work down the back through the lamina groove and across the rhomboids. Finish the strokes just below the rhomboids at about T12.

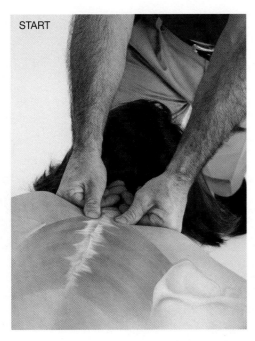
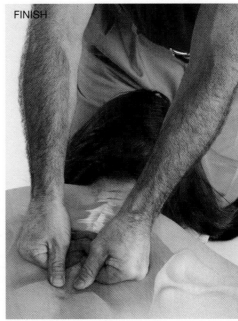

FIGURE 5-42
Myofascial Release, Rhomboids.

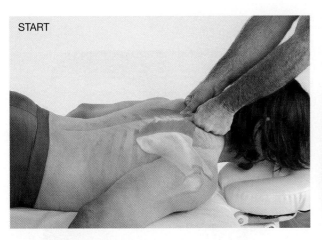
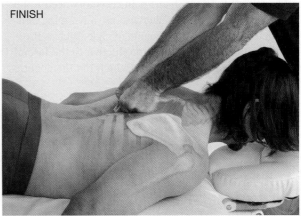

FIGURE 5-43
Reduce Forward Thoracic Curves.

- This may close any open thoracic facet joints due to forward shoulder and neck posture and help correct **kyphosis** (convex thoracic spine) in noncomplicated forward thoracic curves.

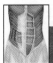

CORE PRINCIPLE

Ischemic muscle pain and trigger points in the middle traps and rhomboids will usually disappear by working and releasing the pectoral muscles, subscapularis, and upper trapezius. This creates balance around the scapula by relaxing the painful, weak, inhibited rhomboids, and middle and lower trapezius.

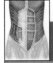

CORE PRINCIPLE

There are no stretching exercises for these muscles as they are weak and inhibited. They need to be strengthened. See the client self-care strengthening section at the end of the chapter.

TRICEPS AND POSTERIOR DELTOID

The posterior deltoid originates on the lower border of the spine of the scapula and inserts on the deltoid tuberosity. It extends and laterally rotates the shoulder. The triceps is a superficial muscle on the back of the arm involved in extension of the elbow and the shoulder.

Usually, the myofascial and neuromuscular pain patterns in these weak muscles are best addressed by releasing and stretching their antagonists—pectoralis major, subscapularis, and biceps. After relaxing the posterior deltoids and triceps, the client would strengthen them as part of self care.

Step 5: Area Preparation

Goal: to prepare the posterior deltoid and triceps prior to performing myofascial release.

 CORE PRINCIPLE

Do *not* use ice during myofascial mobilization, unless there is minor inflammation (heat, redness, or swelling). Ice may cause the fascia to become less mobile and restrict movement. If the pain receptors need to be calmed, apply Biofreeze. Otherwise use a warming ointment that has a viscosity to minimize glide, such as Prossage Heat. Ice may be counterproductive to the fascial mobilizing and healing process, which the therapeutic work is promoting.

The client is prone with the shoulder abducted 90 degrees and arms off the side of the table. If he or she is on a body cushion, place a bolster under the arm.

Step 6: Myofascial Release

Goal: to warm up, soften, and mobilize the fascia and to move the fascial layers back to normal, resting positions.

- Perform myofascial spreading with your fists, palms, or fingers working the triceps from insertion to origin, to relax them (Figure 5-44A ■).
- Work 45 degrees into the tissue, distal to proximal, over the belly of the posterior deltoid, to return the tissue back to where it belongs (Figure 5-44B ■).
- Work across the posterior rotator cuff , across the middle trapezius, and push the erector spinae back onto the spine (especially important in clients with forward thoracic curves and medially rotated shoulders) (Figure 5-44C ■).
- Repeat this several times.
- Then, using the knuckles. palm of the hand, or the pads of the fingers slowly perform cross-fiber gliding strokes

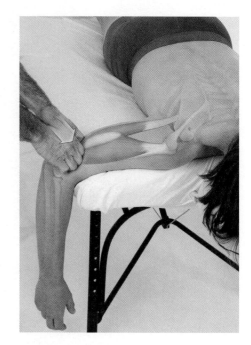

FIGURE 5-44A
Myofascial Release, Triceps.

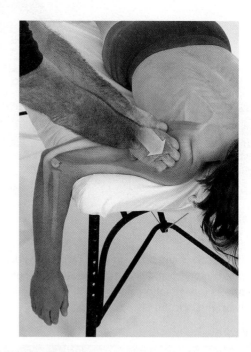

FIGURE 5-44B
Myofascial Release, Triceps and Posterior Deltoid.

working from the distal triceps, across the infraspinatus and teres minor up onto the erector spinae.
- Repeat this several times using progressively deeper strokes, alternating with compressions, to increase the blood flow to the entire area.

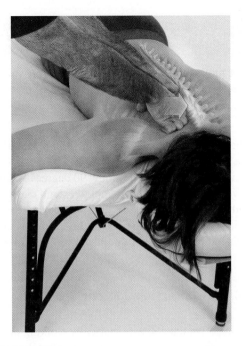

FIGURE 5-44C
Myofascial Release of Posterior Deltoid, Middle Trapezius, and Push Erector Spinae onto Spine.

Step 4: Assess Resisted Range of Motion (RROM)

To assess posterior deltoid RROM:

- The client is prone with the shoulder abducted 90 degrees and with the bent arm off the side of the table.
- Have the client gently attempt to horizontally abduct the shoulder using 20 percent force as you resist.
- If the client experiences pain, ask him or her to point to the specific spot with one finger. It is probable that the pain is at the muscle–tendon junction of posterior deltoid or proximal triceps on the posterior shoulder.

Step 8: Multidirectional Friction

Goal: to soften the collagen matrix by working in multiple directions to prepare for a more functional mobilization of posterior deltoid scar tissue fibers.

CORE PRINCIPLE

If there is not a muscle–tendon strain or ligament sprain, multidirectional friction would *not* be part of the treatment.

Perform multidirectional friction to the specific area for only 20 to 30 seconds each time. Do not overwork the area. Go to the next step.

Step 9: Pain-Free Movement

Goal: to determine if the client can actively perform shoulder horizontal abduction and adduction without pain. If so, this gives permission to proceed with pain-free eccentric scar tissue alignment techniques on the posterior deltoid.

Ask the client to move the shoulder through horizontal abduction and horizontal adduction several times to initiate the process of realigning the strained fibers.

- Pain-free? Proceed to step 10.
- Pain? Repeat step 8, working slower and deeper, but still pain-free. Repeat step 9 and then proceed to step 10 when there is no pain.

Step 10: Eccentric Scar Tissue Alignment

Goal: to apply pain-free eccentric contraction by lengthening an injured posterior deltoid against mild resistance to realign or redirect the scar tissue.

PRECAUTIONARY NOTE

After surgery, do not disrupt the proper healing of scar tissue by beginning this protocol too soon. Consult the client's physician before treatment.

CORE PRINCIPLE

The greatest error during the eccentric alignment procedure is being too aggressive and not keeping the technique pain-free each time. Too much force in opposing directions can cause a new injury or reinjure the site.

Apply eccentric contraction to realign the deeper scar tissue. This must be performed pain-free.

- The client is prone with the shoulder abducted 90 degrees and with the bent arm off the side of the table.
- Have the client lift the arm up off the table.
- Have the client resist gentle horizontal adduction performed by you.

- Tell the client to "barely resist, but let me win."
- Start with a pressure of only two fingers and then have the client increase resistance only if there is no discomfort.
- Repeat this several times, pain-free.

Step 4: Assess Resisted Range of Motion (RROM)

Goal: to re-assess if there is still a posterior deltoid strain present and exactly where it is located.

PRECAUTIONARY NOTE

Do not move too fast, or use too much force while performing a resisted test.

Repeat the posterior deltoid resisted test.

- Pain? Repeat steps 8 through 10. Then perform the resisted test again
- Pain-free. Finish with step 11 when there is no longer any pain.

CORE PRINCIPLE

Do not perform stretches on the weak, inhibited, or over-stretched muscles, as these muscles need to be strengthened, not stretched further.

Step 4: Assess Resisted Range of Motion (RROM)

Goal: to assess if there is a triceps strain present and exactly where it is located.

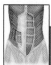

CORE PRINCIPLE

If there is a torn muscle or tendon, it will be treated *last*, after you have balanced out opposing muscle groups and addressed the problems in the muscle belly leading to the muscle tear.

PRECAUTIONARY NOTE

Do not move too fast, or use too much force while performing a resisted test.

- The client is prone with the entire arm off the side of the table.
- Have the client bend the elbow 90 degrees and then have him or her gently attempt to extend the elbow and shoulder using 20 percent force as you resist.
- Pain? Ask the client to point to the specific spot. This indicates a muscle strain and will be worked last.

Step 8: Multidirectional Friction

Goal: to soften the collagen matrix by working in multiple directions to prepare for a more functional mobilization of triceps scar tissue fibers.

CORE PRINCIPLE

If there is not a muscle–tendon strain or ligament sprain, multidirectional friction would *not* be part of the treatment.

- Pain during the resisted test? Ask the client to isolate the painful area by pointing to it.
- Perform multidirectional friction to the specific area to free the scar tissue that is creating the pain.
- Use a supported finger and work for only 20 to 30 seconds.

PRECAUTIONARY NOTE

Do not overwork the area and create inflammation.

Step 9: Pain-Free Movement

Goal: to determine if the client can actively perform elbow extension and flexion without pain. If so, this gives permission to proceed with pain-free eccentric scar tissue alignment techniques on the triceps.

Ask the client to move the elbow through flexion and extension several times to redirect the direction of the injured fibers.

- Pain-free? Proceed to step 10.
- Pain? Repeat step 8, working slower and deeper, but still pain-free. Repeat step 9 and then proceed to step 10 when there is no pain.

Step 10: Eccentric Scar Tissue Alignment

Goal: to apply pain-free eccentric contraction by lengthening an injured triceps against mild resistance to realign or redirect the scar tissue.

PRECAUTIONARY NOTE

After surgery, do not disrupt the proper healing of scar tissue by beginning this protocol too soon. Consult the client's physician before treatment.

CORE PRINCIPLE

The greatest error during the eccentric alignment procedure is being too aggressive and not keeping the technique pain-free each time. Too much force in opposing directions can cause a new injury or reinjure the site.

Apply eccentric contraction to realign the deeper scar tissue. This must be performed pain-free.

- The client is prone with the entire arm off the side of the table.
- Have the client extend their elbow and then gently resist elbow flexion performed by you.
- Tell him or her to "barely resist, but let me win."
- Start with a pressure of only two fingers and then have the client increase resistance only if there is no discomfort.
- Repeat this several times, pain-free.

Step 4: Assess Resisted Range of Motion (RROM)

Goal: to reassess if there is still a triceps strain present and exactly where it is located.

PRECAUTIONARY NOTE

Do not move too fast, or use too much force while performing a resisted test.

Perform the triceps resisted test.

- Pain? Repeat steps 8 through 10. Then perform the resisted test again.

CORE PRINCIPLE

Do not perform stretches on the weak, inhibited, or overstretched muscles, as these muscles need to be strengthened, not stretched further.

SCAPULA REPOSITION

The scapula, or shoulder blade, is located on the upper back. Along with the clavicle it is one of the two bones that make up the shoulder girdle. It is involved in stabilization and movement of the arm. The movements of the scapula include elevation, depression, protraction, retraction, and rotation.

Step 5: Area Preparation

Goal: to prepare the scapula before performing scapular mobilization.

CORE PRINCIPLE

Do *not* use ice during scapular mobilization, unless there is minor inflammation (heat, redness, or swelling). Ice may cause the fascia to become less mobile and restrict movement. If the pain receptors need to be calmed, apply Biofreeze. Otherwise use a warming ointment that has a viscosity to minimize glide, such as Prossage Heat. Ice may be counterproductive to the fascial mobilizing and healing process, which the therapeutic work is promoting.

The client is prone with the arm at the side on the table. Perform several compressions on the scapula to warm the soft tissue up by pumping blood and oxygen into the muscles and fascia that can bind it to the ribcage.

Step 6: Myofascial Release

Goal: to warm up, soften, and mobilize the fascia surrounding the scapula and to move the scapula back to normal, aligned position.

CORE PRINCIPLE

Always perform myofascial release *before* proceeding to deeper, more specific work.

- Check to see if the scapula can move freely.
- Hold onto the inferior lower "v" of the scapula with your thumb and index finger, using evenly displaced pressure. Your other hand stabilizes the anterior shoulder using an open hand and finger pads. Do not press into any bony landmarks.
- Gently rock the shoulder, then rotate the scapula right, giving the supporting muscles and fascia a stretch. This is a lot like driving a bus; the scapula is used almost like a steering wheel to massage all the muscle groups around it.
- Relax the scapula, then rock it and rotate it to the left, gently stretching it. Repeat this sequence, stretching further each time, alternating with compressions.
- Then, gently compress the scapula into the ribcage several times to increase blood flow and release the surrounding fascia.
- Next, place the palm of your hand under the shoulder and lift the shoulder up off the table, stretching the pectoralis major and minor.
- Rotate the inferior and medial scapula, with a deep stretch, back toward the midline (downward rotation), which is the optimum alignment. This will stretch the upper tapezius and relax the rhomboids, middle and lower trapezius, and levator scapula. It also reduces adhesions in this entire area (Figure 5-45A ■).
- Finally, drop your thumb under the spine of the scapula, and use your other hand to traction the hemerus down away from the acromion. This will decompress the bursa and the supraspinatus. This may also reduce subacromial bursitis and supraspinatus impingements symptoms (Figure 5-45B ■).
- Finally, abduct the shoulder to 90 degrees, lower the arm off the table to anchor the scapula at the midline and to keep this position, as you continue the protocol. Perform this work bilaterally to enhance structural balance.

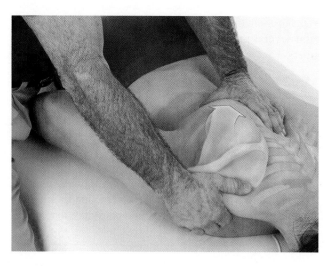

FIGURE 5-45A
Downward Scapular Rotation.

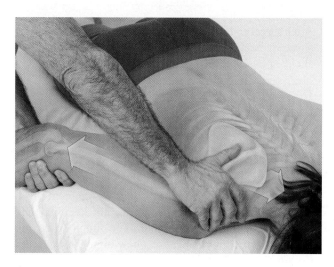

FIGURE 5-45B
Decompress Acromion.

SUPRASPINATUS AND UPPER TRAPEZIUS

The upper trapezius originates on the occiput. Its action is to bilaterally extend the neck, unilaterally rotate the neck to the opposite side, laterally flex the neck, and elevate the scapula. The supraspinatus is located deep to the upper trapezius. It runs under the acromion and attaches to the humerus. Its action is to assist the deltoid with shoulder abduction. It is the only muscle of the rotator cuff group that is not involved with rotation of the shoulder. An impingement of the supraspinatus can occur due to injury, repetitive use, or even be created by an imbalance in the muscles surrounding the shoulder joint. A tight pectoralis minor and subscapularis can twist the anterior humerus medially, which can then impinge the supraspinatus. Typically, the last 20 degrees of abduction is limited and there will be a springy end feel with shoulder impingement.

CORE PRINCIPLE

For effective treatment of supraspinatus impingement and resultant supraspinatus tendinosis, it is imperative to release the pectoralis minor, upper trapezius, and tight subscapularis muscles before working the supraspinatus.

Step 5: Area Preparation

Goal: to position the client for supraspinatus and upper trapezius work.

CORE PRINCIPLE

Do *not* use ice during myofascial mobilization, unless there is minor inflammation (heat, redness, or swelling). Ice may cause the fascia to become less mobile and restrict movement. If the pain receptors need to be calmed, apply Biofreeze. Otherwise use a warming ointment that has a viscosity to minimize glide, such as Prossage Heat. Ice may be counterproductive to the fascial mobilizing and healing process, which the therapeutic work is promoting.

- The client is prone with the shoulders abducted 90 degrees to place the supraspinatus and upper trapezius in a relaxed position.
- The arms are off the side of the table.
- Stand or sit at the head of the table.

Step 7: Cross-Fiber Gliding Strokes/Trigger Point Therapy

CROSS-FIBER GLIDING STROKES

Goal: to tease apart tight muscle bands in contracted, shortened muscle groups.

On one side of the shoulder, lift up the upper trapezius and sink into the underlying supraspinatus. Do cross-fiber gliding strokes with your thumbs and then spread and stretch the fibers, moving your thumbs away from each other. Even if the supraspinatus is not directly palpated, this technique will lengthen that muscle. Work the entire superior portion of the supraspinatus muscle working medial to lateral (Figure 5-46 ■). If the client reports discomfort slow down your strokes while you gently work superficial to deep.

TRIGGER POINT THERAPY

Goal: to release trigger points in the supraspinatus muscle belly, if found.

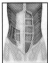

CORE PRINCIPLE

You should primarily perform trigger point work on the contracted, tight muscles, prior to working weak, inhibited muscle groups.

If there is a specific area of pain that radiates or refers when moderate direct pressure is applied, apply trigger point therapy.

- Use direct, moderate pressure for 10 to 12 seconds.

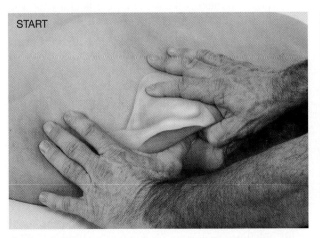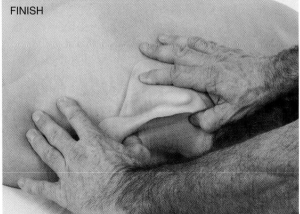

FIGURE 5-46
Cross-Fiber Gliding Strokes/Trigger Point Work, Supraspinatus.

- As the trigger point softens, compress the tissue several times.
- Gently stretch through the tissue (Figure 5-46).

Repeat this work on the client's other shoulder for structural balance.

Step 11: Stretching (During Therapy)

Goal: to create normal muscle resting lengths in shortened or contracted muscle groups. You want to create the normal 30- to 45-degree range of motion of shoulder adduction.

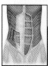

CORE PRINCIPLE

Contracting the muscle against resistance to fatigue the muscle prior to the stretch becomes a muscle resistance test and the client may report pain in a specific area, which is a muscle strain. If so, proceed to multidirectional friction (step 8), pain-free movement (step 9), and eccentric scar tissue alignment (step 10) until the client is pain-free.

SUPRASPINATUS STRETCH 1

- Place the client's bent arm across the back.
- With one hand, hold the client's scapula down onto the ribcage to prevent downward scapular rotation. Place your ring finger and middle finger above and below the spine of the scapula to stabilize it so the scapula does not move. Place your other hand on the client's wrist.
- Have the client push their elbow out toward you into shoulder abduction, against your resistance with 20 percent force for 5 to 10 seconds.
- Have the client relax. Tell him or her to take a deep breath, and then on exhale have the client adduct the arm even further across the back with your assistance for about 2 seconds. Your palm stabilizes the scapula by pushing it down onto the ribcage, in a slightly abducted position, so it doesn't move (Figure 5-47 ■).
- Repeat the contract-relax, contract-antagonist with active assisted stretching several times.

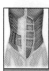

CORE PRINCIPLE

This exercise may also stretch the upper trapezius and middle deltoid, but should minimize any stretch to those muscles to focus on stretching the supraspinatus.

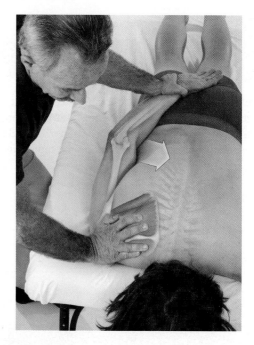

FIGURE 5-47
Supraspinatus Stretch.

SUPRASPINATUS STRETCH 2

If it is uncomfortable or painful for the client to bend their arm across their back, use this stretch instead.

- Have the client place his or her straight arm as close to the body as possible, with a foam wedge or small rolled towel placed between the upper arm and body.
- With one hand, hold the client's distal humerus. Your other hand is on the back of his or her hand.
- Have the client keep his or her arm straight and attempt to push out toward you, attempting abduction, against your resistance with 20 percent force for 5 to 10 seconds.
- Have the client relax. Move your hand from the humerus and place your palm on the scapula, pressing down and rotating the lower border laterally (upward scapular rotation).
- The client takes a breath, and then on the client's exhale, he or she moves the arm closer to the body, with your assistance, for about 2 seconds.
- Your palm holds their scapula against his or her ribcage, in a slightly abducted position, to stabilize it, so it does not move.
- Repeat the contract-relax, contract-antagonist with active assisted stretching several times.

Step 8: Multidirectional Friction

Goal: to soften the collagen matrix by working in multiple directions to prepare for a more functional mobilization of supraspinatus scar tissue fibers.

CORE PRINCIPLE

If there is not a muscle–tendon strain or ligament sprain, multidirectional friction would *not* be part of the treatment.

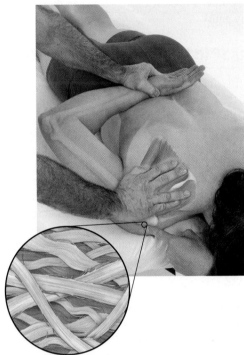

Disorganized scar tissue

FIGURE 5-48
Supraspinatus Muscle Resistance Test.

- Pain during the contraction against your resistance? Ask the client to isolate the painful area by pointing to it (Figure 5-48 ■).
- Put your finger on it and ask if the pain is directly under your finger. It is likely that the pain is under the acromion and is most likely a strain at the muscle–tendon junction, oftentimes secondary to supraspinatus impingement.
- Bring the client's arm into adduction behind the back to allow the supraspinatus tendon to come out from under the lateral edge of the acromion.
- Perform multidirectional friction on the exact spot for only 20 to 30 seconds (Figure 5-49 ■).
- Go to the next step.

PRECAUTIONARY NOTE

Do not overwork the area and create inflammation.

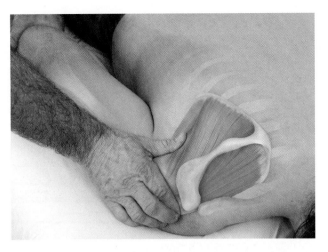

FIGURE 5-49
Supraspinatus Multidirectional Friction.

Step 9: Pain-Free Movement

Goal: to determine if the client can actively perform shoulder adduction and abduction without pain. If so, this gives permission to proceed with pain-free eccentric scar tissue alignment techniques.

With the arm behind the back, ask the client to move the arm through adduction and abduction several times to start realigning the scar tissue. This begins the process of realigning collagen fibers (scar tissue).

- Pain-free? Proceed to step 10.
- Pain? Repeat step 8, working slower and deeper, but still pain-free. Repeat step 9 and then proceed to step 10 when there is no pain.

Step 10: Eccentric Scar Tissue Alignment

Goal: to apply pain-free eccentric contraction by lengthening an injured supraspinatus against mild resistance to realign or redirect the scar tissue.

PRECAUTIONARY NOTE

After surgery, do not disrupt the proper healing of scar tissue by beginning this protocol too soon. Consult the client's physician before treatment.

Apply eccentric contraction to realign the deeper layers of scar tissue. Remember, this is performed pain-free.

- Move the client's arm 20 to 30 degrees of adduction.
- Have the client resist gentle adduction performed by you. Tell them to "barely resist, but let me win" (Figure 5-50 ■).

CORE PRINCIPLE

The greatest error during the eccentric alignment procedure is being too aggressive and not keeping the technique pain-free each time. Too much force in opposing directions can cause a new injury or reinjure the site.

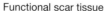

Functional scar tissue

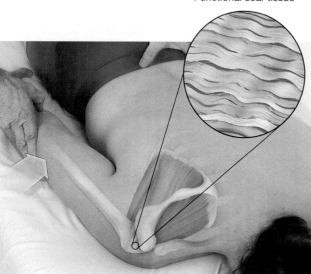

FIGURE 5-50
Supraspinatus Eccentric Muscle Contraction.

- Start with a pressure of only two fingers. If the client has zero discomfort he or she can increase resistance slightly each time.
- Repeat several times, pain-free.

Step 4: Assess Resisted Range of Motion (RROM)

Goal: to reassess if there is still a supraspinatus strain present and exactly where it is located.

PRECAUTIONARY NOTE

Do not move too fast, or use too much force while performing a resisted test.

Repeat the supraspinatus resisted test.

- Pain? Repeat steps 8 through 10. Then perform the resisted test again.

CORE PRINCIPLE

When you finish the resisted test and the client then reports pain in an area other than the supraspinatus, the problem may be in the surrounding supporting muscles.

- Pain-free? Finish with step 11 when there is no longer any pain.

INFRASPINATUS AND TERES MINOR

The infraspinatus and teres minor are two of the four muscles of the rotator cuff. They laterally rotate, adduct, and extend the shoulder. They also stabilize the head of the humerus in the glenoid cavity. Because they are weak, inhibited, and possibly eccentrically contracted, they are easily injured. An example is a common injury to the infraspinatus or teres minor during deceleration of the pitching motion. Throwing a ball at 100 mph involves powerful muscles such as the pectoralis major, subscapularis, and anterior deltoid. This motion must be decelerated and stopped by the small, typically weak infraspinatus and teres minor muscles. Many athletes do not sufficiently strengthen these two muscles, so when they repeatedly stop abruptly during shoulder deceleration, over time they may strain the infraspinatus or teres minor tendons of attachment in the back of the shoulder. This condition over time, due to constant overload, results in tendinosis rather than tendinitis.

CORE PRINCIPLE

An infraspinatus injury could create referral pain in the upper arm—the deltoid area. Perform functional assessment tests to find the specific injured area.

Step 5: Area Preparation

Goal: to prepare the infraspinatus and teres minor for myofascial release.

The client is prone with the arms off the side of the table. Stand or sit at one side of the table.

Step 6: Myofascial Release

Goal: to warm up, soften, and mobilize the fascia and to move the fascial layers back to normal, aligned position.

CORE PRINCIPLE

Always perform myofascial release *before* proceeding to deeper, more specific work.

- Use a myofascial stroke, starting at the lateral edge of the scapula, and continuing all the way across the scapula moving lateral to medial, starting just below the spine of the scapula (Figure 5-51 ■).
- Finish the strokes by going across the rhomboids and pushing the erectors toward the spine. You can use your palm, knuckles, or the back of your hand in a loose fist.
- Repeat the strokes working inferior to the armpit.

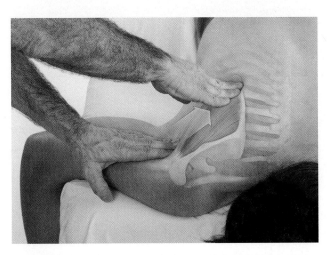

FIGURE 5-51

Infraspinatus and Teres Minor Myofascial Release, Cross-Fiber Gliding Strokes, and Trigger Point Work.

Step 7: Cross-Fiber Gliding Strokes/Trigger Point Therapy

CROSS-FIBER GLIDING STROKES

Goal: to relax the tight muscle bands in the infraspinatus and teres minor.

- Perform cross-fiber gliding strokes over the infraspinatus and teres minor.
- Work lateral to medial, continuing across the middle trapezius and rhomboid muscles, to relax these weak, inhibited, and possibly overstretched muscles. Tender spots are usually found at the lateral border of the scapula.
- This will loosen up tight muscle fibers that often feed and contribute to take out active muscle belly myofascial trigger points, allowing the tissue to move more freely and independently.

- Continue the cross-fiber gliding strokes across the rhomboids and onto the erectors.

TRIGGER POINT THERAPY

CORE PRINCIPLE

You should primarily perform trigger point work on the contracted, tight muscles, before addressing weak inhibited or overstretched muscle groups.

Now that you have brought the infraspinatus and teres minor muscles to to their normal muscle resting lengths, after first releasing the anterior shoulder muscles, there should be minimal tender points. If you do find any tender points they will usually diminish by stretching the pectoralis major, pectoralis minor, upper trapezius, and subscapularis and strengthening the infraspinatus, teres minor, and rhomboids. This is part of the client self-care.

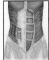

CORE PRINCIPLE

Remember, it is not suggested that you stretch the rhomboids, infraspinatus, and teres mior muscles, as they are weak, inhibited, and eccentrically contracted and do not need to be stretched any further. There are exercises to strengthen these muscles in the client self-care section at the end of the chapter.

Step 4: Assess Resisted Range of Motion (RROM)

Goal: to assess if there is an infraspinatus or teres minor strain present and exactly where it is located.

CORE PRINCIPLE

If there is a torn muscle or tendon, it will be treated *last,* after you have balanced out opposing muscle groups and addressed the problems in the muscle belly leading to the muscle tear.

PRECAUTIONARY NOTE

Do not move too fast, or use too much force while performing a resisted test.

If the initial assessment of the resisted test for the infraspinatus or teres minor was positive, and the client complained of a specific spot of pain, perform the following test:

- The client's shoulder is abducted to 90 degrees with the arm off the side of the table.
- Have the client attempt to laterally rotate the humerus as you resist, or gently try to medially rotate it against their resistance. If the client experiences pain, ask him or her to point to the specific spot, which indicates a muscle strain. It is probable that the injury is at the muscle–tendon junction on the lateral side of the shoulder (Figure 5-52 ■).

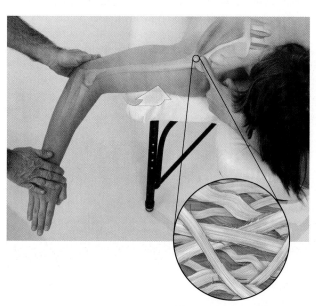

Disorganized scar tissue

FIGURE 5-52
Infraspinatus/Teres Minor Muscle Resistance Test.

Step 8: Multidirectional Friction

Goal: to soften the collagen matrix by working in multiple directions to prepare for a more functional mobilization of scar tissue fibers.

CORE PRINCIPLE

If there is not a muscle–tendon strain or ligament sprain, multidirectional friction would *not* be part of the treatment.

- Pain during the resisted test? Place your finger on the specific spot of pain identified by the client in the resisted test.
- Perform multidirectional friction on the exact spot for only 20 to 30 seconds. If you continue for longer than this, you may cause inflammation (Figure 5-53 ■).

PRECAUTIONARY NOTE

Do not overwork the area and create inflammation.

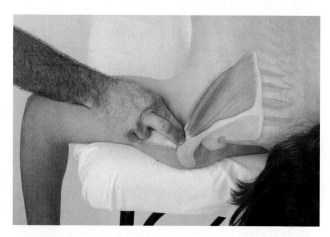

FIGURE 5-53
Infraspinatus Multidirectional Friction.

Step 9: Pain-Free Movement

Goal: to determine if the client can actively perform lateral and medial shoulder rotation without pain. If so, this gives permission to proceed with pain-free eccentric scar tissue alignment techniques.

- The client is prone with the elbow bent 90 degrees.
- Ask the client to move the shoulder through lateral and medial rotation by bringing the hand up toward the head and then back toward the floor.
- Have the client repeat this several times. Scar tissue begins to realign in the direction of movement following friction.
- Pain-free? Proceed to step 10.
- Pain? Repeat step 8, working slower and deeper, but still pain-free. Repeat step 9 and then proceed to step 10 when there is no pain.

Step 10: Eccentric Scar Tissue Alignment

Goal: to apply pain-free eccentric contraction by lengthening an injured infraspinatus or teres minor against mild resistance to realign or redirect the scar tissue.

PRECAUTIONARY NOTE

After surgery, do not disrupt the proper healing of scar tissue by beginning this protocol too soon. Consult the client's physician before treatment.

 CORE PRINCIPLE

The greatest error during the eccentric alignment procedure is being too aggressive and not keeping the technique pain-free each time. Too much force in opposing directions can cause a new injury or reinjure the site.

The client is prone. Apply eccentric contraction to realign the deeper scar tissue. Remember, this must be performed pain-free.

- The client is prone with the arm off the table at 90-degree shoulder abduction.
- Ask him or her to laterally rotate the shoulder by bringing the forearm and hand up toward the head.
- From that position of lateral rotation of the humerus, have the client gently resist medial rotation back to the neutral resting position of the infraspinatus and teres minor performed by you. Tell him or her to "barely resist, but let me win."
- Use only two fingers to create the pressure to begin with and have the client increase resistance only if there is no discomfort (Figure 5-54 ■).
- Repeat this work several times.

 PRECAUTIONARY NOTE

Do not stretch the client's shoulder by moving it into extreme medial rotation. Move it just to where it is perpendicular to the floor (see Figure 5-54).

Step 4: Assess Resisted Range of Motion (RROM)

Goal: to reassess if there is still an infraspinatus or teres minor strain present and exactly where it is located.

 PRECAUTIONARY NOTE

Do not move too fast, or use too much force while performing a resisted test.

Repeat the infraspinatus/teres minor resisted test. The client's shoulder is abducted to 90 degrees with the arm off the side of the table. Have him or her attempt to laterally rotate the arm or resist as you gently attempt to medially rotate it.

- Pain? Repeat steps 8 through 10. Then perform the resisted test again.
- Pain-free? You are finished.

 CORE PRINCIPLE

You do *not* stretch these weak, inhibited, overstretched muscles.

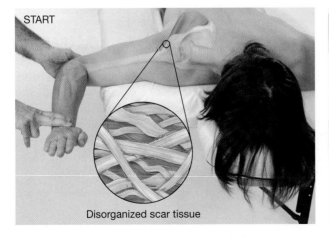

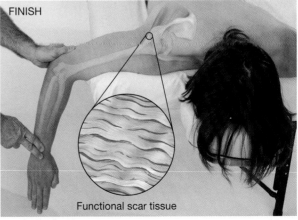

FIGURE 5-54

Eccentric Muscle Contraction, Infraspinatus and Teres Minor.

COMMON CONDITIONS

Thoracic Outlet Syndrome

The following section is as an overview of common clinical conditions of the shoulder that will benefit from the work outlined in this chapter.

Thoracic outlet syndrome is not a single condition. It can include several variations of nerve or vascular compressions near the base of the neck and upper rib cage. It is easily misdiagnosed, due to the difficulty in distinguishing between a cervical rib problem, which is a bony extension of the transverse process of C7, and cervical disc problems.

This text will focus on the portion of thoracic outlet syndrome involving compression at the superior thoracic outlet (Figure 5-55 ■). This common and most understood portion involves compression of the neurovascular bundle passing between the anterior and middle scalenes, also know as anterior scalene syndrome. This part compresses the brachial plexus of nerves and brachial artery. Because the subclavian vein does not pass between the scalene muscles, there are usually only nerve compression symptoms present, such as pain, tingling, and numbness in the arms and hands. We will also focus on nerve and vascular compression between the first rib and clavicle, known as costo-clavicular syndrome; and nerve and vascular compression under a tight pectoralis minor muscle, known as pectoralis minor syndrome. If the treatment in this chapter does not eliminate the nerve compression problems, please refer the client out for additional testing by an orthopedic physician. This may include x-rays and most likely an MRI. For much more detailed information on underlying pathologies and differential diagnosis refer to the text *Orthopedic Assessment in Massage Therapy* by Whitney Lowe.[5]

In review, tight, contracted pectoralis major and pectoralis minor, subclavius, and subscapularis muscles can create forward shoulder posture, also called anterior shoulder rotation. When these muscles, along with the scalenes and sternocleidomastoid (SCM), are contracted they can compress the **brachial plexus** of nerves causing the most common form of thoracic outlet syndrome. The main symptoms are numbness, tingling, and possible pain down the arm.[6] After you balance out the muscles in the shoulder and cervical areas, thoracic outlet syndrome can be relieved. More detailed work on releasing the SCMs and scalenes, and techniques for resolving cervical bony fixations that compress nerves higher up, will be addressed in Chapter 6 on cervical conditions.

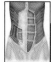

CORE PRINCIPLE

Thoracic outlet syndrome can create symptoms similar to carpal tunnel syndrome. Always look for the source of the pain, don't just rely on the symptoms.

TREATMENT

- Start with the client supine to release the tight anterior shoulder muscles.
- Follow the basic shoulder protocol and the stretches for all of the muscles.
- Then you must also release the tight scalenes and sternocleidomastoid.

PRECAUTIONARY NOTE

If the client has been in a car accident and has not had an MRI, bone scan, or x-ray, *do not* perform the scalene or sternocleidomastoid stretch. If he or she becomes dizzy, disoriented, nauseous, or has blurred vision immediately discontinue this stretch. If the client shows any other inappropriate medical symptoms advise him or her to get a medical exam. Remember, if in doubt, refer out!

PRECAUTIONARY TEST

Before you begin the scalene or sternocleidomastoid stretch you must have the client perform the following precautionary test. This is called the *vertebral artery compression test*.

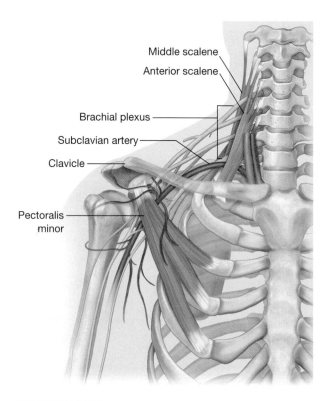

Middle scalene

Anterior scalene

Brachial plexus

Subclavian artery

Clavicle

Pectoralis minor

FIGURE 5-55
Thoracic Outlet Syndrome.

- Ask the client to rotate the neck 45 degrees to the right and then extend the head back to the left (Figure 5-56A ■).
- The client then holds this position for 30 seconds.
- Repeat this test on the other side; rotate the neck to the left, and then extend it back to the right (Figure 5-56B ■).
- Ask the client if he or she feels any of the symptoms listed in the Precautionary Note. If so, *do not* proceed with this work, until cleared from their physician. The client could have vertebral artery compression and vascular insufficiency which decreases vascular flow to the brain.[7]

Step 11: Stretching (During Therapy)

Release and stretch the anterior scalene and sternocleidomastoid (SCM) which is covered in much greater detail in Chapter 6 on cervical spine conditions.

- The client is supine with you supporting the back of the neck with one hand.
- Ask the client to place his or her hands under the hips to keep the shoulders down.

- Traction the client's neck with the hand under the neck, and have the client slowly rotate the head to the tight side as you do a myofascial stretch to the SCM, and then have the client slowly extend the head down and back toward the opposite side with your assistance for 2 seconds (Figure 5-57 ■).
- Repeat this stretch several times. Repeat this stretch on the other side, if needed.

Step 11: Stretching (During Therapy)

To stretch the medial scalene:

- The client is supine on the table, with their hands under their hips to hold the shoulders down.
- Support the back of the neck with one hand using slight cervical traction, and ask him or her to laterally flex the neck away from the shoulder you are working on to stretch. Perform a myofascial glide up the lamina groove on the side being stretched. Assist the stretch (Figure 5-58 ■).

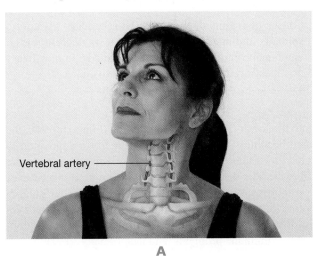

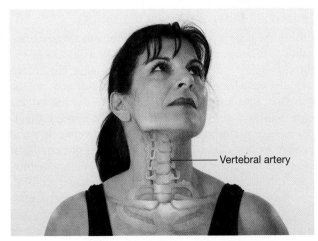

A

B

FIGURE 5-56
Vertebral Artery Compression Test.

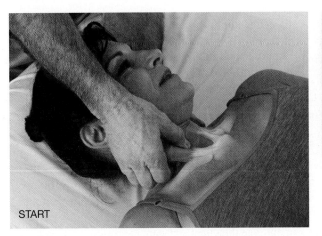

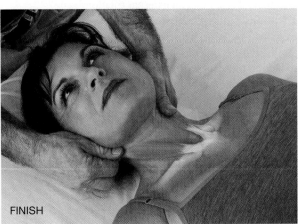

FIGURE 5-57
Myofascial Stretch SCM and Anterior Scalene.

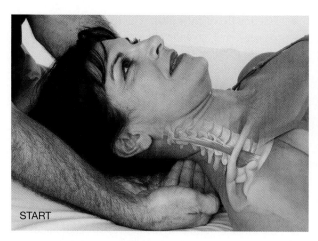
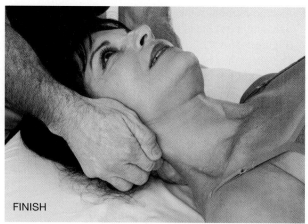

START · FINISH

FIGURE 5-58
Myofascial Stretch, Medial Scalene.

- Repeat this several times to stretch the medial scalene and lateral neck flexors.
- Repeat this stretch on the other side, if needed.

Frozen Shoulder (Adhesive Capsulitis)

Frozen shoulder is commonly used to refer to adhesive capsulitis.[8] However, this section of the book will focus on the distinct clinical pathology of adhesive capsulitis. True frozen shoulder includes a variety of pathologies, that may include adhesive capsulitis, subacromial **bursitis,** tendinosis, **rotator cuff** injuries, and other clinical conditions limiting shoulder motion. Adhesive capsulitis involves loss of active and passive motion due to adhesions within the glenohumeral joint capsule.[9] Refer to the previous section of this chapter, page 156 (adhesive capsulitis), for frozen shoulder protocol.

An accident, trauma, emotional or physical stress, repetitive movements, or overuse (weekend warrior) can lead to immobilization or lack of full range of motion of the shoulder. When this happens, adhesions may build up in the shoulder joint capsule and cause adhesive capsulitis. A client with this condition may have a combination of limited flexion, abduction, or external rotation. The greatest restriction is usually abduction and external rotation.

Early-onset adhesive capsule involvement initially causes a bone-on-bone-like end feel in lateral rotation, and then abduction becomes bone-on-bone-like, usually limiting abduction to about 35 to 45 degrees. The end feel on a passive range of motion test will appear to be bone-on-bone-like. Simple conditions such as supraspinatus impingement and bursitis could lead to frozen shoulder due to prolonged immobility and limited shoulder movement.

Dr. Erik Dalton says that the joint capsule has a considerate amount of slack, loose tissue, so the shoulder is unrestricted as it moves through its large range of motion. However, in clients with a true adhesive capsulitis, inflammation in the joint makes the normally loose (inferior) parts of the joint capsule stick together. In his opinion, this is usually caused by fibrin deposition from dried inflammatory waste products. As gravity slowly pulls the waste products

CORE PRINCIPLE

Causes of frozen shoulder can be secondary to supraspinatus impingement, rotator cuff tears, labrum tears, emotional contributions, prolonged shoulder immobilization, postsurgical complications, and so on.

into the lower (plicated) capsular folds (Figure 5-59 ■), the area becomes dehydrated and causes fibrin deposition to glue down the capsule. The more inflammation, the more fibrosis, thus the capsule slowly fills up until it infiltrates the entire capsule. This seriously limits the shoulder's ability to move, and causes the shoulder to freeze. Dalton believes most frozen shoulders are caused by supraspinatus tendonitis, autoimmune problems, and lack of daily stretching.

TREATMENT

Refer to the section of this chapter (page 156) on joint capsule work.

- Pain-free joint capsule work is imperative for success in treating this condition.
- Start with this and progress through the shoulder protocol, returning to the joint capsule work when necessary. At any point, when you are balancing out the muscle groups of the shoulder, if there is a bone-on-bone-like end feel, perform this revolutionary capsule work.
- Continue to reassess the client's range of motion and each end feel until it is pain-free.
- Have the client stop any strengthening exercises he or she is currently doing except for those for the rhomboids, lower trapezius, infraspinatus, and teres minor, that help stabilize excessive upward scapular movement. See the client self-care exercises at the end of the chapter. Give the client homework in the form of stretches specific to the restricted muscles

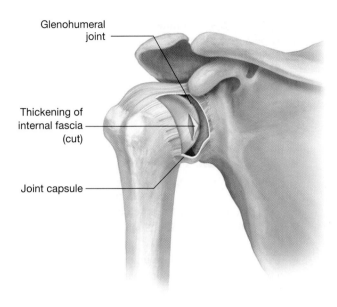

Early Adhesive Capsulitis

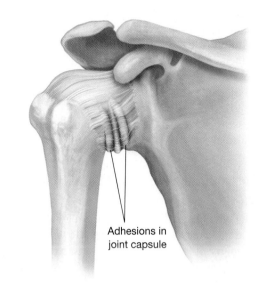

Advanced Adhesive Capsulitis

FIGURE 5-59
Joint Capsule Adhesions.

and pain-free range of motion for neuromuscular reeducation. If the fascial adhesions inside the joint capsule are released, and the fibrosis of the capsule itself is immobilized, the client must take the shoulder through each full range of motion daily to prevent adhesions from forming again. The worst thing to do in clients with adhesive capsulitis is to immobilize their shoulder.

Rotator Cuff Injuries

See treatment protocols in earlier section. Since the rotator cuff involves a group of four muscles, you must perform a thorough assessment to determine which of the muscles are involved: supraspinatus, infraspinatus, teres minor, or subscapularis (pages 152–156). It is not uncommon for an athlete to be diagnosed with a rotator cuff injury and actually have bicipital tendinosis. Muscle resistance testing is vital to determine which muscles are injured as the treatment and rehabilitation will change depending on which muscle groups are involved. The most common muscle to be injured in this group is the supraspinatus, because it is often impinged due to a tight subscapularis, pectoralis minor, upper trapezius, and middle deltoid leading to strained fibers as it moves under the acromion, as well as the teres minor because it is usually weak and inhibited, and placed under extreme eccentric forces during deceleration of the shoulder, especially in athletes.

TREATMENT

- Determine which of the four muscles of the rotator cuff are injured through resisted tests.
- Start the shoulder protocol at the very beginning with the velvet glove technique.

- You must release and balance all of the muscles surrounding the shoulder to properly treat this condition.
- Follow the specific protocol for the injured muscle including myofascial release, multidirectional friction, and eccentric scar tissue alignment.
- Continue to reassess and listen to the client to ensure the treatment is pain-free.

Supraspinatus Tendinosis

Supraspinatus tendinitis is a misleading term, because in many cases by the time the client presents to the therapist he or she does not have inflammation. A better term would be *tendon pain* or *tendinosis*, which is the tearing of tendon fibers in the absence of an inflammatory process.[10] The supraspinatus is usually injured because of heavy demands placed on it during the initiation of abduction such as carrying a briefcase, laptop computer, purse, or baby carrier. It is often impinged under the acromion due to tight pectoralis and tight subscapularis muscles. The client will complain of posterior, superior shoulder pain. Be sure to assess the shoulder in the first 20 to 30 degrees of abduction (see page 154). Movement beyond that is the action of the middle deltoid, which will be painful to a resisted test above 30-degree abduction. Also, the fibers of the supraspinatus tendon can become impinged where it runs under the acromion process, which can cause chronic pain and resultant fiber tears.

TREATMENT

- Start with the basic shoulder protocol.
- After the velvet glove technique release the pectoralis major and minor, subclavius, upper trapezius, middle deltoid, and the subscapularis. It is necessary to release and balance all of the muscles surrounding

the shoulder, especially the pectoralis minor and sub-scapularis, to properly treat this condition.

- Next, follow the specific protocol for the supraspinatus including myofascial release, cross-fiber gliding strokes, trigger point work, multidirectional friction, and eccentric scar tissue alignment (see page 182 to186).
- Reassess and repeat the protocol until the client is pain-free.

Infraspinatus Tendinosis and Teres Minor Tendinosis

This is a common condition seen in both athletes and non-athletes as these muscles tend to be weak, overstretched, and prone to injury. It is a common early season condition seen in baseball players, especially pitchers. Throwing a ball at 100 mph involves powerful muscles such as the pectoralis major, subscapularis, and anterior deltoid. The force of deceleration can be up to ten times greater than acceleration. This motion must be decelerated and stopped by the small, typically weak and inhibited, infraspinatus and teres minor muscles. Many athletes do not sufficiently strengthen these two muscles, so when they repeatedly stop abruptly during deceleration they stress or strain the tendons of attachment in the back of the shoulder over time.

TREATMENT

See pages 186 to 189 on the general shoulder protocol.

- Follow the basic previous shoulder protocol, as you must release the tight, restricted anterior muscles first to allow the weak, inhibited, or overstretched infraspinatus and teres minor to relax. The most important muscle to release prior to treating these muscles is the subscapularis.
- Next, perform the specific previous protocol for these muscles including myofascial work and cross-fiber gliding strokes to bring the muscle back to their normal resting position, multidirectional friction, and eccentric scar tissue alignment.
- Repeat and reassess until the client is pain-free. It is then imperative to strengthen these weak, inhibited, overstretched muscles. See the client self-care section at the end of the chapter.

Subscapularis Tendinosis versus Bicipital and Coracobrachialis Tendinosis

These conditions typically are called tendinitis. A better term for both of these conditions may be *tendon pain* or *tendinosis*, which is the tearing of tendon fibers, due to repeated stress or overload, in the absence of an inflammatory process.[11] It is important to perform muscle resistance testing to determine which of these muscles are causing anterior shoulder pain (page 153). The long head of the biceps tendon and the subscapularis tendon lie next to each other and general palpation may not determine which muscle is creating the tendon pain. Even though the pain may be in the same area, the treatment protocol and the subsequent stretching are both drastically different.

SUBSCAPULARIS TREATMENT

- Follow the shoulder protocol starting at the beginning with the velvet glove technique.
- You will need to release all of the other anterior shoulder muscles—pectoralis major, minor, and subclavius—before you work this muscle.
- Next, follow the specific protocol for the subscapularis including multidirectional friction and eccentric contraction (see page 174).
- This is an extremely rare injury, as this muscle has a broad, flat, wide tendon, that is very deep and well protected. Although this muscle is almost always tight, subscapularis tendinosis is rare.

BICEPS AND CORACOBRACHIALIS TREATMENT

- Start the basic shoulder protocol and release all of the anterior shoulder muscles.
- The client is supine with the arm supinated, with support under the elbow using a bolster or towel. Have the client perform a resisted test with the shoulder flexed to 90 degrees, palm facing up, to pinpoint the injury.
- Follow with the rest of the biceps/coracobrachialis protocol (see pages 166 to 170).
- Continue to reassess and repeat any or all of the protocol until the client is pain-free.

Subacromial Bursitis

The **subacromial bursa** is located underneath the acromion, to prevent compression of soft tissue against the bone. This fluid-filled sac has two major sections and most of it is inaccessible. The more distal portion is the subdeltoid bursa. When the arm is fully abducted, the bursa moves up under the acromion process. The **bursa** can become agitated by repetitive compression of the humerus into the acromion usually due to tight upper trapezius, middle deltoid, and supraspinatus muscles (Figure 5-60 ■). An indicator of bursitis is when shoulder pain begins shortly after initiating shoulder abduction, and continues to about 135 degrees. This is called a painful arc, which happens because the irritated bursa is compressed as the client abducts the shoulder. After about 135 degrees of abduction, the irritated tissue moves proximally under the acronium process and is no longer compressed. The pain is described as being deep within the shoulder joint. There can also be an inflammation to this bursa resulting from autoimmune disease such as rheumatoid arthritis, infection, gout, calcific deposits, or other systemic disorders. If in doubt, always refer out!

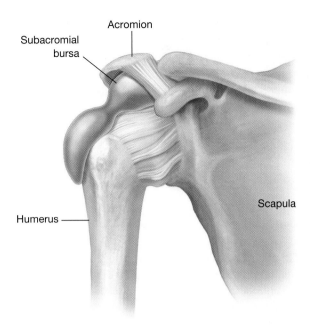

Acromion

Subacromial
bursa

Humerus

Scapula

FIGURE 5-60
Inflamed Bursa.

TREATMENT

- To eliminate bursitis, the most important muscles to work are the anterior shoulder muscles that contribute to shoulder impingement and the upper trapezius, middle deltoid, and supraspinatus muscles, which may be causing the compression on the bursa.
- This will release the tension on the shoulder joint and usually alleviate the symptoms of bursitis.

CORE PRINCIPLE

The actual inflammatory site of bursitis is *never* worked.

Upper Crossed Syndrome

Dr. Vladimir Janda (1928–2002) simplified assessing commonly occurring upper body postural distortions and problems by defining **upper crossed syndrome.** According to Janda, when some upper crossed muscles are placed under stress they become tight. These muscles include pectoralis major, pectoralis minor, subscapularis, sternocleidomastoid, anterior scalenes, upper trapezius, levator scapula, and the suboccipitals. Also, when other upper crossed muscles are placed under the same stress they become weak and inhibited. These muscles are rhomboids, middle and lower trapezius, infraspinatus, teres minor, and neck flexors.[12]

To alleviate chronic upper body pain patterns, every therapist should attempt to create balance between these two

groups, by releasing and stretching the tight muscles to bring the upper body back to postural balance or alignment and then strengthening the weak, inhibited muscles to keep this balance (Figure 5-61).

Step 11: Stretching (Client Self-Care)

Goal: for the client to perform stretches suggested and demonstrated by you to create normal muscle resting lengths in shortened or contracted muscle groups.

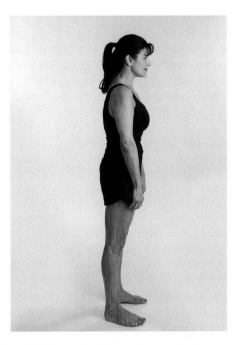

FIGURE 5-61
Forward Head Posture/Upper Cross Syndrome.

PRECAUTIONARY NOTE

In certain states, massage therapists are not allowed to "prescribe" stretches. If you are not competent, or if you feel that suggesting stretches is outside your scope of practice, do not follow this step. Be safe, refer out. Wait until you become competent by becoming certified as a personal trainer or certified in active isolated stretching.

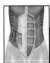

CORE PRINCIPLE

Do not suggest stretches for the weak, inhibited, or overstretched muscles, as these need to be strengthened, not stretched further.

PRECAUTIONARY NOTE

Do not have the client stretch beyond normal range of motion, as this could create hypermobile joints and result in injury.

Emphasis on client self-care! Client self-care is essential for the client to keep the normal muscle balance and range of motion that was created during therapy. Clients must learn these techniques and perform them at home to accustom their minds and bodies to the new pain-free range of motion. Teach the clients active assisted stretching first. Once they understand the stretches and can correctly perform them for you, you can teach them the more advanced PNF stretches. To perform the stretches, the clients need a stretch rope, towel, or long belt.

TECHNIQUES FOR CLIENT SELF-CARE

- Tell the client that the stretches will take only a few minutes a day to perform and are necessary for continued results.
- The client should stretch after exercise or a hot shower when the fascia and muscles are warm.
- Tell the client to not stretch into pain. The client and you need to differentiate between uncomfortable stretching due to tight muscles and painful stretching that can aggravate his or her clinical condition.
- The client starts the stretches with the tightest side first until normal range of motion is achieved. Then he or she continues to stretch both sides for continued balance and symmetry.
- Suggest only two to four stretches, specific for the condition addressed, each time you see a client. Make sure he or she can perform these correctly before suggesting any additional stretches.
- Print copies of the stretches for your clients to take with them for reference.

PECTORALIS MAJOR

- The client is standing with the arms straight out in front of the body and the palms together. Make sure the client keeps the head in the neutral position and the shoulders square to the front.
- He or she exhales and brings the arms back, engaging the rhomboids, squeezing the scapula together, and holding for about 2 seconds.
- Then the client brings the arms forward, takes a deep breath, and raises up the arms 20 degrees. He or she exhales and brings the arms back at this new position and holds for about 2 seconds.

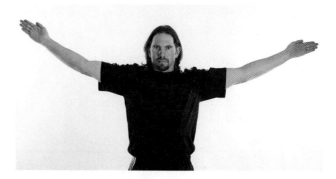

FIGURE 5-62
Pectoralis Major Stretch.

- The client brings the arms forward again, takes a deep breath, and again raises up the arms 20 degrees. He or she repeats the stretch for about 2 seconds at this new position (Figure 5-62 ■).
- On the third stretch ask the client to turn the thumbs outward into forearm supination. This starts to bring the pectoralis minor into the stretch. Repeat this entire sequence two or three times.

PECTORALIS MINOR

1. Have the client perform the following stretch:

   - The client is standing.
   - He or she places the hands behind the head, low on the neck, elbows bent, with the neck slightly extended back.
   - Make sure the client keeps the shoulders square to the front.
   - He or she exhales, brings the elbows back, and up towards the ceiling, and holds the stretch for about 2 seconds (Figure 5-63 ■).

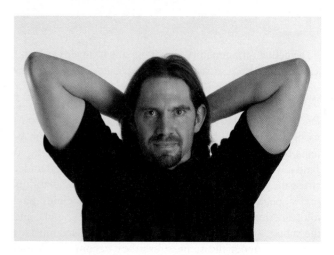

FIGURE 5-63
Pectoralis Minor Stretch.

- The client relaxes, brings the elbows forward, takes a deep breath, and on exhale repeats the stretch again.
- Repeat this stretch 8 to 10 times

2. For clients with very tight pectoralis minor muscles, have them abduct the arm to 135 degrees and keep the head in neutral.

- The action the client needs to visualize is to take the arm across the body toward the opposite hip.
- Ask the client to attempt this against a doorjamb or restrictive barrier to fatigue the muscles for 5 to 10 seconds.
- He or she relaxes, inhales, and on exhale engages the antagonist muscles, pulling the arm back. Then he or she slowly walks forward into the doorjamb and holds this position for about 2 seconds.
- Precaution: The client should *not* lean or bounce into the doorway (Figure 5-64 ■). Moving too quickly, bouncing into the stretch, or doing this stretch too aggressively into the doorway, can initiate a protective stretch reflex and lead to an injury.
- Make sure the client keeps the shoulders square.
- He or she stays at this new position and repeats the contract-relax, contract-antagonist two or three times.
- Have the client repeat this stretch on the other side for balance.

PRECAUTIONARY NOTE

Door stretches should be used for clients with thoracic outlet syndrome. But, be careful, as aggressive stretching can cause injury to muscle fibers and make the client's condition worse.

SUBSCAPULARIS

Have the client hold a stretch rope in one hand, keeping the wrist straight, and loop it around the back and over the outside of the elbow to the other hand that is resting on the hip. The elbow is tucked in at the side. Make sure he or she keeps the shoulders square.

- The client attempts medial rotation, of the shoulder, bringing the arm toward the midline, using the stretch rope as resistance for 5 to 10 seconds.
- He or she relaxes, inhales, and on exhale engages the antagonist muscles (infraspinatus and teres minor) and laterally rotates the shoulder (bringing the arm back) while assisting with the stretch rope for about 2 seconds (Figure 5-65 ■).
- At this new position, repeat this stretch two or three times.
- Have the client perform this stretch on the other side for balance to achieve 80 to 90 degrees of lateral shoulder rotation.

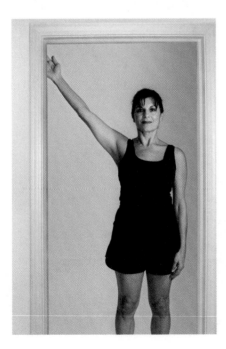
FIGURE 5-64
Pectoralis Minor Stretch into Doorway.

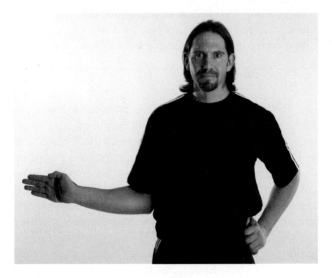
FIGURE 5-65
Subscapularis Stretch.

Step 12: Strengthening (Client Self-Care)

Goal: to strengthen weak, inhibited muscle groups around a joint creating muscle balance throughout the body—structural integration.

CORE PRINCIPLE

The client must stretch the tight, contracted muscles before strengthening the opposing weak, inhibited, or overstretched muscles.

PRECAUTIONARY NOTE

To prevent reinjury after treating a strain, have the client refrain from beginning a strengthening program for approximately 7 to 10 days, or until he or she is pain-free. In the case of weak inhibited muscle groups, to facilitate healing, have the client stretch the tight antagonist muscles, taking the tension off the injured muscles during that time period.

CORE PRINCIPLE

Suggest only two to four strengthening exercises each time you see a client. Make sure he or she can perform these correctly before suggesting any additional exercises.

The final step in the twelve-step approach to pain management is strengthening the weak, inhibited, and sometimes overstretched muscles. These muscles lack blood flow and oxygen, due to the constant eccentric load placed on them, and need to be strengthened to allow complete musculoskeletal balance throughout the body. Strengthening is essential to a client's continued improvement and recovery and prevention of injury. Demonstrate the strengthening exercises for your client and then instruct him or her on how to practice the movements at home. The only item needed is a piece of Thera-Band (resistance) tubing.

TECHNIQUES FOR STRENGTHENING

- Stretch the tight antagonist muscles first.
- Show the client how to control and adjust the amount of resistance on the Thera-Band.
- Make sure the client's movements while performing the exercises are slow and controlled during both the concentric (muscle shortening phase) and eccentric

(muscle lengthening phase) contractions, *placing much more emphasis on the eccentric phase.*
- The optimal timing is to take 2 seconds for the concentric (muscle shortening) contraction and 4 seconds for the eccentric (muscle lengthening) contraction.
- Tell the client that only 5 to 10 minutes per day is needed to perform both stretching and strengthening exercises for addressing any specific clinical condition.
- Empower clients to take responsibility for reeducating their muscles, keeping their body balanced, and participating in their own wellness.

ERECTORS, RHOMBOIDS, AND MIDDLE AND LOWER TRAPEZIUS

- Forward shoulder posture causes the scapula and the erectors to move laterally away from the spine. To correct the forward shoulder posture it is imperative to strengthen the rhomboids.

RHOMBOIDS

- The client is sitting on a mat with a Thera-Band.
- Have him or her secure the middle of the Thera-Band tubing around the feet and hold the ends in their hands.
- His or her shoulders are abducted 90 degrees, with elbows bent at 90 degrees.
- The client tightens the rhomboids, drawing the elbows back and bringing the scapula together, working the last 20 to 30 degrees (Figure 5-66 ■).
- He or she slowly concentrically contracts,the rhomboids, taking two seconds and then eccentrically contracts the rhomboids by slowly releaseing back to the starting position taking about 4 seconds. This is very slow work.
- Have the client repeat this exercise 8 to 10 times.

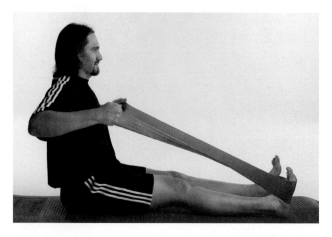

FIGURE 5-66
Rhomboid Strengthening.

CASE STUDY

You are a prominent therapist in the field of clinical massage, and the leading orthopedic surgeon from your local hospital sends you a professional baseball player with a rotator cuff injury in an attempt to avoid surgery. The player is a pitcher and he states in the client history that he felt moderate pain in the back of his shoulder following a game about a week ago. The player has been applying ice to the shoulder. The MRI indicates a problem under the acromion and behind the shoulder blade, near the infraspinatus tendon.

The client does not present with redness, swelling, or inflammation when he arrives in your clinic. He has pain that is mild at rest, but increases with shoulder movement. The orthopedic surgeon has ruled out a labrum tear and is certain there are no muscular ruptures or bone spurs. The shoulder is not hypermobile, indicating good ligament integrity.

You have the client perform active range of motion and note the following:

- Lateral rotation is limited to 45 degrees, indicating tight muscles are limiting full range of motion, especially the pectoralis major and minor and subscapularis.

- Abduction is limited by 20 degrees. At 160 degrees of abduction there is a springy end feel, indicating supraspinatus impingement, with increased pain under the acromion and secondary pain behind the shoulder blade near the end of that movement.

- Internal rotation is also limited and it is uncomfortable for the client to get the arm behind the back.

Passive range of motion evaluation indicates that the end feel in each direction is normal, with the exception of the springy end feel in abduction, but shoulder movement is associated with a little muscular splinting, ruling out adhesive capsulitis.

Muscle resistance testing finds that the only muscle presenting with a strain is the infraspinatus. There is pain at the muscle–tendon junction of the infraspinatus when the client tries to laterally rotate the shoulder against your resistance. The client can isolate the exact spot by pointing to it with one finger. The supraspinatus does not test positive for a strain, indicating an impingement, that has not progressed to supraspinatus tendinosis, probably due to tight pectoralis major and minor and a tight subscapularis.

You start the client face down to create myofascial space in back of the shoulder for muscle groups to move into avoiding working directly on the strain in the teres minor. The strain needs to be worked last after the tight antagonists are released to bring all muscle groups to their normal muscle resting lengths.

You then position the client supine and release and stretch the anterior shoulder muscles from superficial to deep in the following order:

1. Pectoralis major
2. Pectoralis minor
3. Subclavius
4. Biceps and coracobrachialis
5. Upper trapezius and middle deltoid
6. Subscapularis

It is critical to lengthen the subscapularis muscle to its normal resting state, restoring 80 degrees of lateral rotation of the shoulder, to relax the weak, inhibited infraspinatus and teres minor prior to working on the muscle strain behind the shoulder blade.

You perform myofascial work behind the shoulder from lateral to medial to further relax all the weak, inhibited muscle groups such as infraspinatus, teres minor, middle trapezius, and rhomboids, passing over the area of the muscle strain until the final part of the treatment. You then perform another muscle resistance test to the infraspinatus, and the pain is greatly diminished, due to all fibers feeding the tear being in their neutral resting position. But, the client points with one finger to the muscle–tendon junction of the infraspinatus, which indicates a muscle strain.

- You isolate that area and do multidirectional friction for about 30 seconds, pain-free.

- You follow with active medial and lateral rotation of the shoulder, performed pain-free.

- You then apply eccentric contraction to realign the deeper scar tissue by having the client laterally rotate their shoulder and mildly resist gentle medial rotation back to neutral or back to the normal muscle resting length, performed by you.

In the next resistance test the client cannot find the exact spot of pain. You give him the following self-care suggestions:

- Stretch the anterior shoulder muscles to their normal resting lengths with emphasis on stretching the subscapularis to completely relax the infraspinatus for approximately 7 to 10 days.

- When there is no longer any discomfort in the infraspinatus, the client begins to strengthen it using Thera-Band tubing with focus on the eccentric work. Continue this each day after stretching the anterior shoulder muscles first. You suggest that the client stretches the anterior shoulder muscles before and after each game or practice session, and focuses on the eccentric phase of strengthening for the infraspinatus and teres minor at least 3 to 4 days per week.

CASE STUDY

The client is a published author who spends about 6 to 8 hours per day working on her books. This particular client has just gone through menopause and is currently struggling to get any books published. It is obvious there is a lot of stress in her life. You notice that she has extremely tight upper trapezius, extremely forward shoulders, and a forward cervical posture. The client is complaining of tingling, numbness, and pins and needle sensations into her right arm starting from the shoulder down. She has trouble typing and has difficulty coordinating her fingers. Her medical doctor has told her she has carpal tunnel syndrome since she uses her hands every day to type. But her chiropractor thinks she has thoracic outlet, and has been focusing on adjusting her neck and shoulder. The client has had these symptoms for about 9 months now, and this morning when she woke up she was unable to lift her right arm to comb her hair and wash her face. There has been no specific underling trauma that could have contributed to an injury.

The client presents with a low and extremely forward right shoulder. During active range of motion the client has limited lateral rotation of the shoulder to 45 degrees, indicating tight pectoralis muscles and subscapularis. The client can abduct the shoulder to only 135 degrees. Passive range of motion finds a bone-on-bone-like end feel in abduction at 135 degrees and a bone-on-bone-like end feel in lateral rotation at 45 degrees, indicating adhesive capsule problems. The client has been trying to stretch her shoulder into a doorway based on the advice of her medical experts and complains of pain with movement and pain when she stretches near the coracoid process in front of the shoulder. Muscle resistance testing indicates a small strain in the attachment of the pectoralis minor at the coracoid process.

Following pelvic stabilization, you start prone and perform myofascial work behind the shoulder to create space in the back of the shoulder. You then place the client supine and begin to release the anterior shoulder muscles from superficial to deep. After releasing the pectoralis major and the tight fascia, tight muscle fibers, and muscle belly trigger points in the pectoralis minor, you treat the muscle strain in the pectoralis minor with multidirectional friction. After pain-free movement and eccentric muscle contractions to the pectoralis minor, you are able to stretch it pain-free but toward the end of the stretch you feel a bone-on-bone-like end feel. Although the classic frozen shoulder would usually be limited to about 30 to 45 degrees of abduction, you realize this may be an early onset myofascial adhesion within the joint capsule, which is closer to adhesive capsulitis than the multifaceted frozen shoulder condition. You apply the joint capsule technique to the shoulder at the exact place of this fascial–osseous adhesion and the end feel becomes soft or leathery. You then release and stretch the subclavius, SCMs, and scalenes. After working the subscapularis, you find the same bone-on-bone-like end feel at 45 degrees of lateral shoulder rotation. You apply the joint capsule work again and are able to stretch the subscapularis to restore lateral rotation to 80 degrees with a leathery end feel.

Prior to going prone to finish the protocol to the back of the shoulder you realize the client can still abduct the arm to only 135 degrees with a bone-on-bone-like end feel. You apply joint capsule work again and the client begins to cry as she raises her arm pain-free to 180 degrees of abduction. She realizes the arm is moving pain-free and does not feel the tingling and numbness any longer. She also talks to you about the stress in her life in regard to the recent challenges in her career. You allow her to share her concerns and reassure her about the outcome of her shoulder. You respect when she is done talking and then move her prone to complete the shoulder protocol.

At the end of the session you go over her self-care program. You caution her about the postures and ergonomics of her workstation. You teach her to stretch the anterior neck and shoulder muscles, with emphasis on her pectoralis minor, scalenes, and subscapularis. She will not start the pectoralis minor stretch until it is pain-free, and you caution her about doing any form of aggressive stretching into a doorway. You tell her the importance of moving her shoulder through full abduction and lateral rotation daily to prevent the capsule problem from coming back. You wait two weeks and then add the strengthening exercises for the back of the shoulder along with additional stretches for her neck, elbow, and forearms.

CHAPTER SUMMARY

This chapter offers the clinical massage therapist a variety of tools to evaluate, identify, and properly address the most common clinical conditions of the shoulder. The author wants to stress the importance of doing pelvic stabilization first, and taking a close look at cervical conditions, to resolve contributing factors that can cause or mimic complicated shoulder conditions. Compensatory pain coming from other areas of the body are referred to as ascending or descending syndromes. Musculoskeletal problems in the lower body that affect clinical conditions of the neck or shoulder are called ascending syndromes. Musculoskeletal problems that come from cervical conditions, and contribute to thoracic outlet or carpal tunnel, are called descending syndromes. In the case of nerve compression in the neck or shoulder, the client diagnosed with carpal tunnel syndrome would have a descending syndrome referred to as multiple crush phenomenon. This will be addressed in more detail in Chapter 7 as we cover elbow, forearm, wrist, and hand conditions.

Manual therapists should stop using generic catch-all terms like rotator cuff injury or frozen shoulder, and instead start to sort out the multiple possibilities presenting themselves as pain in the shoulder area. The intention of this chapter is to ensure that the clinical massage therapist eliminate any underlying causes of specific conditions of the

shoulder prior to treating the resulting clinical symptoms. In doing soft tissue balancing or preparation work first, what often seems like complicated clinical conditions of the shoulder, can often times be resolved in just a few sessions.

This whole body approach will allow clients to live pain-free, and athletes to achieve peak performance. Please keep in mind that there are a number of shoulder conditions not addressed in this book, that are out of the scope of our practice and need to be referred out to the client's physician. If in doubt, refer out!

REVIEW QUESTIONS

1. Which of the following muscle(s) is most commonly injured in the shoulder?
   a. pectoralis major
   b. bursa
   c. supraspinatus
   d. subscapularis
2. Generally, which of the following should you do to the posterior rotator cuff muscles?
   a. strengthen
   b. stretch
   c. stretch, then strengthen
   d. none of the above
3. Of the following, what is the most common restriction in shoulder range of motion?
   a. extension
   b. horizontal adduction
   c. medial rotation
   d. lateral rotation
4. What is the primary muscle that abducts the shoulder, when the shoulder is at 10 degrees of abduction?
   a. subscapularis
   b. supraspinatus
   c. middle deltoid
   d. subclavius
5. The client is standing, arm bent 90 degrees, with the elbow abducted 10 degrees away from the side. The client laterally rotates the shoulder against your resistance. What specific muscle is being tested?
   a. supraspinatus
   b. infraspinatus
   c. posterior deltoid
   d. biceps
6. In the majority of your clients, which of the following describes the pectoralis minor and major?
   a. short and tight
   b. overstretched and weak

   c. inhibited and strong
   d. overstretched and strong
7. What two muscles must you release first before working on a supraspinatus impingement?
   a. infraspinatus and teres minor
   b. subscapularis and posterior deltoid
   c. subscapularis and pectoralis minor
   d. anterior deltoid and pectoralis major
8. Which of the following muscles action is shoulder lateral rotation?
   a. teres minor and teres major
   b. teres minor and latissimus dorsi
   c. teres minor and supraspinatus
   d. teres minor and infraspinatus
9. Bicipital tendinosis is often misdiagnosed as what injury?
   a. thoracic outlet
   b. adhesive capsulitis
   c. rotator cuff tear
   d. frozen shoulder
10. Which shoulder limitations are most common in frozen shoulder problems?
    a. extreme limitation in shoulder abduction and internal rotation and bone-on-bone-like end feel in both positions
    b. extreme limitation in shoulder abduction and lateral rotation and bone-on-bone-like end feel in both positions
    c. extreme limitation in shoulder adduction and lateral rotation and bone-on-bone-like end feel in either position
    d. extreme limitation in shoulder flexion and internal rotation and bone-on-bone-like end feel in either position

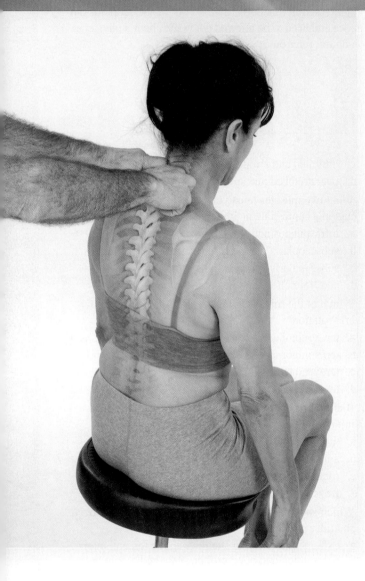

CHAPTER

6 Cervical Spine Conditions

 CHAPTER OUTLINE

Twelve-Step Approach to Cervical Spine Conditions
Cervical Spine Protocols to include:

- Precautionary Tests
- Dura Mater and Dural Sheath Mobilization
- Atlanto-Occipital/Atlanto-Axial Lateral Mobilization
- Atlanto-Occipital/Atlanto-Axial Anterior-Posterior Mobilization
- Velvet Glove Myofascial Release Technique
- Sternocleidomastoid (SCM) and Scalene Release
- Facet Joint Mobilization
- Interspinales, Rotatores, and Intertransversarii
- Suboccipital Muscles
- C1–C2 Rotational Mobilization
- Levator Scapula
- Cervical Decompression

LEARNING OBJECTIVES

Upon completing this chapter the reader will be able to:

- Create structural alignment and balance of the cervical spine muscle groups
- Eliminate the underlying postural and structural cause of common cervical spine conditions before addressing the clinical symptoms
- Restore pain-free normal range of motion of the cervical spine
- Differentiate between soft-tissue problems caused by
  - dural sheath adhesions
  - atlanto-occipital/atlanto-axial fixations
  - myofascial imbalance and myofascial restrictions
  - muscle–tendon tension and imbalance

- myoskeletal alignment problems
- trigger point tension
- joint capsule adhesions
- facet joint fixations
- C1–C2 rotational restrictions
- strained muscle fibers
- scar tissue
- Teach the client self-care stretching and strengthening exercises (if needed) to perform at home to maintain myoskeletal balance and pain-free movement of the cervical spine following therapy.

KEY TERMS

Bony fixation   *208*
Facet joint fixation   *208*

Lateral shearing
  force   *211–212*

The cervical spine work starts at the lumbar and sacral region, as it is highly recommended to begin with pelvic stabilization, to have the best effect on treating clinical conditions of the neck. The myofascial structure of the torso is so powerful you should also release and lengthen the entire superficial front line to be able to effectively work the muscles of the neck. For clients with anterior (forward) shoulder posture, you should also perform the shoulder protocol to bring those muscles into balance prior to working the cervical spine. The term ascending syndrome refers to conditions of the neck that start further down the body. Instability of the pelvis, leg length discrepancies, or extreme imbalance of the shoulders will have a profound effect on cervical conditions.

Repetitive movements, poor posture, injuries, or incorrect body mechanics can lead to tight, contracted muscles and soft-tissue problems (strains or sprains) of the neck. You will learn the difference between stretching the sternocleidomastoid and scalenes versus the levator scapula, as improper release of muscle groups coming from the chest and shoulders can severely compress the cervical spine on the attachment side and limit the result of manual therapy.

Work the restricted side first; typically the dominant side, usually working up the neck to lengthen the spine. Continually traction the neck and then gently release it so it doesn't bounce back and entrap a nerve or a blood vessel, to create space and to improve vascular circulation. The overall goal is to restore normal range of motion, restore normal muscle resting lengths, and reduce pain in the cervical spine. This chapter was written to address common conditions of the cervical spine. It is highly recommended that therapist take hands-on training beyond the information presented in this chapter to treat more complicated cervical conditions.

TWELVE-STEP APPROACH TO CERVICAL SPINE CONDITIONS

The following muscles groups and structures are covered in this chapter:

- Dura mater and dural sheath mobilization
- Atlanto-Occipital/Atlanto-Axial lateral mobilization
- Atlanto-Occipital/Atlanto-Axial anterior-posterior mobilization
- Facet joint mobilization
- Sternocleidomastoid (SCM) and scalenes
- Interspinales rotatores intertransversarii
- Suboccipital muscles
- Levator scapula
- C1–C2 rotational mobilization
- Levator scapula
- Cervical disc decompression

Precautionary Tests

The following are very important precautionary tests:

PRECAUTIONARY NOTE

If the client has been in a car accident and has not had an MRI, bone scan, or x-ray, *do not* perform this work. If the client becomes dizzy, nauseous, disoriented, has blurred vision, or feels like he or she is going to pass out, immediately discontinue treatment. If the client shows any other inappropriate medical or neurological symptoms, advise him or her to get a medical exam. Remember, if in doubt, refer out!

TRANSVERSE ALAR LIGAMENT TEST

This test *must* be performed first. If the client "fails" this test you *must immediately* refer him or her out. This indicates a serious condition!

This is a test for hypermobility or rupture of the alar ligament, caused from trauma to the neck, which subsequently does not protect the spinal cord. It could create the symptoms listed in the Precautionary Note, and can put direct pressure on the spinal cord, causing numbness to shoot down both arms.

The client is seated with the head in neutral position (Figure 6-1 ■). Have him or her place one finger on the chin. Ask the client to move the neck backward (military posture), keeping the head in the neutral plane while gently pressing on their chin (Figure 6-2 ■). If the client reports any symptoms listed in the Precautionary Note, including pain, tingling, numbness, or parasthesia into the extremities, *do not* proceed with the cervical work!

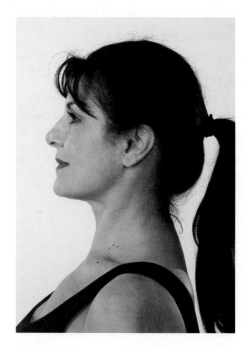

FIGURE 6-1
Neutral Cervical Position.

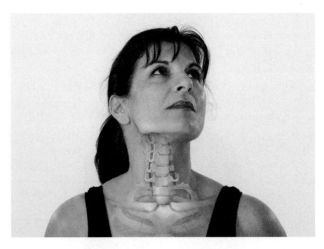

FIGURE 6-3B
Vertebral Artery Compression Test—Left Side.

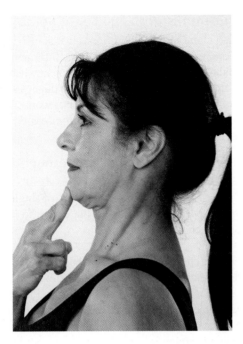

FIGURE 6-2
Alar Ligament Test.

Note: The client may report feeling a "lump" in the back of the throat during this movement. This is due to the pressure of C2 on the throat, and it is normal.

VERTEBRAL ARTERY COMPRESSION TEST

Have the client rotate the neck 45 degrees to the right and then extend it back to the left, but only to where it is comfortable (Figure 6-3A ■). Have him or her hold this position for 30 seconds. Repeat this test on the other side, rotating the neck left and extending back to the right (Figure 6-3B ■).

If the client experiences neurological symptoms like blurred vision, dizziness, nausea, or feels as if he or she is going to pass out, have the client stop immediately and return

the head to neutral. *Do not* proceed with the cervical work; refer the client out. He or she could have *vertebral artery insufficiency* which decreases vascular flow to the brain.[1]

The following extract on vertebral artery syndrome is reproduced with permission from Dr. Erik Dalton:

> Vertebral artery syndrome is commonly referred as vertebrobasilar artery insufficiency (VBI). The vertebral arteries enter the cervical spine at the level of C6–C7 (bilaterally) and make their way headward threading through the intertransverse foramina of each cervical vertebra and exiting at the superior side of the transverse process of C1. Each of these relatively small arteries then wrap themselves around the posterior arch of the atlas, penetrate the posterior occipitoatlantal membrane and tuck up through the foramen magnum to join together to form the basilar artery system. As these arteries make their way to the brain, they may become completely blocked by a clot—resulting in a stroke, or may be temporarily occluded, bruised, or ruptured by certain head on neck movements.[2]

Therefore, a red flag should be raised in clients presenting with severely restricted head and neck rotation, alerting the therapist to the possibility of vertebral artery problems. The vertebral artery test described previously should be performed before introducing any type of rotational movements. Proper referrals should be made if the test proves positive.

CERVICAL COMPRESSION/DECOMPRESSION TEST

This is a *gentle* compression test. The client is seated, with the head in neutral position. Gently lift and traction the head first, for distraction (Figure 6-4B ■). Then, gently press down with both hands on the top of the head for several seconds (Figure 6-4A ■).

Begin with light pressure and then slowly increase the pressure to a moderate level. Ask if the client is experiencing any symptoms like radiating pain, tingling, or numbness in

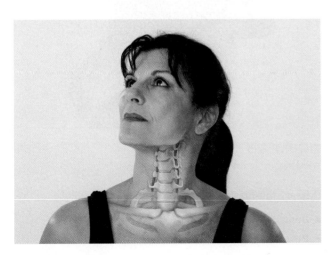

FIGURE 6-3A
Vertebral Artery Compression Test—Right Side.

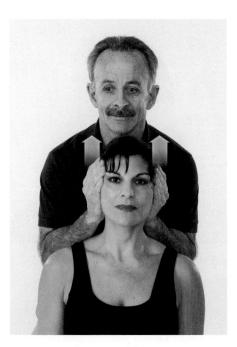

FIGURE 6-4A
Cervical Decompression.

the arm, and determine what side of the neck is involved. If the client has numbness or tingling or radiating pain into the shoulders or arms, this could indicate severe disc degeneration, bulging discs, ruptured discs, spinal stenosis, or bone spurs that compress the spinal nerve roots on the involved side. In this case, *do not* perform the cervical work. Refer the client out to an orthopedic specialist or neurologist. Only if you are cleared by the physician should you perform cervical work on these clients.

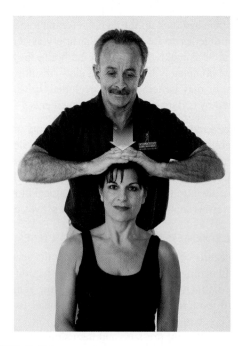

FIGURE 6-4B
Cervical Compression.

Step 1: Client History

A thorough client history will offer valuable insights into a client's condition. In addition to the basic information completed on the client history form, ask the client when, where, and how the problem began. Also ask the client to describe the area of pain and what makes it better or worse. This will give you a starting point from which to assess the client's active range of motion.

Step 2: Assess Active Range of Motion (AROM)

Goal: To assess range of motion degrees of single-plane movements performed solely by the client, to identify tight or restricted muscle groups.

Assess the client's active ROM of the four primary single-plane movements of the cervical spine, pain-free. They are flexion, extension, rotation, and lateral flexion. Please keep in mind the degrees may vary slightly based on different references. Ask the client to keep the shoulders square. Determine if the range of motion is normal. Please understand that the normal degrees for each cervical range of motion will vary with different references. The degrees listed in this text are accurate estimates for healthy clients. If the range of motion is less than average, identify which muscle groups are restricted and therefore preventing normal movement.

If flexion is less than 45 to 50 degrees, work on releasing the extensors (antagonists)—longissimus capitis and cervicis, semispinalis capitis and cervicis, spinalis capitis, splenius capitis and cervicis, and trapezius—to restore normal muscle resting lengths (Figure 6-5 ■).

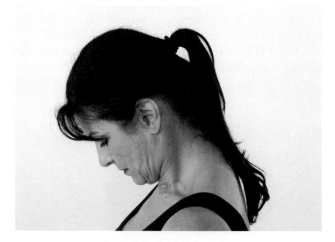

FIGURE 6-5
AROM Cervical Flexion, 45–50 Degrees.

Primary muscles:

- Longus capitis and coli
- Rectus capitis anterior and lateralis
- Scalenes (anterior, medial, posterior)
- Sternocleidomastoid

If extension is less than 75 to 85 degrees, work on releasing the flexors (antagonists)—longus capitis and coli, rectus capitis anterior and lateralis, anterior, medial, and posterior scalenes, and sternocleidomastoid—to restore normal muscle resting lengths (Figure 6-6 ■).

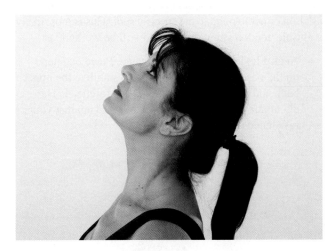

FIGURE 6-6
AROM Cervical Extension, 75–85 Degrees.

Primary muscles:

- Longissimus capitis and cervicis
- Semispinalis capitis and cervicis
- Spinalis capitis
- Splenius capitis and cervicis
- Trapezius

If lateral flexion is less than 40 to 45 degrees, work on releasing the lateral flexors on the other side of the neck (antagonists)—iliocostalis cervicis, levator scapula, longissimus cervicis, multifidus, scalenes, sternocleidomastoid, semispinalis cervicis, and splenius cervicis—to restore normal muscle resting lengths (Figure 6-7A ■ and 6-7B ■).

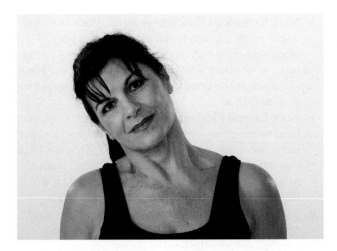

FIGURE 6-7A
AROM Cervical Lateral Flexion, Right 40–45 Degrees.

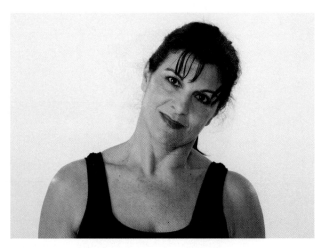

FIGURE 6-7B
AROM Cervical Lateral Flexion, Left, 40–45 Degrees.

Primary muscles:

- Iliocostalis cervicis
- Levator scapula
- Longissimus cervicis
- Multifidus
- Scalenes, SCM
- Semispinalis and splenius cervicis

If rotation is less than 80 to 90 degrees, work on releasing the rotators on the other side of the neck (antagonists)—iliocostalis cervicis (contralateral), levator scapula (contralateral), longissimus cervicis (contralateral), multifidus (ipsilateral), scalenes and sternocleidomastoid (ipsilateral), and splenius cervicis (contralateral)—to restore normal muscle resting lengths. Keep in mind that about 45 degrees of rotation occurs at the atlanto-axial joint, and the remaining 45 degrees within the C2–C7 area (Figures 6-8A ■ and 6-8B ■).

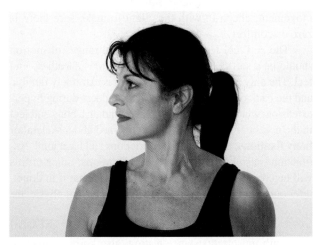

FIGURE 6-8A
AROM Cervical Rotation, Right, 80–90 Degrees.

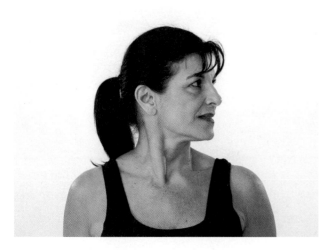

FIGURE 6-8B
AROM Cervical Rotation, Left, 80–90 Degrees.

Primary muscles:

- Iliocostalis cervicis (ipsilateral)
- Levator scapula (ipsilateral)
- Longissimus cervicis (ipsilateral)
- Multifidus (contralateral)
- Scalenes, SCM (contralateral)
- Splenius cervicis (ipsilateral)

Step 3: Assess Passive Range of Motion (PROM)

Goal: to assess range of motion end feel of single-plane movements performed on the client by you. Pain during passive movement predominately implicates inert tissues, but may involve muscles that are being stretched.

Determine the end feel of flexion, extension, lateral flexion, and rotation through passive ROM tests.[3] Ask the client to keep the shoulders square. As you perform each movement, check in with the client to make sure there is zero discomfort.

The end feel for all passive cervical ranges of motion should be a soft-tissue stretch, also known as a leathery end feel. The only exception is when a client is extremely flexible and the back of the head touches the shoulders during hyperextension, which stops the movement. Finding a bony end feel in the neck alerts you to be more concerned about skeletal or **bony fixations,** like atlas–axis restrictions and facet joint dysfunctions, also known as **facet joint fixations.** Some of this will be corrected with this cervical protocol, but if in doubt, refer out to an osteopath, chiropractor, or medical physician.

Step 4: Assess Resisted Range of Motion (RROM)

Pain with muscle resistance testing, also know as manual resistance testing, occurs when there is mechanical disruption of tissue. This indicates a strain to one or more of the

muscles performing the action that you are resisting. The client attempts each of the four single-plane movements of the cervical spine while you apply gentle resistance. For precaution, start the test with minimal contraction by the client, and then slowly increase the reverse resistance to fully recruit the muscle fibers. If the client experiences pain or discomfort, ask him or her to point to the specific spot. This is most likely a muscle–tendon strain or tear, and will be worked last.

- **Neck Flexion:** The client is seated. Place one hand on the base of the client's neck (to stabilize the upper back and neck) and one hand on the forehead. The client attempts to flex the neck forward against your resistance (Figure 6-9 ■).

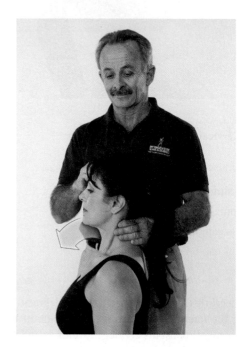

FIGURE 6-9
Resisted Test, Neck Flexion.

- **Neck Extension:** The client is seated. Place one hand on the upper sternum to stabilize the upper body. Then place your other hand on the back of the client's head using a "c" clamp with slight traction, lifting up. He or she attempts to extend the neck against your resistance (Figure 6-10 ■).
- **Neck Lateral Flexion:** The client is seated. Place one hand on the client's left shoulder to stabilize the upper body, and one hand on the left side of the client's head (not over the ear). The client attempts lateral flexion to the left against your resistance (Figure 6-11A ■). Repeat this test on the right side (Figure 6-11B ■).
- **Neck Rotation:** The client is seated. Place one hand on each side of the client's head. He or she gently attempts to rotate the head to the left against your resistance (Figure 6-12A ■). Repeat the rotation test to the right (Figure 6-12B ■).

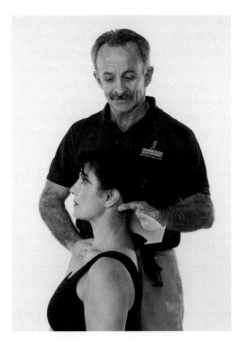

FIGURE 6-10
Resisted Test, Neck Extension.

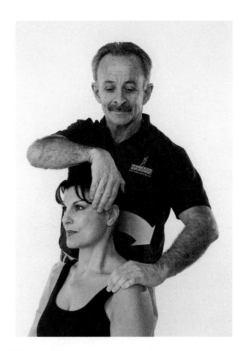

FIGURE 6-11B
Resisted Test, Neck Lateral Flexion—Left.

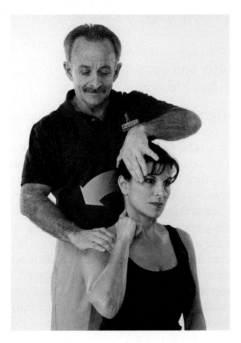

FIGURE 6-11A
Resisted Test, Neck Lateral Flexion—Right.

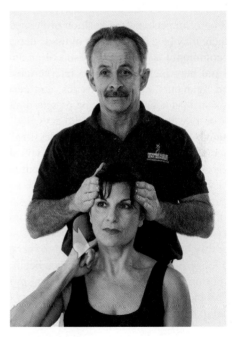

FIGURE 6-12A
Resisted Test, Neck Rotation—Left.

WHIPLASH

It is strongly recommended that any client with a whiplash condition be evaluated first by a physician to rule out serious pathologies that can be compromised by the application of manual therapy techniques. There can be a great number of structures involved, including cervical fractures, torn ligaments, and ruptured discs. The scope of this chapter will focus on balancing out the major and minor muscle groups of the neck to facilitate better bone alignment, and the treatment of minor strains and minor sprains of the cervical spine in the non-acute or chronic phase of this condition.

Whiplash is characterized by a collection of symptoms that occur following damage to the neck, usually because of sudden extension and flexion. However, depending on

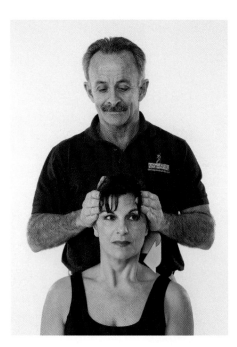

FIGURE 6-12B
Resisted Test, Neck Rotation—Right.

the direction of impact and the position of the neck during impact, there may be a wide variety of tissue damage.[4] The disorder commonly occurs as the result of an automobile accident and may include injury to intervertebral joints, discs, and ligaments, cervical muscles, and nerve roots. Symptoms such as neck pain may be present directly after the injury or may be delayed for several days.[5]

Although most rear-end accidents specifically injure the sternocleidomastoid and the scalenes, typically all of the muscles of the neck are affected. The client may complain of a variety of symptoms including neck pain, stiffness and muscle spasms, headaches, pain in the shoulder or between the shoulder blades, dizziness, ringing in the ears, blurred vision, memory problems, and sleep disturbances.[6] Only after the client has been cleared by his or her physician and is no longer in the acute phase can you begin massage therapy. Perform the entire following cervical protocol, as bringing balance to all of the muscles of the cervical spine is essential to resolving the problem.

CERVICAL SPINE PROTOCOL

Cervical Mobilization

The following four techniques are the result of blending the atlas–axis work taught by by Paul St. John[7] with basic myoskeletal alignment techniques from Dr. Erik Dalton. This particular approach has been modified and slightly simplified. *Training in Posturology with Paul St. John and Randall Clark, and training in Myoskeletal Alignment with Dr. Erik Dalton is highly recommended for a more advanced*

look at this work. The author suggests that dural sheath mobilization, C1–C2 mobilization, and facet joint mobilization be done prior to, or in conjunction with, soft tissue work, especially if there are any bony end feels when evaluating passive movements of the neck. End feel for all cervical movements should be tissue stretch. Thus, if there are fixations in bones of the neck, it will be difficult to release and stretch the tight muscle groups without this work.

Dura Mater and Dural Sheath Mobilization

The dural membrane surrounds the brain and spinal cord to protect the contents and to sustain a barrier to antigens, yet transport nutrients to the central nervous system. The dura mater and the dural sheaths may adhere to the vertebral or neural foramena, or the dural sheaths may adhere to the neurons as they exit. As a result, they may cause stimulation of the nerves and resulting muscle tension patterns associated with these entrapments. Performing the following technique will often result in an overall relaxation response, and may be used in conjunction with other modalities to facilitate the therapist's work. Uneven traction on the dura mater may lead to fascial distortion that encroaches upon the pituitary glands leading to hormonal dysfunction.[8]

Dura Mater and Dural Sheath Mobilization Protocol

- The client is supine with the neck in neutral cervical spine position. Seated at the clients head, the therapist places his or her hands on each side of the head with your fingers around the ears. It is recommended that the therapist bring the heels of his or her hands together, so his or her fingers would be above the ears.
- Keep the cervical spine in perfect neutral without anything placed behind the neck for these techniques. With the heel of the hands together, press the client's cranium directly inferior for approximately 5 seconds. This will shorten the dura mater and muscles along the spinal column. Be certain that the neck does not go into flexion or extension with the pressure, because this buckling will limit the effectiveness of the technique (Figure 6-13A ■).
- Traction the cranium superiorly by hooking the fingers under the nuchal line of the occiput and pulling in a superior direction. Keep the fingertips at a right angle to the occiput as this will provide the most leverage. Be certain not to use the mandibles; this can compress the TMJ causing an excitation of the trigeminal nerve (Figure 6-13B ■). The emphasis is on the traction phase, and each traction should result in more movement as the muscles continue to relax.
- Repeat this compression/decompression sequence five or six times.

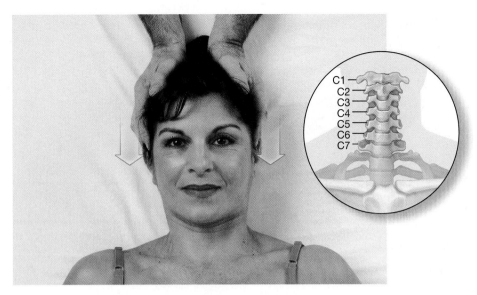

FIGURE 6-13A
Dura Mater and Dural Sheath Mobilization (Compression).

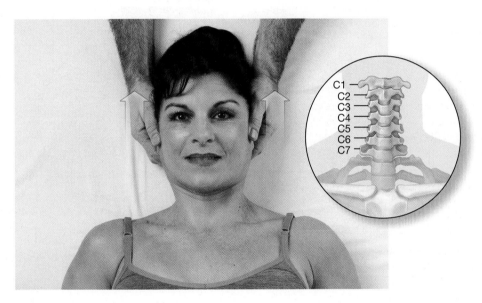

FIGURE 6-13B
Dura Mater and Dural Sheath Mobilization (Decompression).

Atlanto-Occipital/ Atlanto-Axial Lateral Mobilization Protocol

To reduce **lateral shearing forces,** where the C1 cervical vertebrae slides slightly lateral to one side.

- The client is supine with the neck in neutral position. Place one hand along the cervical spine with the palm conformed to the entire neck, and the thenar eminence near lateral border of the SCM against the lateral edge or transverse process of C1. The other hand is just above the opposite ear on the head; this hand stabilizes.
- With no lateral neck flexion or tilting of the head, the therapist should gently push his or her palm on the

cervical spine to see if there is in-line movement to the opposite side. Check for restricted movement to both the client's left (Figure 6-14A ■) and to the client's right (Figure 6-14B ■). The images show C1 sheared to the client's right, limiting lateral movement to the client's left. Because C1 is sheared right limiting movement to the left, the client gently pushes back to the right against your resistance for 5 to 10 seconds. He or she relaxes and then you gently slide the neck sideways into the direction of the restriction, in this case increasing movement to the client's left side. Keep the eyes level during the movement. Make sure the lip line stays horizontal. This is a very gentle muscle energy technique and should be absolutely pain-free.

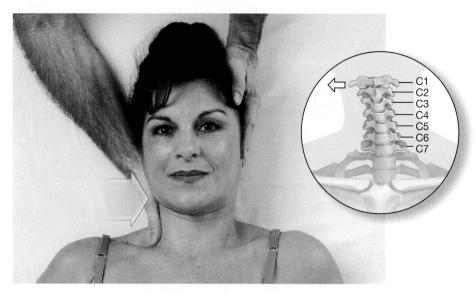

FIGURE 6-14A
Assess/Correct Lateral Shearing Forces—Right.

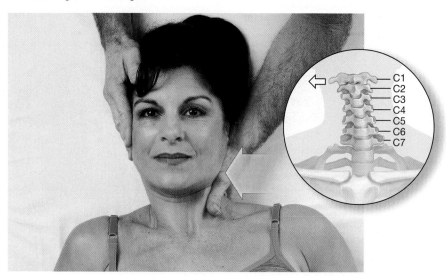

FIGURE 6-14B
Assess/Correct Lateral Shearing Forces—Left.

Atlanto-Occipital/Atlanto-Axial Anterior-Posterior Mobilization Protocol

The client is supine. Have the client move so that the head is off the end of the table but the neck is still slightly supported on the table (Figure 6-15 ▪).

- Once the neck is cradled and the client can relax, have him or her slide up slightly so the shoulders are at the top edge of the table. Place one hand under the neck to support the neck, with slight traction on the sub-occipital ridge. Your other hand supports the forehead. Prevent any cervical flexion and extension, and prevent any lateral flexion during this technique.

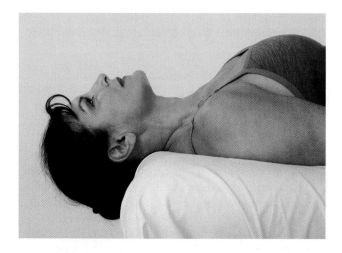

FIGURE 6-15
Beginning Position on Table with Neck Supported to Prevent Hyperextension.

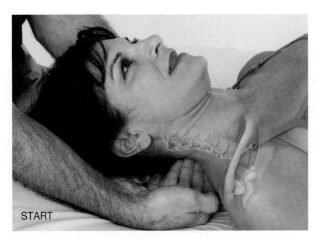
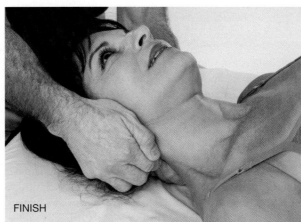

FIGURE 6-23A
Myofascial Stretch Right Medial Scalenes.

Repeat this fascial hook, and deep cross-fiber gliding strokes several times. This will affect the attachments of the medial and posterior scalenes on the posterior tubercles and also the levator scapula on the transverse processes of C1–C4. Make sure to perform this same sequence on the left side of the neck

With the client's hands still under the hips, rotate the client's neck 45 degrees to the left. The therapist's left hand is under the clients head with the fingers in the right lamina groove. The right finger pads starts on the right levator scapula and moves superiorly up and into the lamina groove of the neck to meet the left hand, as you passively laterally flex the neck to the left (chin moves toward opposite shoulder). This mobilization helps release tension in both the right posterior scalene and the right levator scapula (Figure 6-23B).

To perform this on the left posterior scalene and levator, rotate the client's neck 45 degrees to the right. Place the right hand under the head with the fingers on the left lamina groove. The left hand starts on the left levator scapula and moves superiorly up the lamina groove to meet the right

hand, as you passively laterally flex the neck to the right (chin moves toward opposite shoulder).

To finish, stand at the clients head and place both hands under the client's neck with your finger pads in both of the lamina grooves. Move both hands superiorly, bilaterally up the neck as you traction and decompress the neck. By releasing the tension in muscle groups that attach to the cervical transverse processes, it will allow the therapist to easily open and close stuck or stubborn cervical facet joints in a technique later in this chapter.

Step 11: Stretching (During Therapy)

> ## ✋ PRECAUTIONARY NOTE
>
> Before you begin this stretch, repeat the vertebral artery compression test. If the client is uncomfortable, dizzy, or nauseous, do not perform this stretch.

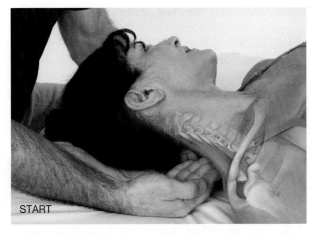
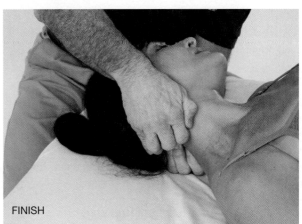

FIGURE 6-23B
Myofascial Stretch Right Levator Scapula and Posterior Scalenes.

✋ PRECAUTIONARY NOTE

Stretching is not suggested for the muscle groups around a hypermobile joint. Strengthening would be more appropriate to stabilize any joint that has excessive movement due to ligamentous laxity.

To stretch the anterior scalene and SCM, the client is supine on the table with you supporting the head. The back of the neck is still supported on the table so he or she cannot hyperextend the neck. Ask the client to place their hands under the hips with palms facing up. This will roll the shoulders posteriorly and help anchor down the shoulders to lengthen the SCM and scalenes.

To stretch and lengthen the anterior scalene and SCM on the right side, gently traction the client's neck and have him or her rotate the head 45 degrees, or only as far as it will go pain-free to the right. He or she exhales and slowly, *actively* laterally flexes the neck to the left with your assistance and traction for about 2 seconds (Figure 6-24A ■). This should be performed only if there is zero discomfort. This is to prevent injury, especially to those clients who have disc or facet pathologies. Repeat this stretch several times.

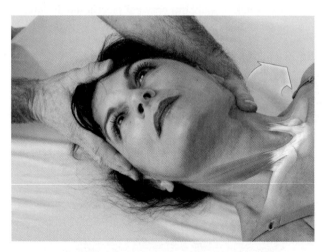

FIGURE 6-24A
Stretch Right SCM and Anterior Scalene.

Next, perform the stretch on the left side. This time, have the client rotate the head 45 degrees to the left. He or she exhales, and slowly, *actively* laterally flexes to the right with your assistance for about 2 seconds. This will effectively stretch the anterior scalenes and the SCM.

Finish with in-line traction to the neck again. Release the neck very slowly and gently.

Step 11: Stretching (During Therapy)

To stretch the right medial scalene, the client is supine on the table with the hands anchored under the hips. Stabilize

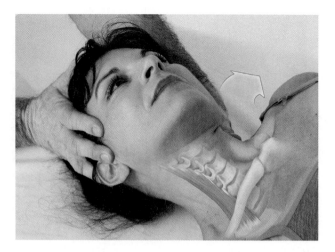

FIGURE 6-24B
Stretch Right Medial Scalene.

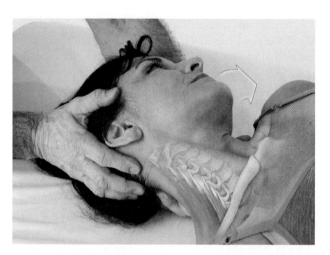

FIGURE 6-24C
Right Posterior Scalene Stretch.

the shoulder down with one hand. Ask the client to laterally flex the neck away from the side you are stretching while you assist the stretch (Figure 6-24B ■). Repeat this several times to stretch the medial scalene and lateral neck flexors. Repeat this on the other side, if needed.

Step 11: Stretching (During Therapy)

To stretch the posterior scalene, the client is supine on the table with the hands anchored under the hips. Stabilize the shoulder down with your hand and ask the client to take the chin toward the opposite shoulder. You assist this posterior scalene stretch (Figure 6-24C ■). Repeat several times and on the other side, if needed.

✋ PRECAUTIONARY NOTE

Do not perform this protocol with clients that have bulging discs without medical clearance and hands on training.

CERVICAL SPINE MOBILIZATION TECHNIQUES

1. **Translation:** Translation involves gently moving the client's cervical vertebrae side to side, individual vertebra by vertebra, to improve joint alignment and joint play. This is *not* lateral flexion. The head stays in the same plane with no movement in the upper cervical vertebrae. Start at C7 and with your finger pads brace each side of the spinous process and try to gently move it side to side (Figure 6-25A ■). Work superiorly up the neck to C2. If a restriction is found during right translation, have the client resist the movement for 5 to 10 seconds and then relax as you perform right translation again. If a restriction is found during left translation, have the client gently resist your movement for 5 to 10 seconds. The client relaxes and you again perform left translation.

2. **Lateral Flexion/Facet Joint Mobilization:** Now perform lateral flexion vertebra by vertebra to soften small intrinsic cervical muscles such as the intertransversarii and improve joint mobilization. This technique can easily open and close stuck facet joints,

without needing high velocity manipulation, because you have already released the tension in the muscle groups that attach to the transverse processes. Place your hands under the client's head with your index finger anterior to the transverse processes between C7 and C6, behind the SCM. Your middle finger is in the lamina groove between C7 and C6. Gently laterally flex the neck left while the right two fingers gently press and lift upward. Then, gently laterally flex the neck right while the left two fingers gently press and lift upward (Figure 6-25B ■). Repeat these techniques as you work up the neck to C2. If a restriction is found during lateral flexion, have the client gently resist this movement for 5 to 10 seconds and then relax. Then try the lateral flexion with finger pad support and bracing again. This work must be pain-free. If in doubt, refer out!

3. **Combination:** Your hands and fingers are in the same position as for lateral flexion. Start at the C7 vertebra and move it side to side, then laterally flex it left and right, and perform slight traction

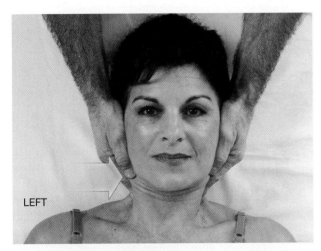
LEFT

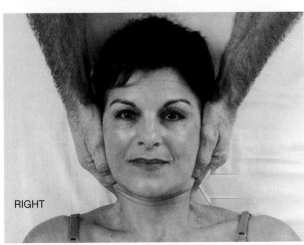
RIGHT

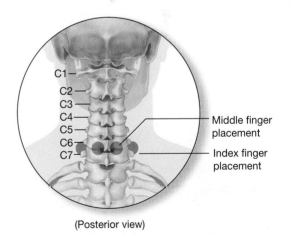
Middle finger placement
Index finger placement
(Posterior view)

FIGURE 6-25A
Translation.

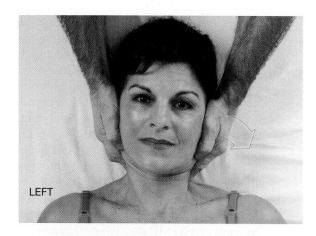

LEFT

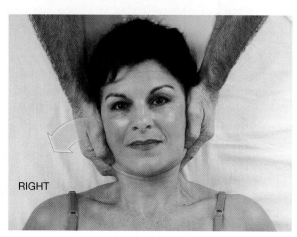

RIGHT

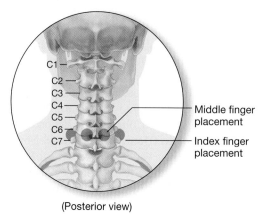

Middle finger placement

Index finger placement

(Posterior view)

FIGURE 6-25B
Lateral Flexion.

(Figure 6-25C ■), sliding up the neck to the next vertebra. Repeat the sequence working each vertebra separately to soften the small intrinsic muscles that will help open and close and mobilize each individual joint.

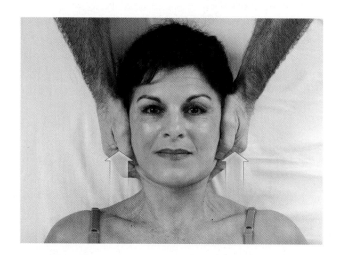

FIGURE 6-25C
Cervical Traction.

INTERSPINALES, ROTATORES, AND INTERTRANSVERSARII

See video clip of this technique at www.myhealthprofessionskit.com.

The next three unique techniques involve releasing groups of short, deep intrinsic muscles in the cervical spine—interspinales, rotatores, and intertransversarii. They are part of the transversospinalis muscles and they lie deep to the erector spinae. You don't need to know their specific names to be able to perform these techniques; however, the more you learn about the muscles, the better your clinical and orthopedic massage treatment will be (Figure 6-26 ■).

These muscles are so deep that they cannot be palpated. Instead, your massage tool will be the movement of the bones against the pressure of your fingers onto the deep muscles. This will allow the massage to occur from the inside out. Perform all of the movements for these three techniques passively and pain-free.

Note: For simplification and easy recall, the following sequences can also be identified by the motion of the client's head: "yes" (flexion), "no" (rotation), "I don't know" (lateral flexion).

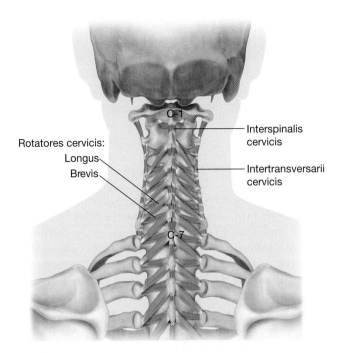

FIGURE 6-26
Cervical and Upper Thoracic Spine.

Interspinales ("Yes")

The interspinales are located between the spinous processes of the cervical, lumbar, and some of the thoracic vertebrae. Their action is extension of the spine and when they are tight they can create compression of the cervical discs. See video clip of this technique at www.myhealthprofessionskit.com.

Step 6: Myofascial Release

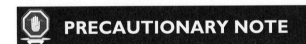

PRECAUTIONARY NOTE

Do not perform this technique if the client has bulging or herniated discs.

Gently traction the client's neck using a "c" clamp grip with one hand. Then place your finger pad or the side of your index finger opposite hand, horizontally, in the gap between the spinous bones of C7 and C6. Gently press up between the spinous processes of C7/C6 while passively moving the client's head through flexion and extension several times, followed by traction. This allows the movement of the spinous processes to massage the interspinales from the inside out. Slowly release the client's head. Then move between C6 and C5 and repeat the traction, press up, flex-extend, and release. You may feel a myofascial release or a crunchy sensation as the neck starts to release and lengthen.

As you move up the neck, it may be harder to find the gap between the bones. If so, bring the client's head into flexion to be able to better palpate the correct location. Continue to work up the neck to the suboccipital ridge finishing with the interspinales muscle located between C3 and C2. The base of the skull limits you from proceeding any further.

Repeat this entire sequence, moving up the neck a couple of times. Start with a very gentle pressure and work deeper as the muscles release, as long as it is pain-free and they do not have a bulging or herniated disc. Finish with in-line traction and a 5-second stretch to the neck again. Release the neck very slowly. See video clip at www.myhealthprofessionkit.com.

Rotatores ("No")

The rotatores are located on all the vertebrae, running from the transverse process to the spinous process above it. They assist the multifidi in extension of the spine and rotation to the opposite side. See video clip of this technique at www.myhealthprofessionskit.com.

Step 6: Myofascial Release

The most predominant myofascial adhesions are found in the rotatores. Work the tight, restricted or dominant side first. Gently traction the client's neck with one hand and curl the finger pads of your other hand under the client's neck and find the lamina groove on the opposite side. Your fingers will press into and glide up the lamina groove while passively moving the client's head through rotation left and right. Perform deep cross-fiber gliding strokes up the lamina groove if you find any fibrosis.

Check also for rotated vertebrae, due to tight muscles. You may feel them as you work up the lamina groove. The goal is a "smooth groove." Repeat this several times and then again on the other side of the neck. This will effectively massage the rotatores from the inside out by the movement of the cervical vertebrae. Traction the neck, stretch for 5 seconds, and release very slowly.

Intertransversarii ("I Don't Know")

These muscles are located between the transverse processes of the cervical, lumbar, and some of the thoracic vertebrae. Their action is lateral flexion of the spine. When these muscles are short and contracted they can lock down the facet joints, causing the facet joints to be locked closed on the tight side. See video clip of this technique at www.myhealthprofessionskit.com.

Step 6: Myofascial Release

This is a repeat of a previous technique, if needed, to better open and close stubborn facet joints in the cervical spine. Traction the client's neck. Place your index finger just behind the SCM and in front of the transverse processes. Place your second finger behind the transverse processes in the lamina groove. With firm pressure passively move the client's head from side to side—lateral flexion. Start between C7 and C6 and move up the client's neck pinning the muscles with direct, firm pressure. The movement of the bones will help release the deep intrinsic tissue, facilitating facet joint movement. Repeat the sequence several times. This work can be done bilaterally as in Figure 6-25B or unilaterally as in the www.myhealthprofessionskit.com video clip. End with traction of the neck for 5 seconds, releasing slowly and gently.

SUBOCCIPITAL MUSCLES

See video clip of this technique at www.myhealthprofessionskit.com.

Note: You must first release the scalenes and SCM, to eliminate the client's forward head posture, before you work the suboccipital muscles.

These muscles are almost always contracted to compensate for the forward head posture in order to keep the eyes level. This is known as the righting reflex. For every action in the body, there will be an opposite and equal reaction. It will be much easier to restore the rotation at C1–C2 if the forward head posture, and compensatory firing of the suboccipital muscles are addressed first. The suboccipital muscles also play an important role in head–eye coordination and postural orientation.[10] These two sets of four muscles are the deepest muscles of the upper posterior neck. On each lateral side are the oblique capitis superior and oblique capitis inferior. Medial to these are the rectus capitis posterior major and rectus capitis posterior minor. The rectus capitis posterior major crosses C1–C2 and can severly limit cervical rotation if tight or restricted. The rectus capitis posterior minor actually connects to the dura mater, the connective tissue that surrounds the spinal cord and the brain, and when restricted can cause vascular, ischemic headaches including migraines[11] (Figure 6-27 ▪).

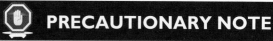

PRECAUTIONARY NOTE

Do not press directly on the soft spot, or on the muscle belly of the rectus capitis posterior minor, below the base of the skull (above C2); the vertebral artery could be compressed.

Clients with forward neck posture (due to tight SCM and scalenes) will compensate by hyperextending their neck, which causes the suboccipitals to contract and close down the articulations of C1 and C2. This can create compression of nerves and blood vessels leading to pain and neuropathy. It can also cause the cervical vertebrae to fuse, wear out, degenerate, herniate, rupture, or create facet joint dysfunction. These myofascial and muscular fusions produce limited neck rotation and the only way to return the neck to normal is to lengthen the muscles of extension and create space between the bones.

Step 6: Myofascial Release

Using your finger pads, perform a sweeping stroke working lateral to medial staying on the suboccipital ridge. Start with deep myofascial spreading and progress to cross-fiber gliding or cross-fiber frictioning, and work progressively deeper. Repeat this several times.

This will soften the attachments of various muscles, including the splenius capitis, semispinalis capitis, oblique capitis superior, and the deeper rectus capitis posterior major and rectus capitus posterior minor. We also suggest releasing the muscle bellies of the oblique capitus superior and oblique capitus inferior. However, the most important muscle that crosses C1–C2 restricting cervical rotation is the rectus capitis posterior major.

Locate the rectus capitis posterior major (RCPM). With the client at 20 degrees of cervical flexion, slide your finger pads up the lamina groove, then move lateral of the midline, at the base of the skull (away from the soft spot). To make sure you are on the RCPM, have the client look upward or slightly extend the upper cervical area..You will feel the RCPM contract or shorten. Traction the neck and take two fingers and apply direct gentle pressure on both of the RCPMs at the base of the skull for several seconds to start to soften the muscles.

Next, place your index and middle fingers at the attachment of the rectus capitis posterior major on C2 spinous process and glide up to the base of the skull. Slide your fingers laterally and perform cross-fiber gliding strokes across the RCPM (Figure 6-28 ▪). Then put the client's head in neutral, traction the client's neck, and have him or her actively tuck the chin as you assist, while gliding laterally on the RCPM. Move at a diagonal angle from origin to insertion: C2 to the attachment on the skull. Keep the neck in-line and the head

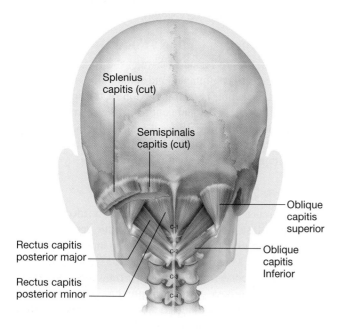

FIGURE 6-27
Suboccipital Muscles.

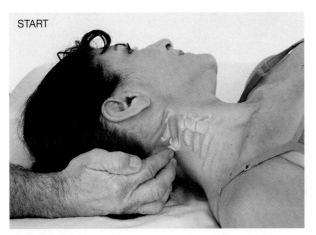
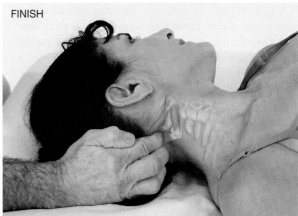

FIGURE 6-28
Rectus Capitus Posterior Major Release.

on the table; this is not neck flexion. This will stretch the rectus capitis posterior major, and help open up C1 and C2 to create disc space and restore cervical rotation. With the head remaining in neutral, repeat the cross-fiber gliding strokes followed by the assisted chin tuck. You can also perform general cross-fiber strokes from C2 to the base of the skull, mobilizing any other restricted tissue, such as the obique capitis superior and rectus capitis posterior minor. Remember not to press into the belly of the rectus capitis posterior minor to avoid pressure to the basilar artery.

If you find any muscle belly trigger points, apply direct pressure for 10 to 12 seconds, compress the area to further soften it, and then gently stretch the tissue. Finish with in-line traction and neck stretch for 5 seconds. Release very slow and gently.

Cervical Joint Capsule Work and C1–C2 Mobilization

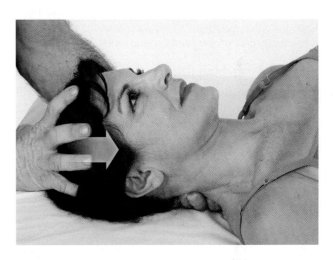

FIGURE 6-29A
Gentle Cervical Compression.

> 🖐 **PRECAUTIONARY NOTE**
>
> Do not perform the compression part of this work on the client if the compression/decompression test (the third precautionary test) was uncomfortable for the client, or if he or she experienced radiating pain, numbness, or tingling.

Cervical joint capsule work can be performed if any ROM end feel was bone-on-bone-like. The client is supine. Support the head by placing one hand under the entire neck, and the other hand on top of the head, using evenly displaced pressure. Gently compress the client's head toward the shoulders (Figure 6-29A ■), then slowly decompress it by pulling it back toward you (Figure 6-29B ■). This is a

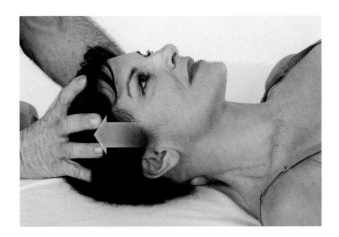

FIGURE 6-29B
Cervical Decompression and Traction.

gentle and slow compression with emphasis on traction or decompression, similar to the technique earlier in this chapter for dura mater and dural sheath mobilization. Again, the intent is to further mobilize the dural sheath, soften any joint capsule adhesions, and decompress the cervical discs, especially high up in the area of C1–C2.

It is imperative that you check in with the client and ask if this is uncomfortable or if he or she feels dizzy or nauseous. There cannot be any pain or neurological symptoms created by this work; if so, stop immediately.

Repeat the gentle compression/decompression several times, mobilizing the deep investing fascia: gently traction, gently compress, and slowly decompress. Make sure the neck stays in perfect neutral during this technique: no flexion, extension, lateral flexion, or rotation. You may feel some popping and releasing of the fascia as you create more freedom in the joints, especially between C1 and C2 helping to restore normal rotation. Remember 45 degrees of the total 90 degrees of cervical rotation occurs at C1–C2. It is critical to perform this work *totally pain-free*, as even minor muscle tension prevents proper joint capsule work.

Step 11: Stretching (During Therapy)

This technique, developed by Dr. Erik Dalton, and will open up the myofascial adhesions between C1 and C2 to allow cervical rotation in clients that had limited rotation with a bony end feel.[12] Flex the client's neck forward 30 to 45 degrees (Figure 6-30A ■). This will help "gap" C1 and C2 to create additional space. Next, using mild in-line traction on the neck to decompress C1 and C2, have the client rotate the head to the right only to the restricted barrier (Figure 6-30B ■). The therapist supports the back of the neck with one hand and the client's forehead with the other hand. The client attempts to rotate to the left, against your resistance, using a minimal force just beyond turning the eyes to the left for about 5 seconds (Figure 6-30C ■). He or she relaxes, takes a deep breath, and on exhale, the therapist

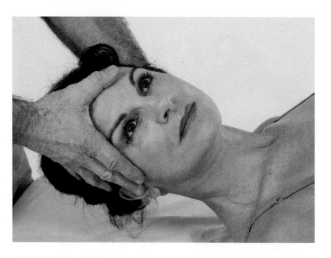

FIGURE 6-30B
C1–C2 Mobilization Technique—Correct Right Rotation Restriction.

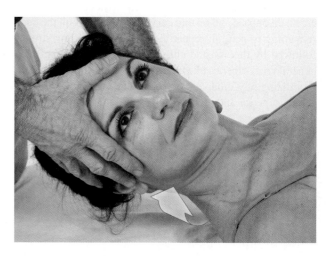

FIGURE 6-30C
C1–C2 Mobilization Correction—Gentle Resisted Left Rotation.

further tractions the neck and has the client slowly rotate to the new restriction to the right for about 2 seconds.

Note: Do not force this movement or overshoot the restricted barrier. Meet the restriction with only a subtle, one-finger pressure stretch.

This stretch is performed with your assistance, with *a lot* of in-line traction, and with a very gentle subtle stretch at the end. At this new position, repeat the contract-relax, contract-antagonist with active assisted stretching two or three times, or until you restore 80 to 90 degrees of right cervical rotation.

Lengthen the spine with cervical in-line traction by leaning back and tractioning the neck bilaterally for 5 seconds. Come out of the stretch extremely slow. Then

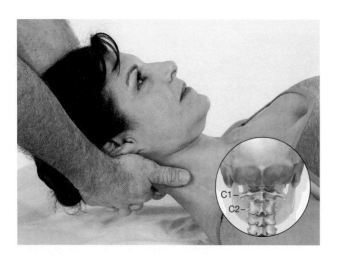

FIGURE 6-30A
C1–C2 Mobilization—30–45 Degrees Cervical Flexion.

repeat the atlas-atlas mobilization technique to the opposite side, if it is needed.

Step 8: Multidirectional Friction

If the client complains of pain during the previous stretches, repeat the resisted test and isolate the exact spot by having the client put a finger on it. Perform multidirectional friction for only 20 to 30 seconds, so you don't create inflammation. If the area is tender, ease up on your pressure. Proceed to the next step.

Step 9: Pain-Free Movement

Have the client slowly rotate the neck in both directions. Repeat this several times. If this is pain-free, proceed with the eccentric work. If the client reports pain during this movement, return to the multidirectional friction working a little deeper, but still pain-free.

Step 10: Eccentric Scar Tissue Alignment

Next, apply eccentric contraction to realign the scar tissue. It must be performed pain-free. Traction the client's neck and have him or her gently resist as you gently lengthen the strained muscles against mild resistance. Tell the client to "barely resist, but let me win." Start with a pressure of only two fingers. Have the client increase the resistance only if it is pain-free. Repeat this several times.

Step 4: Assess Resisted Range of Motion (RROM)

To assess RROM, flex the client's neck forward 30 to 45 degrees. The client attempts to rotate the neck against your resistance. If there is still a specific point of pain, return to the multidirectional friction and then repeat the eccentric work. Continue to evaluate until the client is pain-free and then finish with the stretch.

Step 11: Stretching (During Therapy)

If the client showed limited lateral flexion during the initial assessments, perform this stretch of the lateral neck flexors including the medial scalenes. Have the client tuck his or her hands under the hips, to stabilize his or her own shoulders, and use both of your hands to stretch the neck. Have the client perform lateral flexion to the left to the restricted barrier (Figure 6-31 ■). Then have the client attempt lateral flexion to the right against your resistance at 20 percent force for 10 seconds. He or she relaxes and takes a deep breath, and on exhale engages the antagonists and laterally flexes further to the left with your assistance for about 2 seconds.

At this new position, repeat the contract-relax, contract-antagonist with active assisted stretching two or three times, or until you achieve 40 to 45 degrees of lateral cervical flexion. Traction the client's neck, lean back, and then gently stretch it for 5 to 10 seconds, releasing very slowly. Repeat on the other side, if needed.

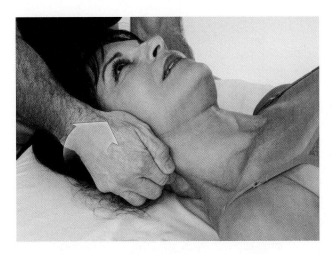

FIGURE 6-31
Stretch Right Lateral Neck Flexors.

Step 8: Multidirectional Friction

If the client complained of pain when he or she contracted against your resistance, have him or her point to the specific spot. Perform pain-free multidirectional friction to the exact area of discomfort for only 20 to 30 seconds.

Step 9: Pain-Free Movement

Ask the client to perform lateral flexion to each side. If there is no discomfort, go to the eccentric work. If the client complained of pain while performing this movement, return to the multidirectional friction work.

Step 10: Eccentric Scar Tissue Alignment

Next, apply eccentric contraction performed pain-free. Traction the client's neck. Ask the client to gently resist as you gently perform lateral flexion away from the injured side. Tell the client to "barely resist, but let me win." Start with a pressure of only two fingers and if there is no pain, have the client increase resistance. Repeat this several times.

Step 4: Assess Resisted Range of Motion (RROM)

To reassess RROM, have the client laterally flex the neck against your resistance. If the client still experiences a specific area of pain, perform the multidirectional friction and pain-free movement again. Then repeat the eccentric work and perform the stretch.

LEVATOR SCAPULA

The levator scapula originates on the transverse processes of C1–C4 and attaches to the superior, vertebral border of the scapula (Figure 6-32 ■). Its action is to unilaterally elevate the scapula, flex the head laterally (to the same side), and rotate the head (to the same side). Bilaterally the levator scapula extends the head. The levator scapula stretch is

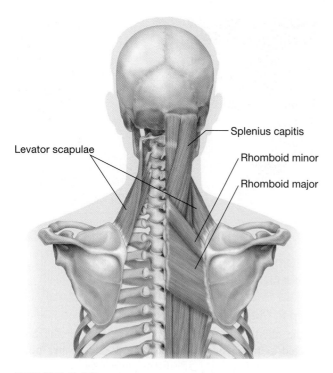

Levator scapulae

Splenius capitis

Rhomboid minor

Rhomboid major

FIGURE 6-32
Cervical and Thoracic Muscle Review.

different than the SCM and scalene stretch and it is important to learn the difference between the various stretches.

Step 11: Stretching (During Therapy)

Stretch only the short, restricted side, not the overstretched side. If the restricted side is on the right, have the client put the right hand under the hip to depress the shoulder. That frees up both of your hands to perform the stretch.

Next, have the client turn the head 45 degrees to the left. In this position, gently traction the neck and have the client exhale and actively flex their neck to the left, for 2 seconds (Figure 6-33 ■). This is performed with your assistance. Repeat the stretch several times. Traction the client's neck 5 seconds. Release slowly.

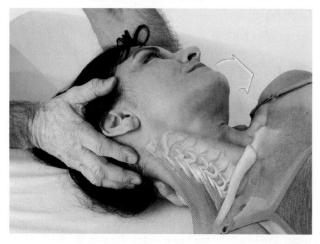

FIGURE 6-33
Right Levator Scapula and Posterior Scalene Stretch.

Step 8: Multidirectional Friction

If the client reported a specific area of pain when performing the levator stretch, have them contract the muscle against your resistance and have him or her point to it. Perform multidirectional friction pain-free for 20 to 30 seconds. Use light pressure if the area is tender.

Step 9: Pain-Free Movement

Ask the client to perform the same movement that created the pain during the stretch; he or she rotates the neck 45 degrees and then flexes laterally. Have him or her repeat this several times. If there is no pain, go to the eccentric work.

Step 10: Eccentric Scar Tissue Alignment

Apply eccentric scar tissue alignment, performed pain-free, to realign the scar tissue. Have the client rotate the neck 45 degrees. Stabilize the shoulder on the side the injured levator attaches. Then ask him or her to gently resist as you flex the neck laterally at a 45-degree angle away from the injured side. Tell the client to "barely resist, but let me win." Start with light pressure and then have the client increase pressure only if there is no discomfort. Repeat this several times.

Step 4: Assess Resisted Range of Motion (RROM)

To assess RROM, have the client rotate the neck 45 degrees and gently laterally flex their neck against your resistance. If there is pain, return to the multidirectional friction, the pain-free movement, and the eccentric work. Finish with the stretch.

UPPER THORACIC WORK

This is a great myofascial finishing technique. The client is seated with the hips and knees flexed 90 degrees and you are standing behind him or her. Place the knuckles of your index and middle fingers in each lamina groove, with wrists straight with the fingers curled under. Use your index fingers and thumbs as guides in the lamina groove. Start high up near the base of the skull at about C2 (Figure 6-34A ■). Ask the client to slowly flex the neck forward, dropping the chin down toward the chest. Start the slow, deep myofascial strokes at the base of the neck and glide downward through the upper trapezius, middle trapezius, and rhomboids to the lower thoracic vertebrae to about T12, as the client slowly continues to flex the thoracic spine forward, Keep the knuckles deep in the lamina groove and have the client's hands drop toward the floor during the entire technique (Figure 6-34B ■). Repeat these myofascial strokes several times to clear out the lamina grooves. This can allow for better closure of the thoracic facet joints, especially with clients that have extreme thoracic kyphosis. It is suggested that you release the superficial fascial front line of the body prior to doing this work. That superficial front line model of therapy was developed by industry pioneers Ida Rolf and Tom Myers, and is not addressed in this book, but is taught in our live seminars.

hands over the client's hands and have him or her bring the elbows slightly back to also stretch the pectoralis minor. He or she takes a breath. As the client exhales, ask him or her to slowly lift the hands upward as you assist (Figure 6-35 ■). Release very slowly. Repeat this slow deep traction several times to decompress the neck.

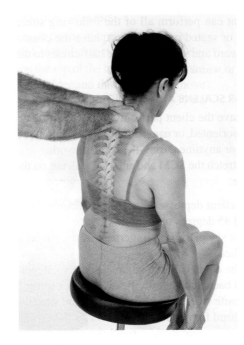

FIGURE 6-34A
Myofascial Release Down Lamina Groove.

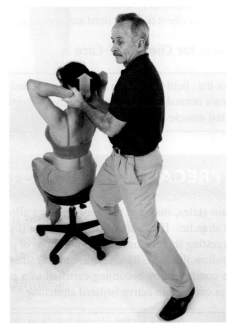

FIGURE 6-35
Cervical Traction.

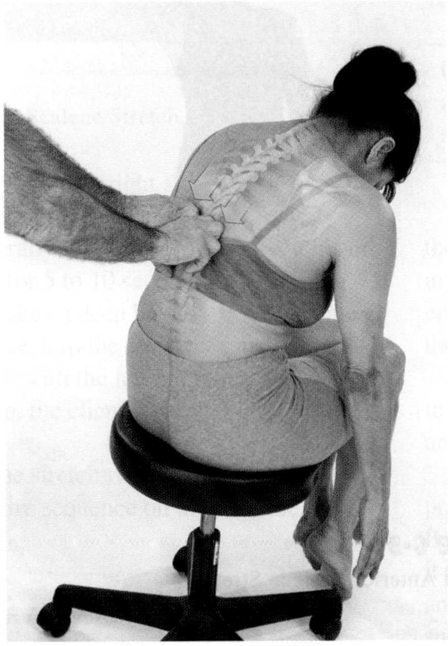

FIGURE 6-34B
Myofascial Release Down Lamina Groove.

NECK DECOMPRESSION

Finish the cervical protocol with a firm neck decompression. The client is seated with the head in neutral. You are standing behind him or her. Have the client place the hands low on the neck, interlocking the fingers. You place your clasped

---

PRECAUTIONARY NOTE

There are many other clinical conditions of the neck that will be better treated by other modalities, or covered in greater detail in our live workshops. The treatments in this book can be complimented by other techniques and disciplines. There are also many clinical conditions of the neck that should be referred out to other health care providers. The author did not cover soft tissue work to the anterior triangle of the neck, a procedure that would be taught in a neuromuscular class, because he feels that work requires much more A&P review. Such work should be supervised in a hands-on training program. Likewise, this book does not go into detail on ascending syndromes, in which cervical compensations result from true leg length discrepancies. The author believes that adding techniques from modalities such as Posturology, Myoskeletal Alignment, and NMT can complement the work demonstrated in this text. For more in depth supervised training in these complimentary modalities, hands-on training is recommended.

Carpal tunnel, thoracic outlet, and whiplash are completely different conditions of the upper body. However, they are initially all treated together by looking at the neck, shoulder, and elbow before addressing the forearm, wrist, and hand conditions. To achieve optimum results, it is highly recommended that you perform pelvic stabilization, and the neck and shoulder protocols, especially if there are nerve conduction problems in the forearm, wrist, or hand. Treatment of elbow, forearm, wrist, and hand conditions follows the same soft-tissue balancing approach. Once you have completed pelvic stabilization, and the neck and shoulder protocols, and restored normal muscle resting lengths, you will get better results when you address specific conditions of the forearm, wrist, and hand such as lateral and medial epicondylosis and **carpal tunnel syndrome.**

> This is based on a term called **multiple crush phenomenon,** where there is more than one region of compression on a nerve trunk. Sections of the nerve distal to the first site of compression become nutritionally deficient because of axoplasmic flow blockage. Consequently, these distal regions are more susceptible to irritation from even a minor degree of compression (becoming the second or third site of crush). For example, with a proximal compression on the brachial plexus in the shoulder area, everything distal to that site is more susceptible to pathology. Even a minor degree of compression on the median nerve in the distal forearm or hand could then become symptomatic. The double (or multiple) crush phenomenon explains why clients might have simultaneous symptoms of thoracic outlet syndrome and carpal tunnel syndrome.[1]

TWELVE-STEP APPROACH TO ELBOW, FOREARM, WRIST, AND HAND CONDITIONS

Repetitive movements, poor postures, trauma, or incorrect body mechanics can contribute to problems related to the elbow, forearm, wrist, and hand. Begin by assessing active, passive, and resisted ranges of motion. You need to focus on the tight, contracted muscle groups that are limiting pain-free movement, not the muscle group creating the movement. Then determine if the problem is myofascial restriction, tight bands, trigger point tension, or scar tissue, and use the specific techniques outlined for each condition. Following are the main conditions that are covered in this chapter:

- Medial epicondylosis (golfer's elbow)
- Lateral epicondylosis (tennis elbow)
- Carpal tunnel syndrome
- Thumb strain or sprain
- Degenerative arthritis
- Trigger finger

Step 1: Client History

The goal is to obtain a thorough medical history including precautions and contraindications for treatment of the client's elbow, forearm, wrist, or hand condition. Ask the client when, where, and how the problem began. Also, ask him or her to describe the area of pain and what makes it better or worse. Find out what type of work he or she does that could lead to repetitive motion problems and poor postures, such as working on the computer all day.

Step 2: Assess Active Range of Motion (AROM)

Assess the client's active ROM, performed pain-free, of the primary single-plane movements of the elbow and wrist. Determine if the range of motion is normal. Please understand that the normal degrees for each elbow range of motion will vary with different references. The degrees listed in this text are accurate estimates for clients with healthy elbows. Range of motion degree estimates may vary slightly depending on the reference. Elbow joint flexion should be 145 to 150 degrees and complete extension 0 degrees. The following are the average ROMs for the wrist and forearm: flexion, 80 to 85 degrees; extension, 70 to 80 degrees; pronation, 80 to 85 degrees; supination, 90 degrees; radial deviation, 15 to 20 degrees; and ulnar deviation, 30 to 45 degrees. Pronation and supination are movements in the forearm that actually occur in the transverse plane at the proximal and distal radioulnar joints. If the ROM is less than average, identify which muscle groups are restricted and therefore preventing normal movement.

You would focus on releasing these restricted, antagonist muscle groups:

- If elbow flexion is less than 145 to 150 degrees, work on releasing the elbow extensors (antagonists)—anconeus and triceps—to restore normal muscle resting lengths.
- If elbow extension is less than 0 degrees, work on releasing the elbow flexors (antagonists)—biceps brachii, brachialis, and brachioradialis—to restore normal muscle resting lengths.
- If wrist flexion is less than 80 to 85 degrees, work on releasing the wrist extensors (antagonists)—extensor carpi radialis brevis, extensor carpi radialis longus, and extensor carpi ulnaris—to restore normal muscle resting lengths.
- If wrist extension is less than 70 to 80 degrees, work on releasing the wrist flexors (antagonists)—flexor carpi radialis, flexor carpi ulnaris, and palmaris longus—to restore normal muscle resting lengths.
- If wrist pronation is less than 80 to 85 degrees, work on releasing the wrist supinators (antagonists)—biceps brachii and supinator—to restore normal muscle resting lengths.
- If wrist supination is less than 90 degrees, work on releasing the wrist pronators (antagonists)—pronator quadratus and pronator teres—to restore normal muscle resting lengths.
- If wrist radial deviation/abduction is less than 15 to 20 degrees, work on releasing the wrist ulnar deviators/adductors (antagonists)—extensor carpi ulnaris and flexor carpi ulnaris—to restore normal muscle resting lengths.
- If wrist ulnar deviation/adduction is less than 30 to 45 degrees, work on releasing the wrist radial deviators/abductors (antagonists)—extensor carpi radialis brevis, extensor carpi radialis longus, flexor carpi

radialis, and palmaris longus—to restore normal muscle resting lengths.

ELBOW JOINT SINGLE-PLANE MOVEMENTS

Elbow joint single-plane movements are as shown in Figures 7-1 ■ and 7-2 ■:

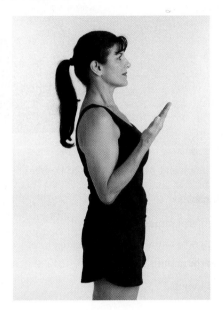

FIGURE 7-1
AROM Elbow Flexion, 145–150 Degrees.

Primary muscles:

- Biceps brachii

- Brachialis, brachioradialis

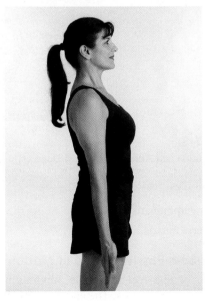

FIGURE 7-2
Elbow Extension, 0 Degrees.

Primary muscles:

- Triceps   • Anconeus

WRIST JOINT SINGLE-PLANE MOVEMENTS

Wrist joint single-plane movements are as shown in Figures 7-3 ■ through 7-8 ■:

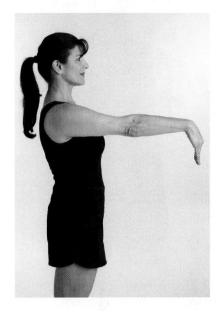

FIGURE 7-3
Wrist Flexion, 80–85 Degrees.

Primary muscles:

- Flexor carpi radialis   • Palmaris longus
- Flexor carpi ulnaris

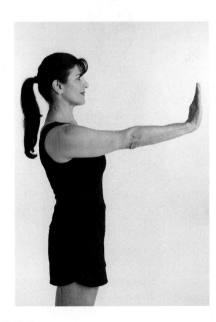

FIGURE 7-4
Wrist Extension, 70–80 Degrees.

Primary muscles:

- Extensor carpi radialis   • Extensor carpi radialis longus
  brevis
                              • Extensor carpi ulnaris

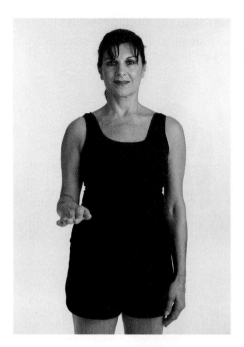

FIGURE 7-5
Wrist Pronation, 80–85 Degrees.

Primary muscles:

- Pronator quadratus
- Pronator teres

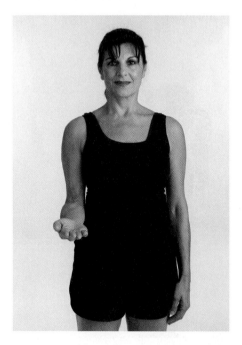

FIGURE 7-6
Wrist Supination, 90 Degrees.

Primary muscles:

- Biceps brachii
- Supinator

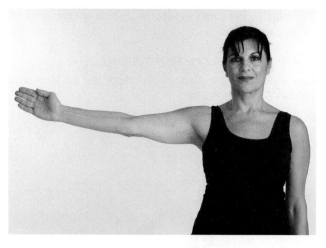

FIGURE 7-7
Radial Deviation and Abduction, 15–20 Degrees.

Primary muscles:

- Extensor carpi radialis brevis
- Extensor carpi radialis longus
- Flexor carpi radialis
- Palmaris longus

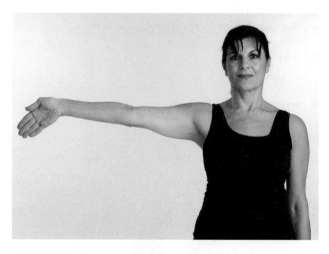

FIGURE 7-8
Ulnar Deviation and Adduction, 30–45 Degrees.

Primary muscles:

- Extensor carpi ulnaris
- Flexor carpi ulnaris

Step 3: Assess Passive Range of Motion (PROM)

Determine the end feel of all the previous movements through passive ROM tests. The end feel for elbow flexion is tissue-on-tissue compression or soft tissue approximation; the forearm comes in contact with the upper arm, and for elbow extension is bone-on-bone. At the wrist, the end feel for flexion, extension, pronation, and supination should be a soft-tissue stretch, which feels leathery. There is a more abrupt, ligamentous end feel to radial and ulnar deviation; also known as a firm tissue stretch end feel.

Step 4: Assess Resisted Range of Motion (RROM)

The client attempts each single-plane movement of the wrist and elbow while you apply resistance. This is done to test for muscle–tendon strains. For precaution, start the test with minimal muscle contraction and then slowly increase the muscle contraction to fully recruit the muscle fibers. If the client experiences pain, ask him or her to point to the specific area. This indicates a muscle strain and this area will be worked last. Muscle strains are most commonly found at the muscle–tendon junctions.

If the client's pain is on the lateral side of the elbow, test the forearm supinator and the wrist extensors. If the client complains of pain on the medial side of the elbow, test the forearm pronators, wrist flexors, and the distal biceps.

The functional assessments discussed previously will help identify which of the following conditions are present and determine which protocol to follow to alleviate the problem.

MEDIAL EPICONDYLOSIS (GOLFER'S ELBOW)

Originally, inflammation was thought to generate the pain in **medial epicondylitis.** However, magnetic resonance imaging (MRI) scans and histology show the presence of microtears in the flexor–pronator tendons without inflammation.[2] Nirsch used the terms *tendinosis* and *angiofibroblastic degeneration* to describe the pathophysiology of medial epicondylitis as microtears in the tendon with a poor healing response.[3]

Medial epicondylosis starts out as a tendon tension problem that leads to injury at the muscle–tendon junction on the anterior medial side of the elbow. It is usually the result of overuse or trauma. The problem is with short, contracted flexor and pronator muscles. The muscles involved in this condition primarily include the pronator teres and the flexor carpi radialis (Figure 7-9).[4]

The flexors are located on the anterior medial surface of the forearm. They originate on the medial epicondyle of the humerus and attach to the base of the second and third

Anterior View

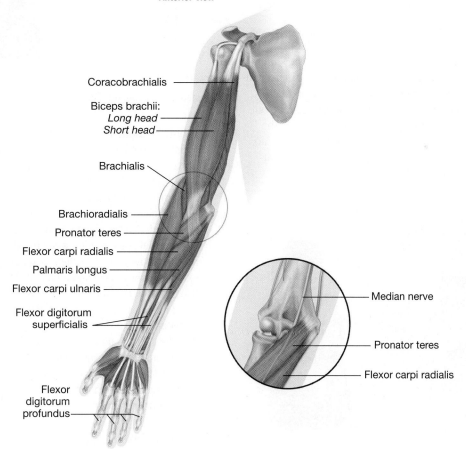

FIGURE 7-9
Forearm Muscle Reference.

metacarpals. The pronator teres is a muscle that runs under the flexors from the medial epicondyle across the ulna to the radius. The median nerve is located under, or runs through the pronator teres and can become compressed and irritated during repetitive movements of the pronator teres or overlying flexors. Pressure on the median nerve, by the pronator teres, can also mimic carpal tunnel symptoms at the wrist. However, ulnar nerve involvement can also occur from compression in the cubital tunnel by the flexor carpi ulnaris muscle. This condition is frequently called golfer's elbow because golfers are most likely to develop this condition due to their swing mechanics, but other populations who engage in repetitive activities are susceptible to this condition.

Step 2: Assess Active Range of Motion (AROM)

Assess each of the client's active forearm wrist movements. Usually, wrist extension and forearm supination will be restricted or limited due to tight wrist flexors and tight pronator teres.

Step 3: Assess Passive Range of Motion (PROM)

The end feel for the wrist, including the limited wrist extension and limited forearm supination, should be soft-tissue stretch.

Step 4: Assess Resisted Range of Motion (RROM)

- **Wrist Flexion:** The client is standing with the shoulder flexed to 90 degrees and the palm facing in toward the body. Grasp the client's palm as if shaking hands and have him or her gently flex the wrist against your resistance. If there is a specific area of pain, ask the client to put a finger on it to pinpoint it. If there is no pain, do *not* friction the tendon as part of your treatment protocol (Figure 7-10 ■).

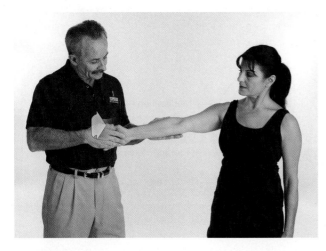

FIGURE 7-10
Resisted Test, Forearm Flexors.

- **Forearm Pronation:** The client is standing with the elbow bent 90 degrees and tucked in at the side. Grasp the client's hand with one hand. Place your other hand

on the client's forearm to stabilize the wrist. The hand on the client's forearm is used for resistance, to protect the ligaments of the wrist. The client then attempts pronation, turning the palm down as you resist. Ask the client to point to the exact area of pain (Figure 7-11 ■).

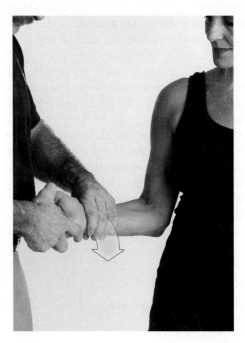

FIGURE 7-11
Resisted Test, Pronator Teres.

- **Elbow Flexion:** This actually tests the bicipital aponeurosis for strained fibers that can scar down the median nerve on the proximal ulnar head. Oftentimes the client who has been diagnosed with carpal tunnel syndrome has a problem higher up in the elbow, shoulder, or neck. Bicipital aponeurosis tendinosis frequently will be missed, and the client will be generically diagnosed with medial epicondylitis when he or she complains of medial elbow pain. The client is standing with the elbow extended. Place one hand on the distal humerus to stabilize it so it does not rotate. Place your other hand on their distal radius and ulna, and stabilize the wrist. Have him or her attempt to flex their elbow against your resistance. Ask the client to point to the specific area of pain. If this tests positive, make sure to restore normal muscle resting length to the biceps, as outlined in the "General Shoulder Protocol" section in Chapter 6, before treating these strained fibers (Figure 7-12 ■).

Step 6: Myofascial Release

To release the flexors, the client is supine with the elbow bent 90 degrees. The forearm is supinated, with the back of the forearm resting on the massage table (you may use a pillow or towel) for support. Stand at the side of the table and start with palmar friction to warm up the forearm. Then perform myofascial spreading at a 45-degree angle into the tissue by

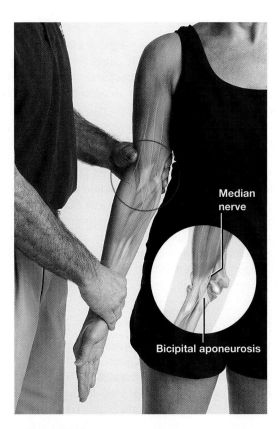

FIGURE 7-12
Resisted Test, Biceps.

hooking into the deep investing fascia moving proximal to distal, from the elbow to the wrist (Figure 7-13A ▪). This will begin to move the tissue back to normal muscle resting lengths. You can use the heels of your hand, knuckles, or finger pads. Expand the connective tissue that surrounds the

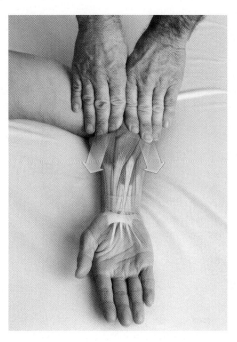

FIGURE 7-13A
Myofascial Spreading, Forearm/Wrist Flexors.

flexor muscles and tendons of the wrist, working slowly and progressively deeper. Alternate the myofascial work with compression broadening strokes, hooking and sinking into the muscle belly. (Figure 7-13B ▪)

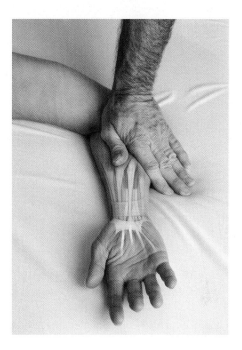

FIGURE 7-13B
Compression Broadening, Forearm/Wrist Flexors.

Step 7: Cross-Fiber Gliding Strokes/Trigger Point Therapy

CROSS-FIBER GLIDING STROKES

Next, perform cross-fiber gliding strokes, working proximal to distal from the elbow to the wrist, releasing the tension on the tendons and loosening any muscle fibers feeding the tight or injured area.

TRIGGER POINT THERAPY

Evaluate the tissue for tight muscle bands or muscle belly trigger points. Pin and traction the skin as you move to more efficiently release the tight bands. If you find a trigger point, apply direct, moderate pressure for 10 to 12 seconds and then gently compress and stretch the area (Figure 7-13C ▪).

FLEXOR RETINACULUM RELEASE

To release the flexor retinaculum, also known as the transverse carpal ligament, the client is in the same position as for the previous step. True carpal tunnel syndrome involves compression of the median nerve under this transverse carpal ligament. To soften or mobilize this structure, place your thumbs over his or her retinaculum, and sink in with moderate pressure. Support the back of the carpal bones with the pads of your fingers to allow deeper pressure into the flexor retinaculum. As you move over the carpal tunnel, ask the client to slowly straighten the fingers and spread them apart while you perform

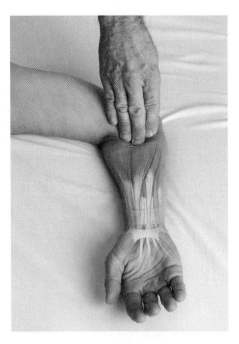

FIGURE 7-13C
Cross-Fiber Gliding Strokes and Trigger Point Work.

myofascial strokes at a 45-degree angle into the tissue. Work across the retinaculum and into the palm of the hand. This may involve 3 to 4 deep strokes as you progress from the distal end of the radius and ulna, across the carpal bones, and into the hand. Hook into the retinaculum and spread the band laterally as you move over the carpal tunnel and into the hand. Active movement, as the client spreads or extends the fingers, facilitates myofascial release and enhances the expansion of the retinaculum (Figures 7-14 ■).

WRIST ARTHROKINETICS

Grasp the client's hand with one hand and stabilize the forearm with the other hand. Gently compress and decompress the wrist using rapid, nonsynchronized movements, several times, to free up any adhesions and decompress the carpal bones. This can also be called joint play, or joint mobilization. Muscle activation or inhibition is a response to joint mobilization. The goal is to distract the client, to eliminate unconscious holding patterns, and can create additional joint space. Repeat the arthrokinetics, then perform slow, deep traction to decompress the wrist. While sustaining moderate traction, gently stretch the wrist into extension with the client actively assisting. Repeat the sequence as needed to restore normal joint space and muscle resting length to the forearm flexors and normal range of motion for wrist extension. (Figures 7-15A ■ and 7-15B ■).

Step 6: Myofascial Release Flexor Tendons

To release the fascial adhesions around the tendons of the wrist and their surrounding sheaths. The client is supine in the same position as for the forearm flexor work. Place your fingertips between the tendons over the top of the carpal tunnel on the forearm side of the wrist. Traction the wrist, and perform passive extension of the wrist, while you glide between each of the tendons, working distal to proximal. Start at the hand and glide across the carpal bones to where tendons become muscle in the forearm. Use the tendons like dental floss, by passively extending the wrist, as you glide between individual tendons to free up adhesions (Figures 7-16A ■). This will allow each individual tendon and it's surrounding sheath to move free and independent of each other.

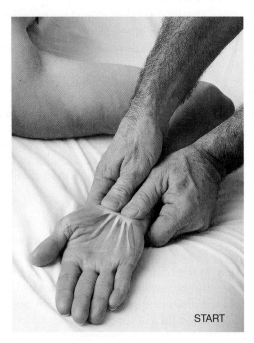
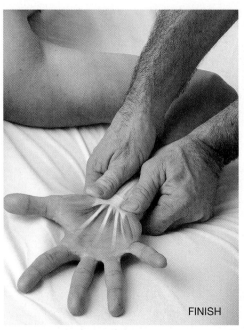

START   FINISH

FIGURE 7-14
Myofascial Spreading, Flexor Retinaculum.

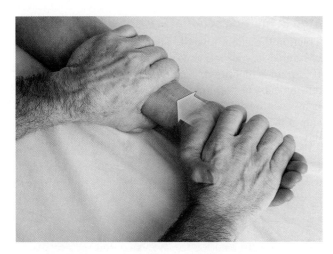

FIGURE 7-15A
Arthrokinetics (Gentle Compression).

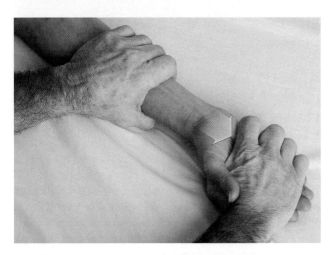

FIGURE 7-15B
Arthrokinetics (Traction).

> ## ✋ PRECAUTIONARY NOTE
>
> Do not jam the carpal bones or hyperextend the wrist.

Next, repeat the traction and passive extension of the client's wrist as you strip through the edges of the tendons using your thumb, working even deeper. You are working on the fascia that binds and sticks the tendons and their surrounding sheaths together.

TENOSYNOVITIS

Tenosynovitis is inflammation or irritation between the wrist tendons and the surrounding synovial sheaths.[5] Tendons in the distal extremities such as the wrist have a synovial sheath around them to reduce friction between the tendons and the retinaculum, or ligament that binds the tendon close to the joint. The tendon must be able to glide freely within the sheath. Chronic overloading and resultant excessive friction leads to adhesions between the tendon and its surrounding protective sheath. The adhesions can result in an inflammatory reaction. You would not do massage directly to the wrist tendons or their sheaths if inflammation is present, but you still need to unload or lengthen the muscle belly of the forearm flexors to reduce the load on those tendons. The symptoms of tendinosis and tenosynovitis are similar. Therefore, excessive load on the forearm flexors can result in tendinosis at the elbow and tenosynovitis at the wrist. For the sake of this protocol, we will refer to tenosynovitis as adhesions within the sheaths of the forearm flexor tendons due to overuse, resulting in constant overload of those tendons. Activities such as working on computers, using power tools, driving cars, or doing massage can result in overuse. The conditions could probably be prevented if the client would stretch their hand and forearm flexors daily. It is the author's experience, and strong opinion, that the therapist should always restore normal muscle resting length to all of the forearm flexors, prior to addressing the tendon sheath problems. This will eliminate the load on the wrist tendons, before treating the adhesions around or within the tendon sheath.

To free up the adhesions within the tendon sheath, pin down one of the wrist tendons with your finger pads, like a guitar string. Once you anchor or mobilize the tendon sheath, draw the tendon slowly through the sheath, by moving the wrist through passive extension and flexion. Perform this with moderate wrist traction to create movement of the tendon inside the sheath. If the muscle belly is relaxed, we believe this technique will decrease the restriction/adhesion of the tendon within the sheath—tenosynovitis—and increase mobility of the tendon within the sheath. Repeat this pin and stretch on all of the tendons you can palpate. If needed, repeat the wrist arthrokinetics again to create additional space for movement before performing the stretch (Figure 7-16B ■).

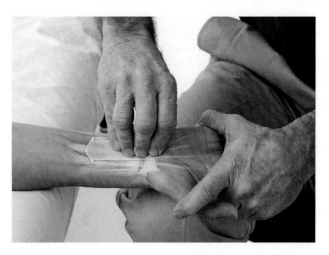

FIGURE 7-16A
Separate Tendon Sheaths.

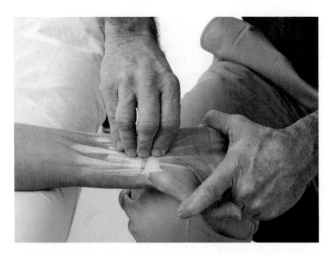

FIGURE 7-16B
Pin Each Tendon Sheath and Passively Extend Wrist.

Step 11: Stretching (During Therapy)

 PRECAUTIONARY NOTE

Stretching is not suggested for the muscle groups around a hypermobile joint. Strengthening would be more appropriate to stabilize any joint that has excessive movement due to ligamentous laxity.

This forearm flexor stretch can be performed with the client's arm in the same position as the myofascial work or with the client's arm supinated at the side. Traction the client's wrist and hold the palm open while slightly extending the wrist with your hand.

Ask the client to flex the wrist at 20 percent force for 5 to 10 seconds while you provide resistance. He or she relaxes, takes a deep breath, and on exhale extends the wrist with your assistance, and traction, for about 2 seconds. Stay at this new stretched position and repeat the contract-relax, contract-antagonist with active assisted stretching two or three times (Figure 7-17 ■). Remember your goal is to restore normal muscle resting length of the forearm flexors, and normal range of motion for wrist extension.

Note: While you are working the flexors, the client may complain of pain in the extensors. As you increase the range of motion in the flexors, there may not be enough myofascial space for the weak, inhibited, or overstretched extensors to shorten and broaden into. If that is the case, start with palmar friction to warm up the back of the arm. Perform myofascial release at a 45-degree angle into the tissue, moving distal to proximal, from the wrist to elbow, to create additional space for the extensors if needed.

Step 8: Multidirectional Friction

Traction the client's wrist. Then have the client flex the wrist against your resistance to find the exact area of pain. If a strain is identified, usually near the medial epicondyle attachments, perform multidirectional friction to this area, pain-free, for only 20 to 30 seconds. Use very light pressure if the area is extremely tender. Then proceed with the next step.

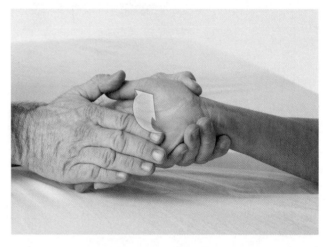

FIGURE 7-17
Forearm Flexor Stretch.

Step 9: Pain-Free Movement

If there is a strain following the friction, ask the client to move the wrist through flexion and extension several times. If there is no pain, perform the eccentric work. If there is discomfort, return to the multidirectional friction, working a little deeper but still pain-free.

Step 10: Eccentric Scar Tissue Alignment

If there is a strain, apply eccentric contraction performed pain-free to realign the scar tissue. Flex the client's wrist, and ask the client to gently resist as you bring his or her wrist from the flexed position into extension. Tell the client to "barely resist, but let me win." Use a resistance of only two fingers to start and then have the client increase the resistance, but only if it is pain-free. Repeat this several times.

Step 4: Assess Resisted Range of Motion (RROM)

To reassess RROM, repeat the wrist flexors resisted test. If there is still pain, return to the multidirectional friction working a little deeper and then repeat the pain-free movement and the eccentric work. If there is no pain, return to the stretch.

Step 6: Myofascial Release

To release the interosseous membrane between the ulna and radius, the client's elbow is bent 90 degrees with the forearm vertical (Figure 7-18 ■). Grasp the ulna and radius

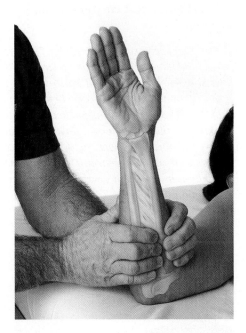

FIGURE 7-18
Myofascial Release of the Interosseous Membrane Using
Radius–Ulna Movement.

distal to the elbow with your thumbs and thenar eminence
on the extensors, or the back of the forearm, and with your
finger pads on the flexors or the front of the forearm. Then
push and pull on the long bones (radius and ulna) with your
finger pads to their end feel in both directions while working distally toward the wrist. When you get to the wrist, use
your finger pads of both hands and glide over the pronator
quadratus, then over the carpal tunnel and into the palm of
the hand. Do not allow pronation and supination of the forearm to occur during this technique.

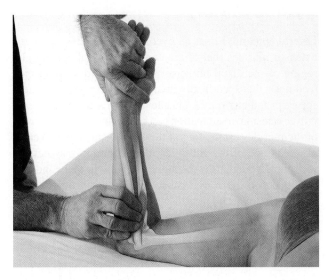

FIGURE 7-19
Pronator Teres Release.

Progressively increase your pressure while performing the push and pull of the radius and ulna. This will create movement and separation to release deep adhesions in
the interosseous membrane between the bones. It will also
create length in the pronator quadratus, at the distal radius
and ulna, which may release tension on the tendons going
through the carpal tunnel. Finally, grasp the client's hand
and traction, and gently rock, the wrist with passive flexion
and extension of the wrist, pain-free. This distraction technique can allow the carpal bones of the wrist to decompress
or even begin to spontaneously align. Repeat this several
times to create more joint space.

Step 6: Myofascial Release

To release the pronator teres, using your finger pads, place
three fingers across the belly of the pronator teres and pin it
down. You are actually pressing the relaxed forearm flexors
into the pronator teres to push it onto the underlying bones.
Then grasp the client's hand and support the wrist while you
passively rotate the forearm through supination and pronation to warm up the muscle (Figure 7-19 ■).

Next, press down on the flexors, pinning the pronator teres onto the underlying bones—ulna and radius—and
stretching into supination and elbow extension. Repeat this
pin and stretch as you move your finger pads, passively gliding through the muscle belly, toward the medial epicondyle.
This stretches and massages the pronator teres from the
inside out to mobilize it and reduce ischemia.

TRIGGER POINT THERAPY

Treat any muscle belly trigger points, if found, with moderate pressure for 10 to 12 seconds, compressions, and a
gentle stretch.

Step 11: Stretching (During Therapy)

To stretch the pronator teres, the client's shoulder is
abducted 90 degrees and elbow is bent 90 degrees with the
palm facing up. Grasp the client's hand. Place three fingers
of your other hand on the flexors and press the pronator
teres onto the underlying radius and ulna. As you extend the
elbow and supinate the forearm, pin and stretch the pronator
teres (Figure 7-20 ■). Keep in mind that the median nerve
runs through this muscle and could be contributing to similar
peripheral median nerve compression symptoms as carpal
tunnel syndrome. This condition, when the median nerve is
compressed by the pronator teres is actually called pronator teres syndrome. Most symptoms of nerve compression
radiate distal to the site of compression. Aching forearm
pain and parastheshia along with pain in median nerve distribution in the hand is likely to be pronator teres syndrome,
and should not be assumed to be carpal tunnel syndrome.
This particular area of median nerve compression at the
elbow can also be compromised by a strain in the bicipital
aponeurosis, a fibrous band that connects the biceps brachii
to the ulna on the forearm. Multiple crush phenomenon, or

compression of the median nerve, in more than one area could also include a third compression of that nerve in the carpal tunnel of the wrist. The clinical massage therapist should evaluate, and treat all three possibilities.

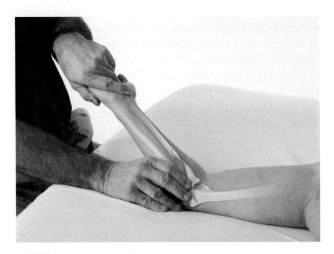

FIGURE 7-20
Stretch Pronator Teres.

Step 8: Multidirectional Friction

Stabilize the client's wrist and forearm. Have the client pronate the forearm against your resistance to find any specific spot of pain. Ask him or her to point to the exact spot. This determines if there is a muscle–tendon strain. Then move the wrist into slight flexion to take the pressure off the muscles. If there is a strain, perform pain-free multidirectional friction for only 20 to 30 seconds. Use light to moderate pressure if the area is extremely tender. Be careful and do not overwork the area.

Step 9: Pain-Free Movement

Ask the client to perform pronation and supination several times. If there is no pain, perform the eccentric work only if there is a strain. If there is discomfort, return to the multidirectional friction.

Step 10: Eccentric Scar Tissue Alignment

Realign the scar tissue, in clients who have a strain, by applying eccentric contraction. It must be performed pain-free. Stabilize the client's wrist and forearm in neutral and ask him or her to gently resist as you perform wrist supination. Tell the client to "barely resist, but let me win." Start with two fingers for resistance and then have the client increase resistance only if it is pain-free. Repeat this several times.

Step 4: Assess Resisted Range of Motion (RROM)

To reassess RROM, repeat the resisted test for the wrist pronator. If the pain is gone, proceed to the stretch. If there is still pain, return to the multidirectional friction, working a

little deeper, and then repeat the pain-free movement and the eccentric work.

Note: Make sure you release the strong short flexors of the forearm, wrist, and hand before treating a strain in the usually weak wrist extensors. You should also usually release the strong short pronators of the forearm before treating the usually weak elbow supinator. This particularly applies to a client working on the computer all day. The position on the computer can shorten the wrist and hand flexors, and shorten the pronators of the forearm. This can cause weakness and inhibition in the client's wrist and hand extensors and forearm supinators (Figure 7-21 ■).

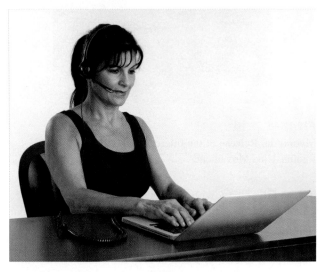

FIGURE 7-21
Observe Workstation Ergonomics.

LATERAL EPICONDYLOSIS (TENNIS ELBOW)

Lateral epicondylitis is an overuse condition involving the extensor muscles that originate on the lateral epicondylar region of the distal humerus. It is more properly termed tendinosis that specifically involves the origin of the extensor carpi radialis brevis muscle.[6–9] Any activity involving wrist extension or supination can be associated with overuse of the muscles originating at the lateral epicondyle. Tennis has been one of the activities most commonly associated with the disorder.[10] In the author's opinion, this condition usually occurs in tennis because the wrist and hand extensors are short, strong, and tight. Therefore, it is the constant stress on the weak wrist extensors, as the player makes contact with the tennis ball repeatedly during the backhand stroke, that causes their extensor tendinosis over time. This condition is more prevalent in the occupational sector, than in tennis players, due to tight wrist and hand flexors and weak, inhibited wrist extensors.

The extensors are a group of four superficial muscles. The supinator is located under the extensors, near the lateral

Posterior View

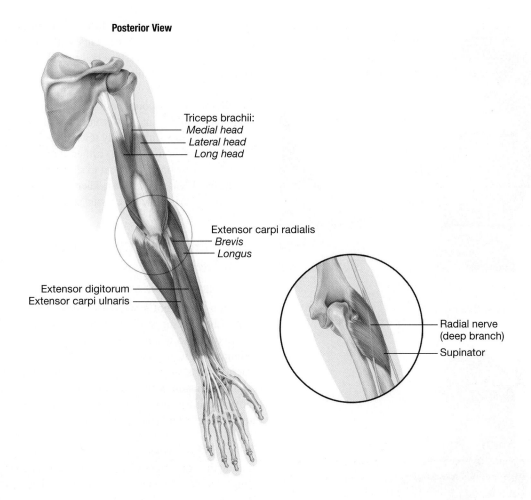

Triceps brachii:
— *Medial head*
— *Lateral head*
— *Long head*

Extensor carpi radialis
— *Brevis*
— *Longus*

Extensor digitorum
Extensor carpi ulnaris

Radial nerve
(deep branch)
Supinator

FIGURE 7-22
Anatomy Reference, Posterior Arm.

epicondyle of the elbow. The radial nerve runs through the belly of the supinator and when compressed can cause a sharp, shooting sensation down the arm (Figure 7-22 ■). This is why both muscle groups must be relaxed to properly treat this condition. It is vital that the therapist first release the wrist flexors and forearm pronators to bring the usually weak, inhibited or overstretched wrist extensors and supinator back to normal resting muscle lengths.

Step 2: Assess Active Range of Motion (AROM)

Assess the client's wrist extension and forearm supination, performed pain-free. The normal range of motion for the wrist extension is 70 to 80 degrees, for forearm supination 90 degrees.

Step 3: Assess Passive Range of Motion (PROM)

The end feel for extension and supination should be soft and leathery.

Step 4: Assess Resisted Range of Motion (RROM)

Note: This would normally be done in the initial assessment if the chief complaint was lateral epicondyle pain or tennis

elbow. It can also be done, as is shown later, with the client on the table at this point in the protocol.

- **Extension:** The client is standing with the elbow straight and the palm facing down. Grasp the back of the client's hand and gently traction the wrist. The client gently extends the wrist against your resistance. If the client reports pain, have him or her point to the exact spot. This injured area should be treated last (Figure 7-23 ■)

- **Supination:** The client's elbow is bent 90 degrees, with the arm tucked in at the side. Grasp the client's hand and stabilize the ligaments of the wrist with one hand, while your other hand stabilizes the forearm. The majority of your resistance comes from the hand stabilizing the forearm, to prevent stressing the ligaments of the wrist. Have the client attempt supination, using only 10 to 20 percent of their strength, as you resist with your hand on the client's forearm. If there is a specific area of pain, have the client point to it (Figure 7-24 ■). Remember, this area of muscle–tendon strain or tendinosis should be worked last, after restoring normal muscle resting length to the muscle belly.

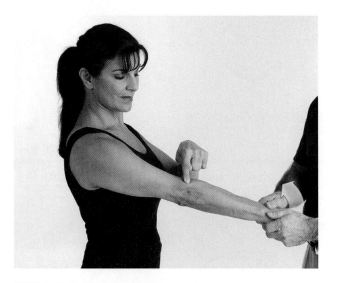

FIGURE 7-23
Resisted Test, Wrist Extensors.

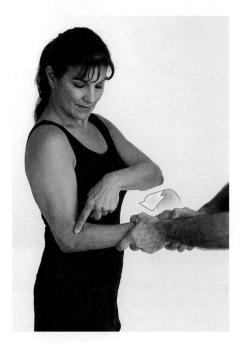

FIGURE 7-24
Resisted Test, Forearm Supinator.

Step 6: Myofascial Release

Note: You must first release the wrist flexors to bring the wrist extensors to normal muscle resting lengths, and take the tension off these weak, inhibited, or overstretched muscles.

To release the wrist extensors, the client is supine with the arm at the side, palm facing down. Warm up the top of the forearm with palmar friction to create superficial heat. Begin myofascial spreading at a 45-degree angle, hooking into the tissue and working from the wrist toward the injured elbow, distal to proximal. Use your finger pads, heels of your hands, or knuckles. Do repeated short strokes to mobilize the deep investing fascia, and minimize glide on the skin (Figures 7-25A ■). This will relax these usually weak, inhibited, or overstretched muscles and return them to normal muscle resting lengths. Check in with the client to make sure you are working pain-free.

Perform gentle compression broadening strokes with the intention of sinking into the tissue at a 45 degree angle toward the bone, and pressing slightly toward the lateral epicondyle. This angle of compression, rather than just compressing directly into the bone, can start to shorten or relax these muscles faster (Figures 7-25B ■). Then return to the myofascial spreading of the connective tissue surrounding the extensors, working even deeper.

Step 7: Cross-Fiber Gliding Strokes/Trigger Point Therapy

CROSS-FIBER GLIDING STROKES

Traction the client's wrist to create space and perform cross-fiber gliding strokes of the extensors, working distal to proximal, to where they attach at the lateral epicondyle (Figures 7-25C ■). To enhance this work, you can pin and traction the skin with one hand as you bring the wrist into slight extension with your other hand. The intention is to move these weak, inhibited, or overstretched muscles back to their normal muscle resting lengths.

TRIGGER POINT THERAPY

During the cross-fiber gliding strokes, treat any muscle belly trigger points, if found, with direct, moderate pressure for 10 to 12 seconds. Then perform compressions over the area again to further broaden and relax the wrist extensors.

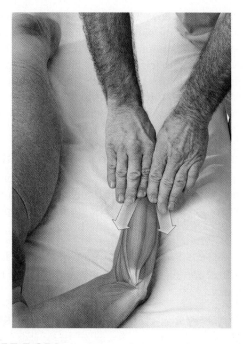

FIGURE 7-25A
Myofascial Spreading, Wrist Extensors.

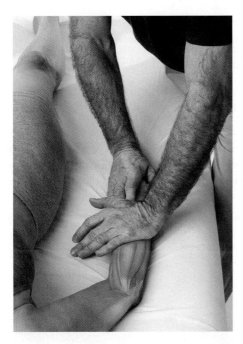

FIGURE 7-25B
Compression Broadening, Wrist Extensors.

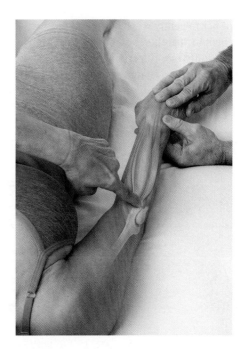

FIGURE 7-26A
Resisted Test, Wrist Extensors.

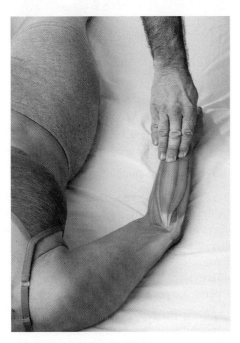

FIGURE 7-25C
Cross-Fiber Gliding Strokes and Trigger Point Work, Wrist Extensors.

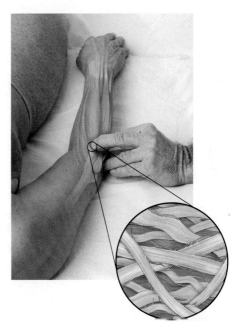

Disorganized scar tissue

FIGURE 7-26B
Multidirectional Friction.

Step 8: Multidirectional Friction

Ask the client to extend his or her wrist against your resistance, to determine if there is pain, associated with a muscle strain, and ask where it is located. Ask the client to point to the exact spot (Figures 7-26A ■). Perform multidirectional friction to the disorganized collagen pain-free for only 20 to 30 seconds. Ease up on your pressure if the area is tender (Figures 7-26B ■).

Step 9: Pain-Free Movement

Ask the client to move the wrist through flexion and extension several times. If there is no pain, perform the eccentric work. If there is some discomfort, return to the multidirectional friction working a little deeper, but still pain-free.

Step 10: Eccentric Scar Tissue Alignment

Apply eccentric contraction to realign the scar tissue. It must be performed pain-free. Have the client extend the wrist, and ask him or her to gently resist as you perform wrist flexion. Tell the client to "barely resist, but let me win." Start with a resistance of only two fingers. The client can then increase the resistance if there is zero discomfort. Repeat this several times, pain-free, to recruit deeper layers of collagen into alignment. (Figure 7-26C ■).

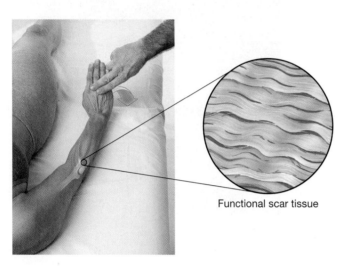

FIGURE 7-26C
Eccentric Muscle Contraction.

Step 4: Assess Resisted Range of Motion (RROM)
To reassess RROM, repeat the wrist extensors resisted test. If there is still pain, return to the multidirectional friction on the extensors, working a little slower and deeper. Then repeat the eccentric work (Figure 7-27 ■).

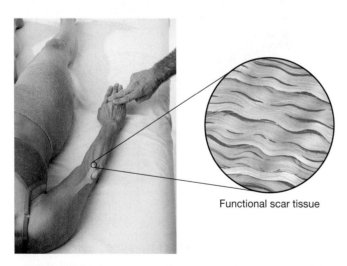

FIGURE 7-27
Resisted Wrist Extension.

Note: Do not stretch the extensor muscles, as they tend to be weak, inhibited, and possibly eccentrically overstretched and do not need to be stretched any further. These muscles must be strengthened to prevent another injury. Strengthening, with emphasis on the eccentric contraction phase, will also

lay down new collagen and realign the existing collagen that was softened through the frictioning part of manual therapy.

Step 6: Myofascial Release

Note: You must work the pronators of the forearm first to return the supinator to its normal resting length.

To release the supinator, locate the supinator by placing your finger pads in the space between two of the forearm extensors. This is between the proximal ulna and radius just distal to the elbow (Figure 7-28 ■).

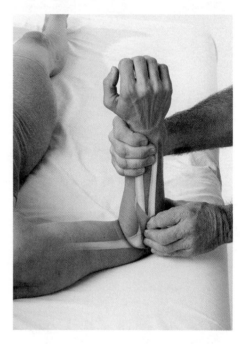

FIGURE 7-28
Myofascial Release, Forearm Supinator.

Bend the elbow 90 degrees, then pin down the supinator and hold with your finger pads while you support the client's distal forearm and passively move it through pronation and supination several times to warm up the muscle. The emphasis is on performing repeated supination to better relax that muscle. This effectively massages the supinator from the inside out.

Next, perform a pin and cross-fiber gliding stroke through the belly of the supinator, moving from distal to proximal several times across that muscle. Once you have relaxed the supinator, test it for a muscle strain by doing a muscle resisted test.

Step 4: Assess Resisted Range of Motion (RROM)
Start by stabilizing the client's wrist and supporting the forearm. Have the client then gently attempt to supinate the forearm against your resistance to find the exact spot of pain. This determines if there is a minor muscle strain or tendinosis. Ask the client to point to the exact spot and then match your finger to that spot (Figure 7-29A ■).

Step 8: Multidirectional Friction
Perform pain-free multidirectional friction for only 20 to 30 seconds. If the area is tender, use only light to moderate pressure (Figure 7-29B ■).

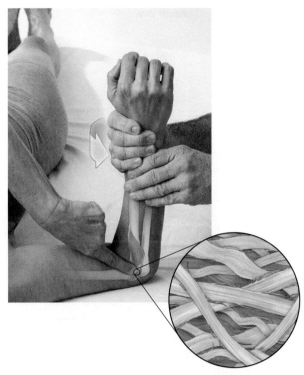

Disorganized scar tissue

FIGURE 7-29A
Resisted Forearm Supination.

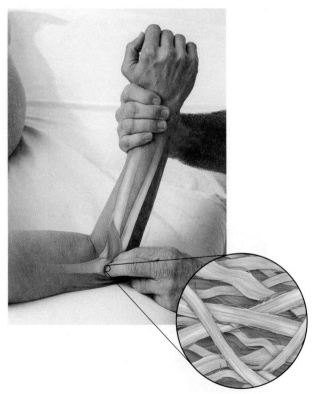

Disorganized scar tissue

FIGURE 7-29B
Multidirectional Friction, Supinator.

Step 9: Pain-Free Movement

Have the client perform supination and pronation several times. If there is no discomfort, perform the eccentric work. If there is some pain, return to the multidirectional friction.

Step 10: Eccentric Scar Tissue Alignment

Realign the scar tissue with eccentric contraction performed pain-free. Have the client supinate the forearm. While you stabilize the client's wrist and forearm, ask him or her to gently resist as you perform wrist pronation, back to the neutral resting position of that muscle. Tell the client to "barely resist, but let me win." Start with a resistance of only two fingers and then if there is no pain the client can increase the resistance to recruit the deeper fibers. Repeat this several times (Figure 7-29C ■).

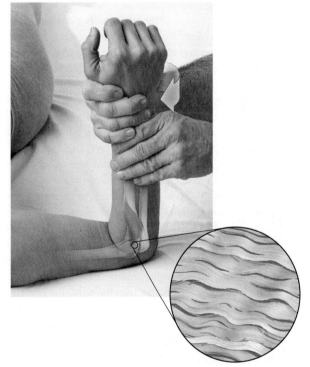

Functional scar tissue

FIGURE 7-29C
Eccentric Muscle Contraction, Supinator.

Step 4: Assess Resisted Range of Motion (RROM)

To reassess RROM, repeat the supinator resisted test. If there is still pain, go back to the multidirectional friction and pain-free movement. Then repeat the eccentric work.

Note: Do not typically stretch the supinator muscle, as it tends to be weak, inhibited, and possibly eccentrically contracted or overstretched. Thus, it does not need to be stretched any further. This muscle must usually be strengthened to prevent reinjury.

CARPAL TUNNEL SYNDROME

Classical carpal tunnel syndrome involves compression of the median nerve under the flexor retinaculum, also called the transverse carpal ligament. Keep in mind there can be many other contributing factors in this condition, such as Guyon's canal syndrome where ulnar nerve compression is possible in a tunnel on the medial side of the wrist called Guyon's canal. The author suggests the clinical massage therapist refer to textbooks such as *Orthopedic Assessment in Massage Therapy* by Whitney Lowe for greater detail on differential diagnosis and additional testing.

Strong wrist flexors and pronators can create carpal tunnel syndrome. Overuse of the wrist flexors leads to overdevelopment of the nine tendons that pass under the sheath of the retinaculum on the anterior side of the wrist. This compresses the median nerve and causes pain, weakness, tingling, and numbness.[11] This can also contribute to tenosynovitis, which is inflammation or adhesions of the tendon sheath. Strong flexors, and biomechanical forces of the wrist, can displace the carpal bones creating discomfort, nerve compression, and an adhesive problem. This book focuses on releasing the forearm and wrist tension and adhesions so the tendons move freely. It will also cover techniques to decompress, mobilize, and facilitate spontaneous alignment of the carpal bones.

Often, clients will complain about pain at the medial epicondyle—at the tight wrist flexors, and forearm pronator attachments—and have numbness and tingling into the wrist, hand, and fingers. Carpal tunnel could be called the "never-just-at-the-wrist syndrome." The pronator teres also passes over the median nerve and can also be a contributing culprit causing symptoms similar to carpal tunnel. A contracted pronator quadratus can restrict tendon movement at the wrist and also contribute to pressure in the carpal tunnel. There are also thoracic outlet and nerve compression problems in the shoulder and neck that can be involved and confused as carpal tunnel. With multiple crush phenomenon, the median nerve does not do well if the nerves that feed the wrist and hand are already compressed higher up in the neck, shoulder, and elbow areas. Be a healing detective and find the cause or source of the pain and treat it wherever it is; don't just rely on the symptoms.

Note: The author cautions therapists and clients against strengthening the wrist and hand flexor muscles by squeezing an exercise ball. Those muscles are usually strong, short, and tight already, and further strengthening places additional tension on the already tight muscles.

Strengthening exercises for wrist and hand flexors can lead to overload on the tendons of the elbow and wrist and often only exacerbates the problem. Cortisone injections, and wrist and elbow braces, may only mask the symptoms; they do *not* eliminate the cause of the problem (Figure 7-30 ■).

Start with and follow the entire protocol for medial epicondylosis, since this is the beginning of the treatment for carpal tunnel and must be performed before you proceed to the next step.

Step 6: Myofascial Release

For myofascial release of the hand, start with myofascial spreading strokes across the client's palm in opposite directions to open it up. Hook into the tissue and work medial to

Palmar View

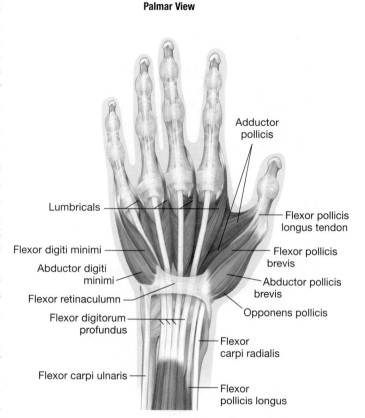

FIGURE 7-30
Anatomy Reference, Wrist and Hand.

lateral across the hand. Then sink into the tissue and work from the base of the palm, across the thenar eminence, working up toward the thumb. Alternate with gentle compressions into the tissue (Figure 7-31A ■).

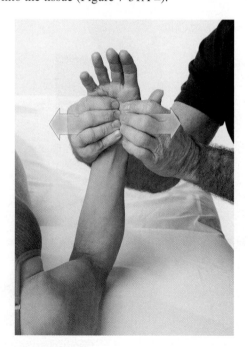

FIGURE 7-31A
Myofascial Release and Compression Broadening.

Perform cross-fiber gliding strokes between each metacarpal to create space and increase blood flow. Spend extra time on the adductor pollicis and thenar eminence, working from midpalm outward toward the thumb.

Next, place your finger pads on the client's palm and your thumbs on the back of the client's hand. Push and pull on the bones of the metacarpals in opposing directions, to their end feel, to allow movement and separation in the interosseous membranes. Work proximal to distal, gliding over the tissue with your finger pads as you push and pull the bones to help release tissue and create joint space (Figure 7-31B ■).

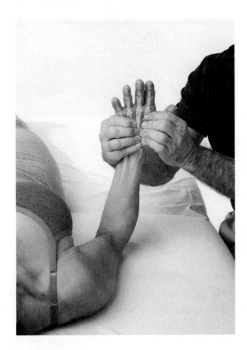

FIGURE 7-31B
Stretch Deep Fascial Layers Using Metacarpals.

Step 11: Stretching (During Therapy)

Have the client open the hand with the fingers in extension. Place one hand over the client's fingers and thumb. Traction the client's wrist, with your other hand on the back of the client's hand as a pivot. Ask the client to attempt to close his or her hand by flexing the fingers and thumb as you resist for 5 to 10 seconds. He or she relaxes and then actively performs finger extension with your assistance for about 2 seconds. Repeat this contract-relax, contract-antagonist with active assisted stretching several times. The muscles of the hand are very strong, short, and tight, and should be stretched by the client daily (refer to Figure 7-35C).

WRIST CIRCLES

Grasp the client's distal end of the ulna and radius bones with both hands. Make sure you stay off the carpal bones. Gently compress the distal end of the ulna and radius together and have the client make three big, slow circles with the wrist, keeping the fingers straight. This can begin to mobilize the carpal bones and help correct minor bony fixations.

Have the client circle the wrist in the other direction and repeat the previous movements. This will allow the carpal bones to be mobilized, and it is not unusual to hear popping sounds and movement in the joints resulting in carpal bone mobility, decompression, and possible spontaneous alignment (Figures 7-32A ■, 7-32B ■, and 7-32C ■).

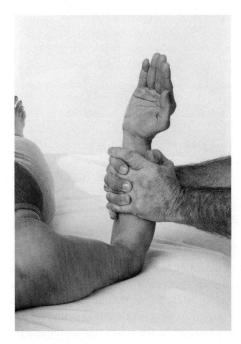

FIGURE 7-32A
Carpal Bone Mobilization.

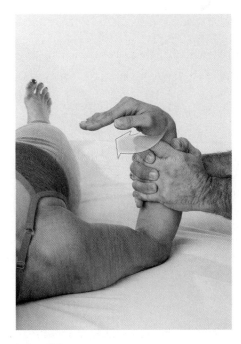

FIGURE 7-32B
Carpal Bone Mobilization.

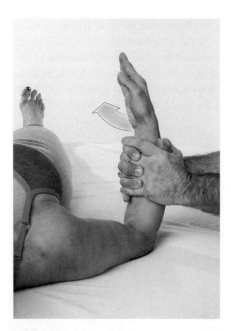

FIGURE 7-32C
Carpal Bone Mobilization.

WRIST MOBILIZATION

Perform a series of movements to create more space in the wrist joint. With the client's palm facing down, place your thumbs on the distal end of the radius and ulna, on the carpal bones. Next, grasp the client's thumb with one hand while your other hand is on the other side of the client's hand. Move the client's wrist to neutral with traction and then into ulnar deviation with traction, stretching the hand and thumb toward the little finger side slowly for 2 seconds. Then return to the neutral position with traction (Figure 7-33A ■).

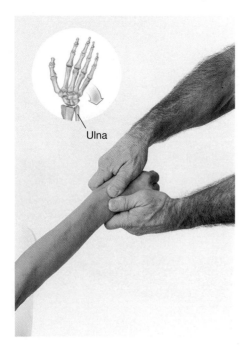

FIGURE 7-33A
Carpal Bone Mobilization—Ulnar Deviation.

Traction the client's wrist and move it into flexion, to open up the wrist, while slowly pressing down onto the carpal bones for 2 seconds. Then move the wrist to the neutral position with traction (Figure 7-33B ■).

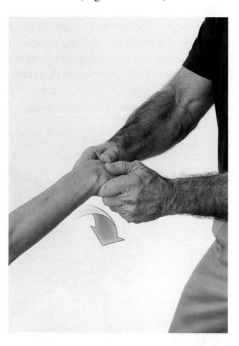

FIGURE 7-33B
Carpal Bone Mobilization—Wrist Flexion.

Next, move the wrist into extension along with traction, again slowly pressing your thumbs down onto the carpal bones for 2 seconds (Figure 7-33C ■). Move the wrist back to neutral with traction and then into radial deviation with traction, stretching the hand toward the thumb side slowly for

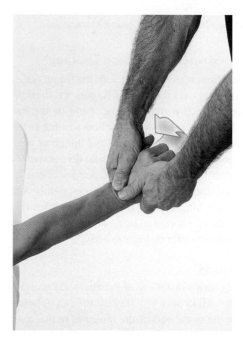

FIGURE 7-33C
Carpal Bone Mobilization—Wrist Extension.

2 seconds. Perform in-line traction and gentle lengthening stretches of the client's wrist several times (Figure 7-33D ■).

Finally, place your finger pads of both hands between the ulna and radius bones starting on the wrist flexors, with your thumbs on the wrist extensors. Gently curl your finger pads in and glide proximal to distal through the carpal tunnel and into the hand, as you passively traction and extend the wrist. Repeat this several times, with progressively deeper pressure as you glide across the carpal tunnel each time. (Figure 7-33E ■).

THUMB STRAIN OR SPRAIN

Anyone who performs repetitive or excessive motions with their hands, including massage therapists, are susceptible to strains or sprains of the thumb. The most common injury is to the muscles or tendons that are located between the thumb and the index finger.

Step 6: Myofascial Release

Release the forearm flexors first. Perform the epicondylosis protocol for the flexors explained in the "Medial Epicondylosis" section. Then follow the instructions for the wrist and hand myofascial release listed under carpal tunnel syndrome.

Step 4: Assess Resisted Range of Motion (RROM)

After you have achieved soft-tissue myofascial release and balance of the muscles of the forearm, wrist, and hand, perform a resisted test to find a possible strain in the thumb area. Place your thumb and index finger between the client's thumb and index finger.

Have the client attempt to move his or her thumb and index finger closer together—adduction—as you apply resistance. Then, have them also gently flex their thumb against your resistance. If there is a specific area of pain during the resisted test, indicating a minor strain, ask the client to point to it. Proceed to the next step (Figure 7-34A ■).

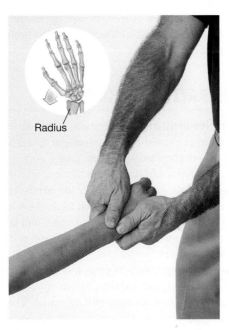

FIGURE 7-33D
Carpal Bone Mobilization—Radial Deviation.

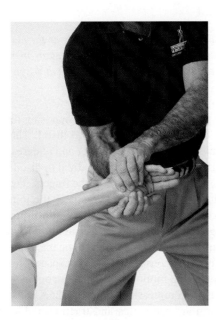

FIGURE 7-33E
Deep Gliding Strokes Through Carpal Tunnel.

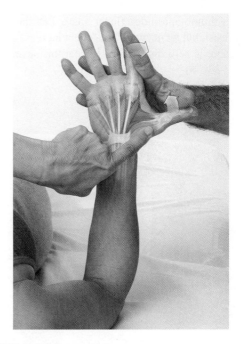

FIGURE 7-34A
Resisted Test, Thumb Strain.

Step 8: Multidirectional Friction

Perform multidirectional friction pain-free to the specific spot of pain for 20 to 30 seconds to soften the collagen matrix. Ease up on your pressure if the client indicates that the area is tender (Figure 7-34B ■).

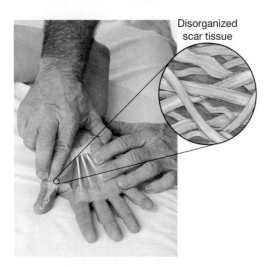

Disorganized scar tissue

FIGURE 7-34B
Multidirectional Friction, Thumb Strain.

Step 9: Pain-Free Movement

Ask the client to move the thumb toward the index finger, and little finger, and back apart several times. If there is no pain, perform the eccentric work. If there is some discomfort, repeat the multidirectional friction work.

Step 10: Eccentric Scar Tissue Alignment

Perform eccentric contraction to realign the scar tissue. Have the client gently resist as you perform abduction, moving his or her thumb and index finger apart. Tell the client to "barely resist, but let me win." The client increases pressure only if there is zero discomfort. Repeat this several times (Figure 7-34C ■).

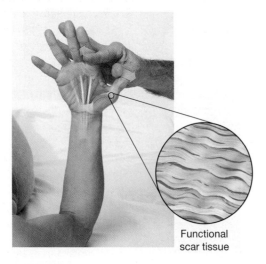

Functional scar tissue

FIGURE 7-34C
Eccentric Contraction, Thumb Strain.

Step 4: Assess Resisted Range of Motion (RROM)

To reassess RROM, repeat the resisted test on the thumb. If there is still pain, return to the multidirectional friction, working a little deeper. Then repeat the eccentric work. When there is no longer any pain, proceed to the stretch.

Step 11: Stretching (During Therapy)

Have the client attempt to bring the thumb and index finger together at 20 percent force for 5 to 10 seconds while you provide resistance. He or she relaxes, takes a deep breath, and then on exhale actively abducts the thumb away from the index finger while you assist the stretch for about 2 seconds. Stay at this new range of motion and repeat the contract-relax, contract-antagonist with active assisted stretching two or three times.

DEGENERATIVE ARTHRITIS

Degenerative arthritis, also known as osteoarthritis, is a type of arthritis caused by inflammation, breakdown, and eventual loss of the cartilage of the joints. Among the over 100 different types of arthritic conditions, osteoarthritis is the most common, affecting usually the hands, feet, spine, and large weight-bearing joints such as the hips and knees. It is also called *degenerative joint disease,* and is typically characterized by swelling, redness, pain, and restriction of motion in the fingers.[12]

Massage therapy can be a great way to ease the pain and stiffness associated with arthritis, and many doctors recommend massage to their patients with arthritis.[13] The best way to treat arthritis is to create joint decompression and space by releasing the muscles and tendons that are pulling on the bones and restricting the pain-free movement.

Treatment

Note: You must treat, stretch, and balance the muscles of the forearm and wrist first to be able to better open the hand. Follow the protocol described in the "Medial Epicondylosis" section.

Push and pull on the metacarpals in opposing directions to their end feel, working proximal to distal. Then perform myofascial spreading on each finger and release of the muscles of all the fingers, moving proximal to distal.

Next, assess the flexibility of the fingers. Tight muscles of both the forearm and hand compress the joints and can create degeneration and joint arthritis. Perform arthrokinetics on any tight or fixated joints. Use rapid, nonsynchronized gentle joint compression and then subtle traction movements to soften any adhesions and create joint space. This looks like a gentle pumping motion using gentle compressive forces followed by decompression (Figures 7-35A ■ and 7-35B ■).

Perform arthrokinetics and traction and stretch each individual finger into extension or neutral alignment, as needed, to increase the space between the joints and to

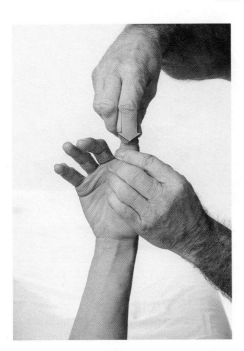

FIGURE 7-35A
Arthrokinetics (Gentle Compression).

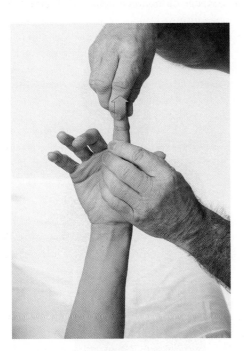

FIGURE 7-35B
Arthrokinetics (Traction or Decompression).

improve vascular circulation. Pivot the back of the finger over one of your fingers as a lever. Stretch an individual finger into extension or neutral alignment, as needed. Use a supported thumb as a lever underneath it.

Next, perform arthrokinetics followed by gentle lateral flexion of any restricted joint. Then perform arthrokinetics followed by gentle rotation of that joint. This can help reduce calcification or bone spurs. As stated earlier, bone spurs (osteophytes) are bony projections that develop along the edges of bones. The bone spurs themselves are not painful, but they can rub against nearby nerves and bones, causing pain.[14]

Repeat the myofascial work as needed and then gently traction the wrist and stretch the fingers again. This will effectively decompress the individual joints to allow pain-free movement, especially hand and finger extension to return (Figure 7-35C ■).

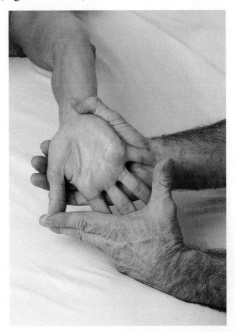

FIGURE 7-35C
Stretch Hand Muscles.

TRIGGER FINGER

Trigger finger, also known as stenosing tenosynovitis, is a condition in which one of the fingers or thumbs catches in a bent position. "This condition develops when a fibrous nodule or thickening develops on the surface of the tendon and prevents smooth gliding action."[15] The finger or thumb may straighten with a snap, like a trigger being pulled and released. If the condition is severe, the finger may become locked in a bent position. Often painful, trigger finger is caused by a narrowing of the tendon sheath that surrounds the tendon in the affected finger. It is usually the thick part of the tendon sheath proximal to the MCP joint of the finger. People whose work or hobbies require repetitive gripping actions are more susceptible.[16] The entire forearm, hand, and wrist protocol may help address the underlying cause of this condition. Treat the tight muscles in the forearm and hand prior to addressing the cyst or scar buildup on the tendon. This eliminates a great portion of the cause of trigger fingers. When manual therapy and stretching fail to help this condition, surgical release of the retinaculum-like sheath may be performed with a simple office procedure.

Step 11: Stretching (Client Self-Care)

Client self-care is important to maintain the soft-tissue balance that was restored by therapy. As the client goes back to normal day-to-day activities, muscle groups (usually the wrist flexors, hand flexors, and forearm pronators) will become short and tight and the antagonists (usually the forearm supinator and wrist extensors) will become weak and inhibited. Daily stretches and therapeutic exercise will help keep those muscle groups in balance.

WRIST FLEXORS

- The client's arm is stretched out with the elbow straight and palm facing up.
- He or she places the thumb of the other hand under the wrist: four fingers on the palm of the hand.
- The client brings the hand upward against his or her own resistance for 5 to 10 seconds.
- He or she exhales, then actively tractions and extends the wrist down and assists with the other hand for 2 seconds.
- The client repeats the stretch two or three times, or until normal range of motion is achieved (Figure 7-36 ■).

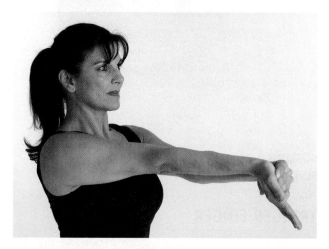

FIGURE 7-36
Forearm/Wrist Flexors Stretch.

HAND FLEXORS

- The client's forearm is supinated with fingers extended and palm up.
- He or she tries to close the hand gently against the resistance of the other hand for 5 to 10 seconds.
- He or she takes a deep breath, then actively extends the fingers back, assisting the stretch with the other hand for 2 seconds. (Figure 7-37 ■)

PRONATOR TERES

- The client's elbow is bent 90 degrees against his or her body with palm up.
- He or she places the palm of the other hand on the back of this hand, with the index finger between the thumb and the index finger of the hand to be stretched.

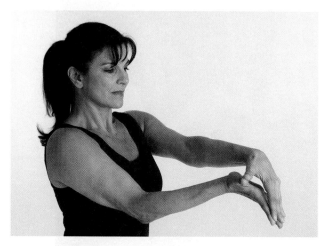

FIGURE 7-37
Hand Flexors Stretch.

- The client tries to gently turn the palm down (pronates) for 5 to 10 seconds against his or her own resistance.
- He or she exhales, then actively supinates (turns palm up) for 2 seconds, gently assisting the stretch.
- The client repeats the stretch two or three times or until normal range of motion is achieved (Figure 7-38 ■).

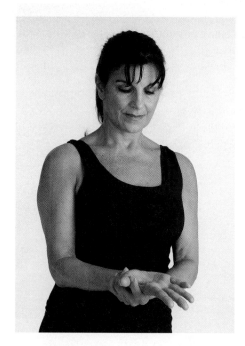

FIGURE 7-38
Pronator Teres Stretch.

Step 12: Strengthening (Client Self-Care)

WRIST AND HAND EXTENSORS

- The client's elbow is bent at 90 degrees along the side of the body.
- He or she wraps a Thera-Band around the involved hand, both ends anchored with the other hand.

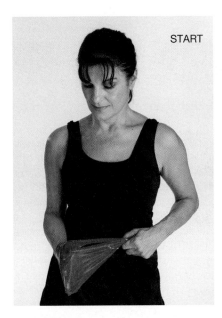

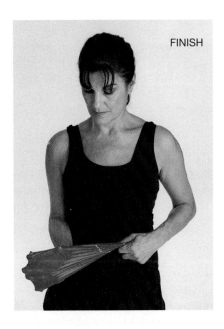

FIGURE 7-39
Strengthen Hand and Wrist Extensors.

- The client slowly extends the fingers and then the wrist from the neutral position taking 2 seconds (concentric contraction).
- He or she slowly returns the fingers and wrist back to the neutral position taking 4 seconds (eccentric contraction) (Figure 7-39 ■).
- The client repeats this exercise 8 to 10 times.

Note: The client should spend more time on eccentric contraction (lengthening phase), since that is more beneficial. For muscle strains, collagen is laid down and scar tissue realigns while eccentrically strengthening the usually weak extensors.

FOREARM SUPINATOR

- The client wraps a Thera-Band around one hand, with elbows bent 90 degrees and hands shoulder-width apart.
- With palms facing each other, he or she slowly turns the exercising hand up (supinates), taking 2 seconds, until the hand is parallel to the floor and ceiling.
- The client slowly returns to starting position, taking 4 seconds, with emphasis on this eccentric phase. (Figures 7-40 ■).
- He or she repeats the exercise 8 to 10 times.

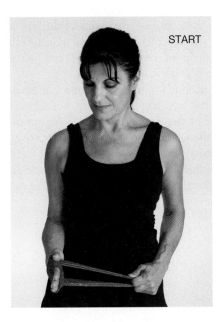

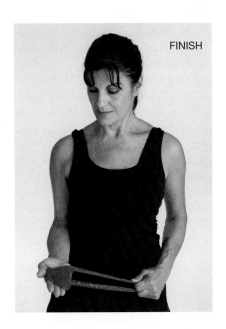

FIGURE 7-40
Strengthen Forearm Supinator.

CASE STUDY

A 30-year-old female office worker is sent to your office with a diagnosis of carpal tunnel syndrome in her right wrist. Your experience and knowledge of the multiple crush phenomenon tells you to evaluate the neck, shoulder, elbow, forearm, wrist, and hand for descending syndromes.

The client history indicates that your client holds the phone in her right ear by laterally flexing her neck to the right most of the day. You find limited range of motion in right rotation and extremely tight SCM and scalenes on the right. You release the right SCM and the scalenes. You then find the right shoulder medially rotated, with only 45 degrees of lateral rotation. You also release and stretch the right subscapularis and pectoralis minor to address possible thoracic outlet problems.

The client also has only 45 degrees of supination of the forearm from working in pronation on the computer all day. You release the forearm flexors, pronator teres, and flexor retinaculum to address possible pronator teres syndrome and carpal tunnel syndrome. The client says that the tingling, numbness, and parasthesia in the forearm, wrist, hands, and fingers is gone. That tells you the pronator teres was probably one of the many causes of the median nerve compression along with the tight flexor tendons and flexor retinaculum.

You educate your client about proper ergonomics at her work station and specific stretches of tight muscles of the neck, shoulder, elbow, forearm, wrist, and hand. The client learns daily stretches for the SCM, scalenes, pectoralis minor, subscapularis, pronator teres, and wrist and hand flexors. You tell her that after learning better the importance of posture and creating proper ergonomics at her work station, some of the stretches may not be necessary.

At a later date you evaluate what stretches she needs to keep doing and teach her a few strengthening exercises for weak, inhibited muscles, to better balance out the neck, shoulder, elbow, forearm, wrist, and hand. The client sends you a number of other people that have nerve compression problems over the next month, and you make sure to look at all possible causes of multiple crush phenomenon.

CHAPTER SUMMARY

This chapter was written to offer the clinical massage therapist a variety of tools to evaluate, identify, and properly address the most common clinical conditions of the elbow, forearm, wrist, and hand. The author wants to stress the importance of performing pelvic stabilization first, and taking a close look at neck and shoulder imbalance to resolve contributing factors that can cause or contribute to complicated elbow, forearm, wrist, and hand conditions.

Myoskeletal conditions coming from the lower part of the body, that effect clinical conditions of the neck or shoulder, are called ascending syndromes. Musculoskeletal problems that come from cervical conditions, and contribute to conditions such as thoracic outlet or carpal tunnel, are called descending syndromes. In the case of nerve compression in the neck or shoulder, the client diagnosed with carpal tunnel syndrome would have a descending syndrome referred to as multiple crush phenomenon. Manual therapists should start to sort out the multiple possibilities presenting themselves as pain in the elbow, forearm, wrist, and hand areas.

The intention of this chapter was to ensure that the clinical massage therapist eliminate any underlying causes of specific conditions of the elbow, forearm, wrist, and hand, prior to treating the resulting clinical symptoms. In performing soft tissue balancing or preparation work first, what may seem like complicated clinical conditions of the elbow, forearm, wrist, and hand, can often be resolved in just a few sessions. This whole body approach will allow clients to live pain-free, and athletes to achieve peak performance.

Please keep in mind that there are a number of elbow, forearm, wrist, and hand conditions not addressed in this book. Some of these other conditions are out of the scope of our practice, or respond better to other modalities or manual therapy disciplines. If you are not getting good results with this work, your client needs to be referred out to other manual therapists or the client's physician. If in doubt, refer out!

REVIEW QUESTIONS

1. If the hand is in neutral and you turn the palm up, which of the following occurs?
   a. pronation
   b. lengthening of the supinator
   c. shortening of the pronator
   d. shortening of the supinator

2. When the wrist flexors and pronator teres are strained over time near the elbow, what condition do they cause?
   a. medial epicondylosis
   b. lateral epicondylosis
   c. tarsal tunnel syndrome
   d. bicipital tendinosis

3. With a doctor's diagnosis of carpal tunnel syndrome, the client experiences pain and tingling in the hand and fingers. Besides your obvious focus of massage on the wrist area, what other structures should be assessed?
   a. Focus the massage on the wrist only; the doctor is usually correct.
   b. Focus the massage on the wrist and assess the forearm for tight flexors and pronator teres.
   c. Assess the wrist and forearm only, as carpal tunnel can be described as "only at the wrist" syndrome.
   d. Assess the forearm, elbow, shoulder, and the neck for tight muscles that may be compressing the nerves creating the tingling in the hands and fingers.

4. What are the two main muscles associated with the pain of lateral epicondyle?
   a. wrist extensors and supinator
   b. wrist extensors and flexors
   c. wrist extensors and pronators
   d. wrist supinator and shoulder flexors

5. Normal range of motion for radial deviation/abduction is _____.
   a. 45 degrees
   b. 15 degrees
   c. 80 degrees
   d. 60 degrees

6. To help decompress the median nerve, starting with a neutral hand, how do you stretch the pronator teres?
   a. turn the palm up
   b. turn the palm down
   c. pronate
   d. flex the wrist

7. The distal biceps attaches at the elbow and when tight can limit what movement?
   a. supination
   b. wrist flexion
   c. pronation
   d. shoulder flexion

8. Trigger finger is described as _____.
   a. a ligament sprain
   b. a muscle strain
   c. stenovitis
   d. narrowing of a tendon sheath

9. Which of the following is a suggested treatment for degenerative arthritis of the fingers?
   a. create joint decompression and joint space
   b. massage to release muscles that are restricting movement
   c. arthrokinetics
   d. all of the above

10. If you work on a computer all day with the palms turned down, what muscle at the elbow could be causing carpal tunnel symptoms?
    a. extensors
    b. pronator quadratus
    c. pronator teres
    d. supinator

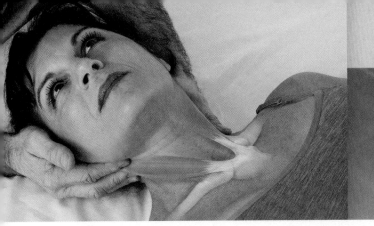

End-of-Chapter Questions—Answer Key

CHAPTER 1

1. b
2. c
3. d
4. a
5. d
6. c
7. b
8. b
9. a
10. c

CHAPTER 2

1. b
2. a
3. c
4. a
5. d
6. b
7. c
8. d
9. b
10. a

CHAPTER 3

1. a
2. c
3. c
4. d
5. b
6. b
7. a
8. d
9. d
10. c

CHAPTER 4

1. b
2. c
3. b
4. d
5. a
6. c
7. c
8. a
9. a
10. d

CHAPTER 5

1. c
2. a
3. d
4. b
5. b
6. a
7. c
8. d
9. c
10. b

CHAPTER 6

1. a
2. b
3. d
4. d
5. c
6. b
7. a
8. c
9. a
10. b

CHAPTER 7

1. d

2. a

3. d

4. a

5. b

6. a

7. c

8. d

9. d

10. c

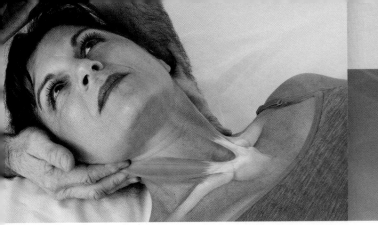

APPENDIX B

Notes

CHAPTER 1

1. Cyriax, J. *Textbook of Orthopaedic Medicine.* 8th ed. Vol. 1, *Diagnosis of Soft Tissue Lesions.* London: Bailliere Tindall, 1982.

2. Rolf, Ida P. *Rolfing: Reestablishing the Natural Alignment and Structural Integration of the Human Body for Vitality and Well-Being.* Rev. ed. Rochester, VT: Healing Arts Press, 1989.

3. Dalton, E. *Myoskeletal Alignment Techniques.* Oklahoma City, OK: E. Dalton: Freedom From Pain Institute, 2005.

4. Cyriax, *Textbook of Orthopaedic Medicine.*

5. Mennell, John. *Joint Pain: Diagnosis and Treatment Using Manipulative Techniques.* Boston: Little Brown, 1964.

6. Gehlsen, G., L. R. Ganon, and R. Helfest. "Fibroblast Responses to Variation in Soft Tissue Mobilization Pressure." *Medicine & Science in Sports & Exercise* 31, no. 4 (1999): 531–35.

7. Travell, Janet, David Simons, and Lois Simons. *Myofascial Pain and Dysfunction: The Trigger Point Manual.* 2nd ed. 2 vols. Baltimore, MD: Williams & Wilkins, 1999.

8. Ibid.

9. Chaitow, Leon, Walker DeLany, Judith, *Clinical Application of Neuromuscular Techniques Volume 1: Upper Body,* Philadelphia, PA: Churchill Livingstone/Elsevier, 2000.

10. Ibid.

11. Travell, *Myofascial Pain and Dysfunction: The Trigger Point Manual.*

12. Davenport, T., K. Kulig, Y. Matharu, and C. Blanco. "The EDUReP Model for Nonsurgical Management of Tendinopathy." *Physical Therapy,* Vol. 85, No. 10, 1093–1103, November, 2005.

13. Mattes, A. *Active Isolated Stretching.* Sarasota, FL: Aaron L. Mattes, 1995.

14. Ibid.

15. Page, Phil, and Todd Ellenbecker. *Strength Band Training.* Champaign, IL: Human Kinetics, 2005.

16. Woodley, B., R. Neusham-West, and D. Baxter. "Chronic Tendinopathy: Effectiveness of Eccentric Exercise," *British Journal of Sports Medicine,* 2007, 41:188–198.

17. Khan, K., J. Cook, J. Taunton, and F. Bonar. Part 1, "Overuse Tendinosis, Not Tendinitis: A New Paradigm for a Difficult Clinical Problem," *The Physician and Sports Medicine* 28, no. 5 (May 2000).

18. Cook, J., K. Khan, N. Maffulli, and C. Purdam. Part 2, "Overuse Tendinosis, Not Tendinitis: Applying the New Approach to Patellar Tendinopathy," *The Physician and Sports Medicine* 28, no. 6 (June 2000).

19. Khan, "Overuse Tendinosis, Not Tendinitis: A New Paradigm for a Difficult Clinical Problem." and Cook, "Overuse Tendinosis, Not Tendinitis: Applying the New Approach to Patellar Tendinopathy."

20. Ibid.

21. Ibid.

22. Almekinders, L. C., and J. D. Temple. "Etiology, Diagnosis, and Treatment of Tendonitis: An Analysis of the Literature." *Medicine & Science in Sports & Exercise* 30. no. 8 (1998): 1183–90.

23. Khan, "Overuse Tendinosis, Not Tendinitis: A New Paradigm for a Difficult Clinical Problem" and Cook, "Overuse Tendinosis, Not Tendinitis: Applying the New Approach to Patellar Tendinopathy."

24. Niesen-Vertommen, S. L., J. E. Taunton, D. B. Clement, and R. E. Moser. "The Effect of Eccentric versus Concentric Exercise in the Management of Achilles Tendonitis." *Clinical Journal of Sports Medicine* 2, no. 2 (1992): 109–13.

25. Curwin, S. L., and W. D. Stanish. *Tendinitis: Its Etiology and Treatment.* Toronto: Collamore Press, 1984.

26. Holmich, P., P. Uhrskow, L. Ulnits, et al. "Effectiveness of Active Physical Training as Treatment for Long Standing Adductor Related Groin Pain in Athletes: Randomized Trial." *Lancet* 1999; 353 (9151): 439–443.

27. Alfredson, H., T. Pictila, P. Jonsson, et al. "Heavy Load Eccentric Calf Muscle Training for the Treatment of

Chronic Achilles Tendinosis." *American Journal of Sports Medicine,* 1998 26 (3), 360–366.

28. Leadbetter, W. B. "Cell-Matrix Response in Tendon Injury." *Clinical Journal of Sports Medicine* 11, no. 3 (1992): 533–78.

29. Vilarta, R., and B. C. Vidal. "Anisotropic and Biomechanical Properties of Tendons Modified by Exercise and Denervation: Aggregation and Macromolecular Order in Collagen Bundles." *Matrix* 9, no. 1 (1989): 55–61.

30. Khan, "Overuse Tendinosis, Not Tendinitis: A New Paradigm for a Difficult Clinical Problem" and Cook, "Overuse Tendinosis, Not Tendinitis: Applying the New Approach to Patellar Tendinopathy."

31. Ibid.

CHAPTER 2

1. SpineUniverse. "What Is Degenerative Disc Disease?" http://www.spineuniverse.com.

2. Edelson, Stewart. *Save Your Aching Back & Neck: A Patient's Guide.* 2nd ed., San Diego, CA: SYA Press and Research, 2002.

3. Mayo Clinic. http://www.mayoclinic.com/health/bone-spurs/DS00627.

4. Schneider, John H. "Bone Spurs (Osteophytes) and Back Pain." http://www.spine-health.com/topics/cd/spurs/spurs01.html.

5. Bachrach R. M., J. Micelotta, and C. Winuk. "The Relationship of Low Back Pain to Psoas Insufficiency." *Journal of Orthopaedic Medicine* 13 (1991): 34–40.

6. Lavine, Ronald. "Iliotibial Band Friction Syndrome." *Current Reviews in Musculoskeletal Medicine* 3 (October 2010): 18–22.

CHAPTER 3

1. Lowe, Whitney. *Orthopedic Assessment in Massage Therapy.* Sisters, OR: Daviau Scott, 2006, 102.

2. Ibid., 105.

3. Ibid., 106.

4. Ibid., 107.

5. Ibid., 108.

6. Ibid., 106, 108.

7. Ibid., 94, 98.

8. Cyriax, J. *Textbook of Orthopaedic Medicine.* 8th ed. Vol. 1, *Diagnosis of Soft Tissue Lesions.* London: Bailliere Tindall, 1982.

9. Khan, K., J. Cook, J. Taunton, and F. Bonar. Part 1, "Overuse Tendinosis, Not Tendinitis: A New Paradigm for a Difficult Clinical Problem," *The Physician and Sports Medicine* 28, no. 5 (May 2000).

10. http://www.mayoclinic.com/health/patellar-tendinitis/DS00625.

11. http://orthopedics.about.com/cs/meniscusinjuries1/a/meniscus.htm.

12. Werner, Ruth. *A Massage Therapist's Guide to Pathology.* Baltimore, MD: Lippincott, Williams & Wilkins, 2002, 134.

13. http://emedicine.medscape.com/article/90661-overview.

CHAPTER 4

1. Khan, K., J. Cook, J. Taunton, and F. Bonar. Part 1, "Overuse Tendinosis, Not Tendinitis: A New Paradigm for a Difficult Clinical Problem." *The Physician and Sports Medicine* 28, no. 5 (May 2000).

2. http://www.mayoclinic.com/health/Achilles-tendinitis/DS00737.

3. Lowe, Whitney. *Orthopedic Assessment in Massage Therapy.* Sisters, OR: Daviau Scott, 2006, 76.

4. Shiel, William C., Jr. Available at MedicineNet.com Web site: http://www.medicinenet.com/shin_splints/article.htm.

5. Lowe, Whitney. *Orthopedic Assessment in Massage Therapy.* Sisters, OR: Daviau Scott, 2006, 56.

6. Lowe, Whitney. *Orthopedic Assessment in Massage Therapy.* Sisters, OR: Daviau Scott, 2006, 56–57.

7. Werner, Ruth. *A Massage Therapist's Guide to Pathology.* Baltimore, MD: Lippincott, Williams & Wilkins, 2002, 489.

8. Ibid., 22.

9. WebMD. http://www.webmd.com/a-to-z-guides/Flat-foot-Pes-Planus-Topic-Overview.

10. Penn Medicine Health Encyclopedia. http://www.pennmedicine.org/encyclopedia/em_DisplayArticle.aspx?gcid=001262&ptid=1.

11. Dalton, E. *Myoskeletal Alignment Techniques.* Oklahoma City, OK: E. Dalton: Freedom From Pain Institute, 2005, 93.

12. Plantar Fasciitis Organization. "Plantar Fasciitis, Heel Spurs, Heel Pain," http:www.plantar-fasciitis.org.

13. Werner, *A Massage Therapist's Guide,* 124.

14. Mayo Clinic. http://www.mayoclinic.com/health/bone-spurs/DS00627.

15. http://www.foot-pain-explained.com/bone_spur.html.

16. http://www.webmd.com/a-to-z-guides/bunions-topic-overview.

17. Werner, *A Massage Therapist's Guide,* 66–67.

18. Cluett, Jonathan. "Ankle Sprain: What Is a Sprained Ankle?" http://orthopedics.about.com/cs/sprainsstrains/a/anklesprain.htm.

19. eMedicineHealth. http://www.emedicinehealth.com/ankle_sprain/article_em.htm.

20. Werner, *A Massage Therapist's Guide,* 107.

21. http://orthopedics.about.com/cs/otherfractures/a/stress-fracture.htm.

CHAPTER 5

1. Werner, Ruth. *A Massage Therapist's Guide to Pathology.* Baltimore, MD: Lippincott, Williams & Wilkins, 2002,134.

2. Vinik, Aaron. "How Is Frozen Shoulder Associated with Diabetes?" *Diabetes Health,* November 1, 1999, http://www.diabeteshealth.com/read/1999/11/01/1702/how-is-frozen-shoulder-associated-with-diabetes/.

3. Lowe, Whitney. *Orthopedic Assessment in Massage Therapy.* Sisters, OR: Daviau Scott, 2006, 218.

4. Cyriax, J. *Textbook of Orthopaedic Medicine.* 8th ed. Vol. 1, *Diagnosis of Soft Tissue Lesions.* London: Bailliere Tindall, 1982.

5. Lowe, 187–188.

6. Werner, 147.

7. Dalton, E. *Myoskeletal Alignment Techniques.* Oklahoma City, OK: E. Dalton: Freedom From Pain Institute, 2005, 218.

8. Werner, 134.

9. Lowe, 216–218.

10. Khan, K., J. Cook, J. Taunton, and F. Bonar. Part 1, "Overuse Tendinosis, Not Tendinitis: A New Paradigm for a Difficult Clinical Problem." *The Physician and Sports Medicine* 28, no. 5 (May 2000).

11. Ibid.,10.

12. Janda, V. "Muscle Weakness and Inhibition in Back Pain Syndromes," Grieve GP, ed. *Modern Manual Therapy of the Vertebral Column,* Edinburg, UK: Churchill Livingstone, 1986.

CHAPTER 6

1. Dalton, E. *Myoskeletal Alignment Techniques.* Oklahoma City, OK: E. Dalton: Freedom From Pain Institute, 2005, 218.

2. Ibid., 218.

3. Cyriax, J. *Textbook of Orthopaedic Medicine.* 8th ed. Vol. 1, *Diagnosis of Soft Tissue Lesions.* London: Bailliere Tindall, 1982.

4. Werner, Ruth. *A Massage Therapist's Guide to Pathology.* Baltimore, MD: Lippincott, Williams & Wilkins, 2002, 132.

5. http://www.ninds.nih.gov/disorders/whiplash.htm.

6. Mayo Clinic. http://www.mayoclinic.com/health/whiplash/DS01037.

7. Neurosomatic Educations Inc. http://www.neurosomaticeducators.com.

8. Ibid.

9. Core Institute, http://www.coreinstitute.com.

10. Myers, Thomas. *Anatomy Trains.* Philadelphia, PA: Churchill Livingstone Elsevier, 2009, 87.

11. Dalton, 271.

12. Ibid., 210.

CHAPTER 7

1. Lowe, Whitney. *Orthopedic Assessment in Massage Therapy.* Sisters, OR: Daviau Scott, 2006, 14.

2. Putnam, M. D., and M. Cohen. "Painful Conditions Around the Elbow." *Orthopedic Clincs of North America* 30, no. 1 (January 1999): 109–18 [Medline].

3. Nirschl, R. P. "Etiology of Tennis Elbow" [letter]. *The Journal of Sports Medicine* 3, no. 5 (September–October 1975): 261–63 [Medline].

4. Gabel, G. T., and B. F. Morrey. "Medial Epicondylitis." In *The Elbow and Its Disorders,* 3rd ed., edited by B. F. Morrey, 537–42. Philadelphia: W. B. Saunders, 2000.

5. http://www.nlm.nih.gov/medlineplus/ency/article/001242.htm.

6. Cyriax, J. H. "The Pathology and Treatment of Tennis Elbow." *The Journal of Bone and Joint Surgery* 18 (1936): 921–40.

7. Nirschl, R. P. "Tennis Injuries." In *The Upper Extremity in Sports Medicine,* 1995, 789–803.

8. Faro, F., and J. M. Wolf. "Lateral Epicondylitis: Review and Current Concepts." *The Journal of Hand Surgery* [American Vol.] 32, no. 8 (October 2007): 1271–79 [Medline].

9. De Smedt, T., A. de Jong, W. Van Leemput, D. Lieven, and F. Van Glabbeek. "Lateral Epicondylitis in Tennis: Update on Aetiology, Biomechanics and Treatment." *British Journal of Sports Medicine* 41, no. 11 (November 2007): 816–19 [Medline].

10. http://orthoinfo.aaos.org/topic.cfm?topic–a00068.

11. National Institute of Neurological Disorders and Strokes. "Carpal Tunnel Syndrome," http://www.ninds.nih.gov/disorders/carpal_tunnel/carpal_tunnel.htm.

12. MedicineNet.com. Definition of Degenerative Arthritis, http://www.medterms.com, March 26, 1998.

13. www.articlesbase.com/diseases-and-conditions-articles/ease-the-pain-of-osteoarthritis-with-massage-205703.html.

14. Mayo Clinic. http://www.mayoclinic.com/health/bone-spurs/DS00627.

15. Mayo Clinic. http://www.mayoclinic.com/health/trigger-fingerDS00155.

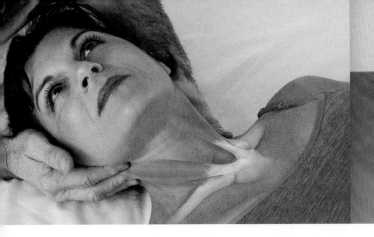

CHAPTER 1

Cyriax, J. *Textbook of Orthopaedic Medicine.* 8th ed. Vol. 1, *Diagnosis of Soft Tissue Lesions.* London: Balliere Tindall, 1982.

Cyriax J. *Textbook of Orthopaedic Medicine.* 10th ed. Vol. 2, *Treatment by Manipulation, Massage and Injection.* London: Balliere Tindall, 1980.

Dalton, Erik. *Myoskeletal Alignment Techniques.* Oklahoma City, OK: Freedom From Pain Institute, 2005. http://www.erikdalton.com.

Mattes, Aaron. *Active Isolated Stretching: The Mattes Method.* Sarasota, FL: Aaron L. Mattes, 1995. http://www.stretchingusa.com.

Myers, Thomas. *Anatomy Trains.* Philadelphia, PA: Churchill Livingstone/Elsevier, 2009.

Travell, Janet, and David Simons. *Travell & Simons' Trigger Point Flip Charts* (Spiral-bound). Baltimore, MD: Lippincott Williams & Wilkins, 1996.

Travell, Janet, David Simons, and Lois Simons. *Myofascial Pain and Dysfunction: The Trigger Point Manual.* 2nd ed. 2 vols. Baltimore, MD: Williams & Wilkins, 1999.

Lowe, Whitney. *Orthopedic Assessment in Massage Therapy.* Sisters, OR: Daviau Scott, 2006.

Waslaski, James. *Advancements in Event and Clinical Sports Massage, Center for Pain Management,* 2011. http://www.orthomassage.net.

Waslaski, James. *Client Self Care Stretch and Strengthen: Rehabilitation Manual,* Center for Pain Management, 2008. http://www.orthomassage.net.

CHAPTER 2

Barnes, John. http://www.myofascialrelease.com.

Benjamin, Ben. http://www.benbenjamin.net.

Biel, Andrew. *Trail Guide to the Body.* 3rd ed. Boulder, Colo.: Books of Discovery, 2005.

Chaitow, Leon. http://www.leonchaitow.com.

Dalton, Erik. *Myoskeletal Alignment Techniques.* Oklahoma City, OK: Freedom From Pain Institute, 2005. http://www.erikdalton.com.

DeLany, Judith. http://www.nmtcenter.com.

Kent, David. http://www.kenthealth.com.

King, Bob. http://www.performancemassagetraining.com.

Kousaleos, George. http://www.coreinstitute.com.

Lowe, Whitney. *Orthopedic Assessment in Massage Therapy.* Sisters, OR: Daviau Scott, 2006.

Mattes, Aaron. *Active Isolated Stretching Therapy.* Sarasota, FL: Aaron Mattes Therapy, 1995. http://www.stretchingusa.com.

Myers, Thomas. *Anatomy Trains.* Philadelphia, PA: Churchill Livingstone, 2009. http://www.anatomytrains.com.

St. John, Paul. http://www.neurosomaticeducators.com.

Travell Janet, David Simons, and Lois Simons. *Myofascial Pain and Dysfunction: The Trigger Point Manual.* 2nd ed. 2 vols. Baltimore, MD: Williams & Wilkins, 1999.

Upledger, John. http://www.upledger.com.

Waslaski, James. *Advancements in Event and Clinical Sports Massage, Center for Pain Management,* 2011. http://www.orthomassage.net.

Waslaski, James. *Client Self Care Stretch and Strengthen: Rehabilitation Manual,* Center for Pain Management, 2008. http://www.orthomassage.net.

Werner, Ruth. *A Massage Therapist's Guide to Pathology.* 2nd ed. Baltimore, MD: Lippincott Williams & Wilkins, 2002.

CHAPTER 3

Cyriax, J. *Textbook of Orthopaedic Medicine.* 8th ed. Vol. 1, *Diagnosis of Soft Tissue Lesions.* London: Balliere Tindall, 1982.

Cyriax J. *Textbook of Orthopaedic Medicine.* 10th ed. Vol. 2, *Treatment by Manipulation, Massage and Injection.* London: Balliere Tindall, 1980.

Dalton, Erik. *Myoskeletal Alignment Techniques.* Oklahoma City, OK: Freedom From Pain Institute, 2005. http://www.erikdalton.com.

Mattes, Aaron. *Active Isolated Stretching: The Mattes Method.* Sarasota, FL: Aaron L. Mattes, 1995. http://www.stretchingusa.com.

Travell, Janet, and David Simons. *Travell & Simons' Trigger Point Flip Charts* (Spiral-bound). Baltimore, MD: Lippincott, Williams & Wilkins, 1996.

Travell, Janet, David Simons, and Lois Simons. *Myofascial Pain and Dysfunction: The Trigger Point Manual.* 2nd ed. 2 vols. Baltimore, MD: Williams & Wilkins, 1999.

Lowe, Whitney. *Orthopedic Assessment in Massage Therapy.*Sisters, OR: Daviau Scott, 2006.

Waslaski, James. *Advancements in Event and Clinical Sports Massage, Center for Pain Management,*2011. http://www .orthomassage.net.

Waslaski, James. *Client Self Care Stretch and Strengthen: Rehabilitation Manual,* Center for Pain Management, 2008. http://www.orthomassage.net.

CHAPTER 4

Benjamin, Ben. http://www.benbenjamin.net.

Biel, Andrew. *Trail Guide to the Body.* 3rd ed. Boulder, Colo.: Books of Discovery, 2005.

Dalton, E. *Myoskeletal Alignment Techniques.* Oklahoma City, OK: Freedom From Pain Institute, 2005. http://www .erikdalton.com.

Lowe, Whitney. *Orthopedic Assessment in Massage Therapy.* Sisters, OR: Daviau Scott, 2006. http://www.omeri.com.

Mattes, Aaron, *Active Isolated Stretching Therapy.* Sarasota, FL: Aaron L. Mattes, 1995. http://www.stretchingusa.com.

Travell Janet, David Simons, and Lois Simons. *Myofascial Pain and Dysfunction: The Trigger Point Manual.* 2nd ed. 2 vols. Baltimore, MD: Williams & Wilkins, 1999.

Waslaski, James. *Advancements in Event and Clinical Sports Massage, Center for Pain Management,* 2011. http:// www.orthomassage.net.

Waslaski, James. *Client Self Care Stretch and Strengthen: Rehabilitation Manual,* Center for Pain Management, 2008. http://www.orthomassage.net.

Werner, Ruth. *A Massage Therapist's Guide to Pathology.* 2nd ed. Baltimore, MD: Lippincott Williams & Wilkins, 2002.

CHAPTER 5

Biel, Andrew. *Trail Guide to the Body.* 2nd ed. Boulder, Colo.: Books of Discovery, 2001.

Dalton, Erik. *Myoskeletal Alignment Techniques.* Oklahoma City, OK: Freedom From Pain Institute, 2005. http://www .erikdalton.com.

Mattes, Aaron. *Active Isolated Stretching.* Sarasota, FL: Aaron L. Mattes , 1995. http://www.stretchingusa.com.

Lowe, Whitney. *Orthopedic Assessment in Massage Therapy.* Sisters, OR: Daviau Scott, 2006.

Waslaski, James. *Advancements in Event and Clinical Sports Massage, Center for Pain Management,* 2011. http:// www.orthomassage.net..

Waslaski, James. *Client Self Care Stretch and Strengthen: Rehabilitation Manual,* Center for Pain Management, 2008. http://www.orthomassage.net.

CHAPTER 6

Biel, Andrew. *Trail Guide to the Body.* 2nd ed. Boulder, Colo.: Books of Discovery, 2001.

Dalton, Erik. *Myoskeletal Alignment Techniques.* Oklahoma City, OK: Freedom From Pain Institute, 2005. http://www .erikdalton.com.

Lowe, Whitney. *Orthopedic Assessment in Massage Therapy.* Sisters, OR: Daviau Scott, 2006.

Waslaski, James. *Advancements in Event and Clinical Sports Massage, Center for Pain Management,* 2011. http:// www.orthomassage.net.

Waslaski, James. *Client Self Care Stretch and Strengthen: Rehabilitation Manual,* Center for Pain Management, 2008 http://www.orthomassage.net.

Werner, Ruth. *A Massage Therapist's Guide to Pathology.* 2nd ed. Baltimore, MD: Lippincott Williams & Wilkins, 2002.

CHAPTER 7

Biel, Andrew. *Trail Guide to the Body.* 3rd ed. Boulder, Colo.: Books of Discovery, 2005.

DeLany, Judith. http://www.nmtcenter.com.

Kent, David. http://www.kenthealth.com.

Lowe, Whitney. *Orthopedic Assessment in Massage Therapy.* Sisters, OR: Daviau Scott, 2006.

Mattes, Aaron. *Active Isolated Stretching Therapy.* Sarasota, FL: Aaron L. Mattes, 1995. http://www.stretchingusa.com.

Waslaski, James. *Advancements in Event and Clinical Sports Massage, Center for Pain Management,* 2011. http:// www.orthomassage.net.

Waslaski, James. *Client Self Care Stretch and Strengthen: Rehabilitation Manual,* Center for Pain Management, 2008. http://www.orthomassage.net.

Werner, Ruth. *A Massage Therapist's Guide to Pathology.* 2nd ed. Baltimore, MD: Lippincott Williams & Wilkins, 2002.

Glossary

Accessory motion The amount of movement at the end range that goes beyond the client's active movement, but remains within normal anatomical limits. When performing passive range of motion the joint is moved all the way through normal and accessory motion. The sensation felt at the end of accessory motion is called the end-feel. Abnormal joint end-feel is an important indicator of joint or soft tissue pathology.

Active assisted stretching The therapist gently assists a stretch performed actively by a client.

Active isolated stretching The process of using agonists and synergists to dynamically move the joint into a range of motion. This form of stretching increases motor-neuron excitability, creating reciprocal inhibition of the muscle being stretched

Active range of motion (AROM) Each specific joint has a normal range of motion expressed in degrees. In active range of motion, the client uses the muscles surrounding the joint to determine the motion possible, within the client's comfort level, prior to doing any tests that may further stress the involved tissues. The therapist will focus on muscle groups limiting each joint movement.

Active trigger point A trigger point that actively refers pain either locally or to another location (most trigger points refer pain elsewhere in the body along predictable nerve pathways).*

Adhesive capsulitis An accident, repetitive movements, or overuse can lead to loss of range of motion, allowing adhesions to build up inside of the shoulder or hip joint capsule. This is also sometimes called a frozen shoulder or frozen hip. However, a true frozen shoulder or frozen hip is a much more aggressive and complicated form of adhesive capsulitis.

Anterior cruciate ligament (ACL) sprain The ACL attaches to the anterior tibia and posterior femur. The ACL's primary function is to prevent hyperextension of the knee and to keep the tibia from sliding forward in relation to the femur. Damage to the ACL is a common sports injury, particularly with activities that involve deceleration, twisting, rapidly changing directions, or jumping. It is common to have concurrent damage to the ACL, MCL, and medial meniscus, which is also called triad injury.

Anterior drawer test A test for anterior cruciate ligament rupture. This test is performed with the client supine with the knee bent at 90 degrees. The therapist places one hand behind the proximal gastrocnemius, the other hand on the thigh above the knee, and attempts to gently pull the tibia forward. There should be very little movement and a ligamentous end feel.

Apley compression test A test to differentiate knee pain caused by meniscal injuries from pain caused by ligament sprains. The test is performed with the client prone and the knee flexed to 90 degrees. With the femur stabilized, the leg is distracted and rotated internally and externally. An axial load is then applied to the leg. Pain produced only when the leg is compressed indicates a meniscal lesion.

Apley distraction test A test to differentiate knee pain caused by meniscal injuries from pain caused by ligament sprains. The test is performed with the client prone and the knee flexed to 90 degrees. With the femur stabilized, the leg is distracted and rotated internally and externally. An axial load is then applied to the leg. Pain produced only when the leg is distracted indicates ligament trauma.

Arthrokinetics Joint movement to create joint space and mobilization.

Atlas–axis mobilization Creating proper functional movement of the atlas–axis bony articulations, using movement and soft tissue techniques to prevent resorting to manipulative therapy.

Bony fixation When articulating bones at the joint are not moving properly, they are stuck or fixated. This is usually because of muscle imbalance, joint tension, or forces that create improper alignment of those particular bones.

Brachial plexus Made up of spinal nerves C5 to T1 that supply the arm. They run from the neck, under the clavicle, and then beneath the pectoralis minor down into the arm.

Bulging disc Formed when the soft, spongy center of the disc, the nucleus pulposus, pushes out and places pressure on the annulus fibrosis that contains the center. Unlike a herniated disc, the bulging disc still contains the nucleus material.

Bunion Swelling of the joint between the big toe and the first metatarsal bone. You will often also see abnormal joint alignment and find a joint fixation.

Bursae Small fluid-filled sacs that provide cushioning to reduce friction between adjacent tissue.

Bursitis Inflammation of the bursa. When these fluid-filled sacs are irritated they generate excess fluid, which creates pain and limits range of motion.

Carpal tunnel syndrome A condition caused by compression of the median nerve in the carpal tunnel and characterized especially by weakness and pain in the hand and fingers.

Chondromalacia Degeneration of cartilage on the underside of the patella, resulting in pain and a grating sensation.

Collagen A protein that is the principal constituent of connective tissue. It is found in tendons, ligaments, bone, cartilage, and skin.

Contralateral Movement to the opposite side.

Coracoid process Small, anterior extension of the scapula, located inferior to the clavicle.

Cross-fiber gliding strokes Gentle gliding strokes performed along the length of a muscle while crossing back and forth over tight fibers to loosen tight muscle bands using the pads of the fingers, fingertips, or thumbs. Work is performed superficial to deep, evaluating for the presence of muscle belly trigger points.

Degenerative arthritis Typically onset during middle age; characterized by degenerative and sometimes hypertrophic changes in the bone and cartilage of one or more joints and a progressive wearing down of opposing joint surfaces usually with pain, swelling, and stiffness (also called osteoarthritis).

Deltoid tuberosity A bump located on the lateral side of the humerus at the halfway point. The deltoid muscle attaches here.

Dorsiflexion The backward flexion of the ankle, away from the sole of the foot. The foot moves toward the tibia.

Eccentric contraction A muscle contraction in which the muscle lengthens.

Eccentric muscle contraction When a muscle tendon lengthens against mild resistance; this is what aligns scar tissue after multidirectional friction is applied to soften the scar.

End-feel When assessing passive range of motion, the joint is moved passively by the therapist all the way through normal and accessory motion. The sensation felt at the end of accessory motion of the joint is called the end-feel.

Eversion Movement of the ankle when the sole of the foot is turned outward.

Facet joints The joint that occurs between facets of the superior and inferior articular processes of adjacent vertebra.

Facet joint fixation The cervical facet joints are not opening and closing properly; stuck open or stuck closed.

Fixated fibular head dysfunction Also referred to as tibiofibular head dysfunction and is fairly common. An injured or tight biceps femoris can pull the head posteriorly causing a proximal fibular head fixation.

Frozen shoulder An advanced or more complicated case of adhesive capsulitis. It involves a more advanced stage of fibrosis in the actual joint capsule. A variety of pathologies that may be involved with a true frozen shoulder include subacromial bursitis, calcific tendonitis, rotator cuff pathology, and other conditions, such as shoulder impingement, limiting shoulder motion.**

Hammer toe A deformity of the toe caused by fixed flexion of the first joint.

Hamstring strain Trauma to the hamstring caused by violent contraction or excessive forcible stretch.

Herniated disc A disc that extrudes into the spinal canal. It is also referred to as a bulging disc, ruptured disc, or slipped disc.

Hyperemia Increased blood flow.

Hypothesis A tentative theory, assumption, or concept based on extensive experience and results that are not yet verified through traditional research such as double-blind studies.

Iliotibial band friction syndrome An inflammatory overuse syndrome caused by mechanical friction between the iliotibial band (ITB) and the lateral femoral condyle. Pain is manifested over the lateral aspect of the knee along the iliotibial band with no effusion of the knee.

Inversion Movement of the ankle when the sole of the foot is turned inward.

Ipsilateral Movement to the same side.

Ischemia Local anemia due to a mechanical obstruction of blood supply.

Kyphosis A deformity of the spine, characterized by extensive flexion. Convex thoracic spine.

Latent trigger point A trigger point that exists, but does not yet refer pain actively along predictable nerve pathways, but may do so when pressure or strain is applied to the myoskeletal structure containing the trigger point. Latent trigger points can influence muscle activation patterns, which can result in poorer muscle coordination and balance.***

Lateral collateral ligament (LCL) Ligament on the outer side of the knee that connects the femur to the fibula.

Lateral epicondylosis An injury at the muscle–tendon junction on the lateral side of the elbow. It is usually the result of overuse or trauma.

Lateral shearing force Usually when C1–C2 slide to the right or the left of each other.

LCL sprain test The client is seated on the table with one leg straight. Stabilize the medial joint line with one hand and gently press against the medial side of the knee with that hand while gently pulling down on the upper gastrocnemius with the other hand. If the client reports pain at the lateral joint line it can be a positive test for an LCL sprain.

Ligament sprain   Trauma to ligaments that causes pain and disability depending on the degree of injury to the ligaments.

Lower crossed syndrome   Postural imbalance, also termed lumbo-pelvic hip disorder, usually presents as a unilateral dysfunction in low back and hip pain. The following muscles are tight/short on one side only: iliopsoas, rectus femoris, adductors, piriformis, and lumbar erectors. The weak, inhibited muscles permitting the asymmetry are gluteus maximus/medius, biceps femoris, tranversus abdominus, internal obliques, multifidi, and some pelvic floor muscles.

MCL sprain test   The client is seated or supine with the leg straight. Press against the lateral side of the knee with one hand while gently pulling back toward you on the medial side of the proximal gastrocnemius with your other hand. If the client reports pain at the medial side of the knee it may be a positive test for an MCL sprain.

Medial collateral ligament (MCL)   Ligament on the inner side of the knee that connects the femur to the tibia.

Medial epicondylosis   An injury at the muscle–tendon junction on the medial side of the elbow. It is usually the result of overuse or trauma.

Meniscus   A "c" shaped fibrous cartilage located in the knee joint between the femur and the tibia. It provides shock absorption and reduces the friction between the contacting bones.

Migraine headaches   Begin with extreme vasoconstriction followed by vasodilation. The excess pressure creates excruciating pain. Women get migraines more than men.

Multiple crush phenomenon   There is more than one region of compression on a nerve trunk. In the case of carpal tunnel syndrome, for example, if the nerves are already compressed in the neck, shoulder, or elbow areas, the distal nerves in the wrist area are more susceptible to irritation from even a minor degree of compression.[†]

Muscle strain   Trauma to the muscle or the musculotendinous unit from violent contraction or excessive forcible stretch.

Muscle–tendon junction   Location where muscles transition and attach to tendons.

Myofascial release   Work performed on the fascia intended to stretch and influence the fascia, to eliminate fascial restrictions.

Myofascial trigger point   Janet Travell describes myofascial trigger point as a hyperirritable spot in skeletal muscle that is associated with a hypersensitive palpable nodule in a taut band. This spot is painful on compression and can give rise to characteristic referred pain, referred tenderness, and autonomic phenomena.[‡]

Neuroma   A benign tumor growing on a peripheral nerve.

Passive range of motion (PROM)   The therapist moves the the client's joint through the available comfortable range of motion, with no effort from the client. Passive range of motion focuses primarily in inert tissues because contractile tissues are not employed during passive movement. The therapist pays attention to pain patterns, accessory movement, and the sensation felt at the end of accessory movement known as joint end-feel.

Patellar tendinosis   Damage to a tendon of the patella at a cellular level.

Patellar tendinitis   Inflammation of a tendon of the patella.

Patello femoral compression test   While the client is seated, press on the patella as he or she flexes and extends the knee. If the client experiences grating sounds and discomfort under the knee he or she may have chondromalacia.

Pathology   The study and diagnosis of disease. General pathology is a broad and complex scientific field, which seeks to understand the mechanisms of injury to cells and tissues, as well as the body's means of responding to and repairing injury.

Periosteal junction   Location where tendons transition and attach to the bone.

Plantar fascia   Thick connective tissue on the plantar surface of the foot.

Plantar flexion   The bending of the ankle downward, toward the sole of the foot.

Posterior cruciate ligament (PCL) sprain   The PCL attaches to the posterior tibia and anterior femur. Its primary function is to prevent hyperflexion of the knee and to keep the tibia from sliding backward in relation to the femur when the knee is flexed. It is stronger and less subject to sports injury than the ACL. The majority of injuries result from the tibia being thrust in a posterior direction, such as when the tibia hits the dash of a car on impact.

Posterior drawer test   A test for posterior cruciate ligament (PCL) rupture. The client is supine with the knee bent 90 degrees. The therapist places both hands just below the knee and gently presses the proximal end of the tibia posteriorly. There should be a ligamentous end feel and very little movement.

Post isometric relaxation   Contracting a muscle produces an inhibition of nerve impulses, resulting in muscle relaxation.

Proprioceptive neuromuscular facilitation (PNF)   A stretching technique where a muscle is passively stretched (contract agonist), then contracts isometrically against resistance (contract antagonist), then passively stretched again to facilitate increased range of motion.

Proprioceptors   Found in the nerve endings of muscles, tendons, and joints. They detect the body's position and movement.

Reciprocal inhibition   When a muscle contracts on one side of a joint (agonist) the muscle on the other side of the joint relaxes (antagonist), resulting in a stretch without tension or possible injury.

Reciprocal inhibition is decreased neural drive and muscle spindle cell excitation. When one group of muscles contracts, a message is sent to the antagonists to relax to allow for a better stretch.

Resisted range of motion (RROM) Also known as manual resistive tests or resisted isometric movements, because they require an isometric muscle contraction. The purpose of manual resistance testing is to evaluate proper function of the contractile tissues (muscle and tendon). This test can determine if there is disruption of soft tissue, and is the best method to determine if the client has a muscle–tendon strain, which is also referred to as tendinosis in this text.

Retinaculum A strong, fibrous band, or thickened fascia, that holds the tendons of muscle groups in place as they cross a joint. An example is the flexor retinaculum, (also know as *transverse carpal ligament*) that holds the flexor tendons of the digits in place as they cross over the carpal bones.[†††]

Rotator cuff A group of four muscles in the shoulder: subscapularis, infraspinatus, teres minor, and supraspinatus. The function of these muscles is to stabilize the glenohumeral joint. They also function to control and assist in shoulder movement.

Scar tissue New tissue that is created to replace damaged and dead cells at the site of an injury.

Sheathed tendon A tendon with a protective covering that is lubricated to help it glide smoothly during movement.

SLAP tear A shoulder injury to the glenoid labrum (fibrocartilaginous rim attached around the margin of the glenoid cavity). SLAP is an acronym for superior labral tear from anterior to posterior.

Sprain An injury to a ligament.

Strain An injury to a muscle or tendon.

Strain-counterstrain was developed by Lawrence Jones D.O. and is also known as positional release. This is where the therapist identifies a point of maximum pain, called a tender point. Monitoring the tender point the therapist positions the patient to maximally relieve the discomfort. The therapist holds the client in the maximally released position and then slowly returns the passive client to a neutral body position. Success of treatment is evaluated by reassessing both the tender point and any accompanying loss of range of motion.

Structural integration A protocol to align and balance the muscles and joints of the body, promoting good posture and allowing greater ease of movement with less or no discomfort.

Subacromial bursa Located underneath the acromion. This fluid-filled sac has two major sections and most of it is inaccessible.

Tendinitis Inflammation of muscles and of muscle–tendon attachments.

Tendinosis Tearing of muscle or muscle–tendon fibers in the absence of an inflammatory process.

Tendon tension Tight tendons in opposing muscle groups that are out of balance.

Tenosynovitis The inflammation of a tendon sheath.

Thoracic outlet syndrome Tight anterior neck and shoulder muscles produce symptoms of pressure on blood vessels and the brachial plexus of nerves. It is characterized by numbness, tingling, weakness, and pain down the arm. The anterior and posterior scalenes and pectoralis minor are the main culprits of this condition.

Trigger point Pain related to a discrete, irritable point in skeletal muscle or fascia, not caused by acute local trauma, inflammation, degeneration, neoplasm, or infection. The painful point can be felt as a nodule or band in the muscle, and a twitch response can be elicited on stimulation of the trigger point. Palpation of the trigger point reproduces the patient's complaint of pain, and the pain radiates in a distribution typical of the specific muscle harboring the trigger point. This term was coined in 1942 by Dr. Janet Travell. This text focuses primarily on active and latent muscle belly myofascial trigger points.[§]

Upper crossed syndrome Postural muscle imbalance of the upper body characterized by tight pectoralis major/minor, upper trapezius, levator scapula, sternocleidomastoid, anterior scalenes, and suboccipitals and weak, inhibited rhomboids, infraspinatus, teres minor, lower/middle trapezius, latissimus dorsi, and neck flexors.

Vascular headaches Caused by excessively dilated blood vessels in the meninges. They are characterized by a pain that throbs with the client's pulse.

NOTES

* http://en.wikipedia.org/wiki/Trigger_point.

** Lowe, Whitney. *Orthopedic Assessment in Massage Therapy.* Sisters, OR: Daviau Scott, 2006.

*** http://en.wikipedia.org/wiki/Trigger_point.

[†] Lowe, Whitney. *Orthopedic Assessment in Massage Therapy.* Sisters, OR: Daviau Scott, 2006.

[‡] Travell, Janet, David Simons, and Lois Simons. *Myofascial Pain and Dysfunction: The Trigger Point Manual.* 2nd ed. 2 vols. Baltimore, MD: Williams & Wilkins, 1999.

[†††] http://en.wikipedia.org/wiki/Retinaculum.

[§] http://en.wikipedia.org/wiki/Trigger_point.

INDEX

A

Abductor digiti minimi, 252
Abductor pollicis brevis, 252
Achilles tendinosis, 120
Achilles tendon, 5, 118
ACL. *See* Anterior cruciate ligament (ACL)
ACS. *See* Anterior compartment syndrome (ACS)
Active assisted stretching, 26–27
Active muscle belly trigger points, 21
Active range of motion (AROM), 7, 14
Adductor brevis, 42, 56, 58
Adductor longus, 4, 42, 56, 58
Adductor magnus, 4, 42, 56, 58
Adductor pollicis, 252
Adhesive capsulitis, 44, 148, 192–193
Advanced clinical massage therapy,
    definition of, 4
Ankle decompression, 122, 136
Ankle distraction and traction, 124
Ankle dorsiflexion, 119
Ankle eversion, 119, 120
Ankle inversion, 119
Ankle inversion sprain, 137–140
Antagonistic muscle groups, 31
Anterior compartment syndrome (ACS), 131–136, 144
Anterior cruciate ligament (ACL) instability, 86–91
Anterior cruciate ligament (ACL) sprain, 86
Anterior drawer test, 86
Anterior talofibular ligament, 137
Anterolateral shin splints, 136–137
Apley compression test, 90, 104
Apley distraction test, 90, 104
Area preparation, 18–19
AROM. *See* Active range of motion (AROM)
Arthritis, degenerative, 256–257
Arthrokinetics
    ankle, 121–122
    definition of, 122
    toe, 130–131
Ascending syndromes, 128

Atlanto-axial anterior-posterior mobilization
    protocol, 212–214
Atlanto-axial lateral mobilization protocol, 211–212
Atlanto-occipital anterior-posterior mobilization
    protocol, 212–214
Atlanto-occipital lateral mobilization protocol, 211–212

B

Biceps brachii, 4, 5, 239
Biceps femoris, 4, 5, 41, 118
Biceps protocol, 166–170
Bicipital tendinosis, 194
Body map, to identify pain areas, 10
Body mechanics, therapist, 15–18
Bone-on-bone end feel, 14
Bone-on-bone-like end feel, 14
Bony fixations, 118, 208
Brachial plexus, 190
Brachialis, 4, 5, 239
Brachioradialis, 239
Bulging disc, 40
Bunion, 128, 131
Bursitis, 192
    subacromial, 194–195

C

Calcaneofibular ligament, 137
Calcaneus, 118
Capsulitis, adhesive, 44, 148, 192–193
Carpal tunnel syndrome, 4, 236, 251–255
Case study
    anterior compartment syndrome, 144
    meniscus tears, 112
    multiple crush phenomenon, 260
    shoulder pain, 199
    thoracic outlet syndrome, 200
    whiplash, 232

Cervical compression/decompression test, 206–207
Cervical mobilization, 210
Cervical spine protocol, 210–217
Chondromalacia, 91
Client draping, 35, 36
Client history
    definition of, 7
    in pain management, 8–13
    in pelvic stabilization, 41
Client self-care
    strengthening in, 28
    stretching in, 27–28
Clinical massage therapy, advanced, definition of, 4
Collagen, 23
    disorganized, 25
    organized, 25
Collagen fibers, 25
Contraction
    concentric, 30–31
    eccentric, 28, 54
Coracobrachialis, 239
Coracobrachialis protocol, 166–170
Coracobrachialis resistance test, 153
Coracobrachialis tendinosis, 194
Coracoid plexus, 153
Corticosteroid injection, for tendinosis, 30
Cross-fiber gliding strokes, 20–21, 22

D

Deep Six, 61, 62
Degenerated disc, 40
Degenerative arthritis, 256–257
Deltoid, 4, 5, 170–175
Deltoid muscle resistance test, 155
Depth, body alignment and, 16
Disc
    bulging, 40
    degenerated, 40
    herniated, 40
    thinning, 40
Dorsiflexion, 119
Draping, 35, 36
Dura mater mobilization, 210, 211
Dural sheath mobilization, 210, 211

E

Eccentric contraction, 25, 54
Eccentric scar tissue alignment, 25–26
Elastic resistance training (ERT), 28
Elbow extension, 237

Elbow flexion, 237, 240
"End feel," 14
Epicondylosis
    lateral, 239
    medial, 239–246
Erector spinae, 50–56, 51, 78–79
ERT. *See* Elastic resistance training (ERT)
Eversion, 119
Extensor carpi radialis, 247
Extensor carpi ulnaris, 247
Extensor digitorum longus, 118
Extensor hallucis longus, 118
Extensor retinaculum, 118
External oblique, 4, 5

F

Facet joint fixation, 208
Facet joints, 53
Fallen arches, 128
Fascia
    effect of ice on, 19
    in tendinosis, 29
Fibular head, 118
Fixated fibular head dysfunction, 88
Flat feet, 128
Flexor carpi radialis, 23, 239, 252
Flexor carpi ulnaris, 239, 252
Flexor digiti minimi, 252
Flexor digitorum longus, 118
Flexor digitorum profundus, 239, 252
Flexor digitorum superficialis, 23, 239
Flexor hallucis longus, 118
Flexor pollicis brevis, 252
Flexor pollicis longus, 23, 252
Flexor pollicis longus tendon, 252
Flexor retinaculum, 252
Forearm
    pronation, 240
    trigger points in, 23
Fracture, leg stress, 140–143
Frontalis, 4, 5
Frozen shoulder, 44, 148, 192–193

G

Gastrocnemius, 4, 5, 111, 118
Gastrocnemius protocol, for Achilles tendon
    pain, 120–123
Gastrocnemius stretch, 122, 141
Gemellus inferior, 42, 56, 57
Gemellus superior, 42, 56, 57

Gluteus maximus, 4, 5, 41, 42, 56, 57
Gluteus maximus lateral fibers, 111
Gluteus medius, 4, 42, 56, 57
Gluteus minimus, 42, 56, 57
Golfer's elbow, 239–246
Gracilis, 4, 42, 58

H

Hammer toe, 128
Hamstrings, 72–81, 110–111
Headaches
    migraine, 159
    vascular, 159
Heat, moist, 18
Herniated disc, 40
Hip adduction, 42
Hip anatomy, 43, 44
Hip extension, 41
Hip flexion, 41
Hip joint capsule, 43–50
Hip joint capsule mobilization, 45
Hip joint capsule work, 44–46
    prone, 59
Hip rotation
    external, 42
    internal, 42
Hip rotators, 56–66
    lateral, 59–63
History, 7, 8–13
Hyperemia, 159
Hypothesis, 31

I

Ice, on muscle belly, 19
Iliacus
    in hip anatomy, 43, 44
    in pelvic stabilization, 43–50
    in range of motion assessment, 41
    release, 47
    stretching, 48–49, 78
Iliocostalis thoracis, 51. *See also* Erector spinae
Iliopsoas, 4
Iliotibial band, 66–71, 118
Iliotibial band friction syndrome, 104–107
Iliotibial band friction test, 104
Iliotibial band stretch, 79–80
Iliotibial tract, 57
Imaging, of tendinosis, 30
Infraspinatus, 4, 5, 186–189
Infraspinatus muscle resistance test, 155

Infraspinatus tendinosis, 194
Inguinal ligament, 43
Interspinales, 222–224
Intertransversarii, 222–224
Inversion, 119
Inversion ankle sprain, 137–140
Ischemia, 27

J

Joint play
    ankle, 121–122
    definition of, 122
    toe, 130–131

K

Knee flexion test, 92
Knee traction, 96
Kyphosis, 176

L

Lachman test, 86
Lamina groove, 52, 55
Lateral collateral ligament (LCL), 88
Lateral collateral ligament (LCL) sprain, 107–112
Lateral collateral ligament (LCL) sprain test, 88
Lateral epicondylosis, 246–251
Lateral hip rotators, 79
Lateral malleolus, 118
Lateral meniscus, 101, 112
Lateral meniscus injury, 107–112
Lateral shearing force, 211–212
Latissimus dorsi, 4, 5
LCL. *See* Lateral collateral ligament (LCL)
Levator scapula, 227–232
Ligament sprain, 94
Ligamentous end feel, 14
Longissimus thoracis, 51. *See also* Erector spinae
Lumbricals, 252

M

Massage therapy, advanced clinical, definition of, 4
Masseter, 4, 5
MCL. *See* Medial collateral ligament (MCL)
Medial adductors, 63–66
Medial collateral ligament (MCL), 88, 101
Medial collateral ligament (MCL) sprain, 101–104

Medial collateral ligament (MCL) sprain test, 102
Medial epicondylosis, 239–246
Medial malleolus, 118
Medial meniscus, 112
Medial meniscus injury, 101–104
Medial rotators, 63–66
Median nerve, 239
Meniscus, 90, 101
Migraine headaches, 159
Morton's neuroma, 128
Multiple crush phenomenon, 236, 260
Muscle groups, antagonistic, 31
Muscle resistance test
    ankle strain, 138, 139
    anterior compartment, 134
    biceps, 153
    deltoid, 155
    infraspinatus, 155
    pectoralis major, 154
    pectoralis minor, 153
    pronator teres, 240
    rhomboid major and minor, 155
    soleus, 123
    subscapularis, 153
    supraspinatus, 154
    teres minor, 155
Muscle strain, 91
Muscle-tendon junction, 15
Myofascial release, 19–20
Myofascial spreading, 22

N

Neck extension, 208, 209
Neck flexion, 208
Neck lateral flexion, 208, 209
Neck rotation, 208, 209
Neuroma, 128

O

Obturator externus, 42, 56
Obturator internus, 42, 56, 57
Ointments, heating, 18
One-legged knee flexion test, 92
Opponens pollicis, 252
Osteophytes, 40–41

P

Pain management, 5–29, 31–33
Palmaris longus, 23, 239

Passive range of motion (PROM), 14
Patellar ligament, 118
Patellar tendinosis, 91, 110
Patellar tendinosis test, 92
Patellar tendinitis, 91
Patello femoral compression test, 91
Pathology, 15
PCL. *See* Posterior cruciate ligament (PCL)
Pectineus, 4, 42, 58
Pectoralis major, 4, 5, 159–161
Pectoralis major resistance test, 154
Pectoralis minor, 161–165
Pectoralis minor resistance test, 153
Pelvic stabilization
    active range of motion in, 41–42
    erector spinae in, 50–56
    hamstrings in, 72–81
    hip rotators in, 56–66
    iliacus release in, 47
    iliotibial band in, 66–71
    knee and, 86
    lateral hip rotators in, 59–63
    medial adductors in, 63–66
    medial rotators in, 63–66
    multidirectional friction in, 53–54
    myofascial release in, 52, 55, 59–60
    passive range of motion in, 43, 56
    psoas release in, 48
    quadratus lumborum in, 50–56
    quadriceps in, 66–69, 71–72
    resisted range of motion in, 43, 55, 59, 62–63
    stretching in, 48–49, 53
    trigger point therapy in, 52
Periosteal junction, 15
Peroneus brevis, 118, 140
Peroneus longus, 4, 5, 118, 140
Peroneus tertius, 118
Pes planus, 128
Piriformis, 42, 56, 57
Plantar fascia, 129
Plantar fasciitis, 129–133
Plantar flexion, 119
Plantaris, 111, 118
Plantaris strain, 96–98
PNF. *See* Proprioceptive neuromuscular facilitation (PNF)
Popliteus strain, 98–101
Posterior cruciate ligament (PCL) instability, 86–91
Posterior cruciate ligament (PCL) sprain, 86
Posterior deltoid, 177–181
Posterior drawer test, 86–88
Posterior talofibular ligament, 137
Posteromedial shin splints, 126–128
Post isometric relaxation, 27
Posture, ideal, 4, 5

Preparation, area, 18–19
Pressure, body alignment and, 16
PROM. *See* Passive range of motion (PROM)
Pronation, 128
Pronator teres, 23, 239
Proprioceptive neuromuscular facilitation (PNF), 26
Proprioceptors, 27
Psoas
    in hip anatomy, 43
    in pelvic stabilization, 43–50
    in range of motion assessment, 41
    release, 48
    stretching, 48–49, 78

Q

Quadratus femoris, 42, 56, 57
Quadratus lumborum, 50–56, 78–79
Quadriceps
    in knee protocol, 91–96
    in pelvic stabilization, 66–69, 71–72
    stretching, 79, 95

R

Radial abduction, 238
Radial deviation, 238
Radial nerve, 247
Range of motion
    active, 7, 14, 42
    passive, 14
    resisted, 15
Reciprocal inhibition, 27
Rectus abdominis, 4, 5
Rectus femoris, 4, 41
Release, myofascial, 19–20
Resistance training, elastic, 28
Resisted range of motion (RROM), 15
Retinaculum, 134
Rhomboid major, 4
Rhomboid major muscle resistance test, 155
Rhomboid minor muscle resistance test, 155
Rhomboids, 176–177
Rotator cuff, 192, 193
Rotatores, 222–224
RROM. *See* Resisted range of motion (RROM)

S

SAG test, 86
Sartorius, 4, 5, 41, 42
Scalenes, 217–222

Scapula reposition, 181–182
Scapula stabilization, 17
Scar
    eccentric alignment of, 25–26
    multidirectional, 24
    tissue, 21
Sciatic nerve, 56, 57
Semimembranosus, 4, 41
Semitendinosus, 4, 41
Serratus anterior, 4, 5
Sheathed tendon, 135
Shin splints
    anterolateral, 136–137
    definition of, 126
    posteromedial, 126–128
Shoulder, frozen, 192–193
Shoulder abduction, 150
Shoulder adduction, 150
Shoulder extension, 150
Shoulder flexion, 150
Shoulder horizontal abduction, 151
Shoulder horizontal adduction, 151
Shoulder joint capsule work, 156–157
Shoulder lateral/external rotation, 151
Shoulder medial/internal rotation, 151
Shoulder protocol, 156–159
Soft/leathery end feel, 14
Soleus, 4, 5, 118
Soleus protocol, 123–126
Soleus stretch, 124, 141
Spinalis thoracis, 51. *See also* Erector spinae
Sprain, 23
    ankle inversion, 137–140
    anterior cruciate ligament, 86
    ligament, 94
    medial collateral ligament, 101–104
    thumb, 255–256
Springy block end feel, 14
Sternocleidomastoid, 4, 5, 217–222
Strain, 23, 24
    muscle, 91
    plantaris, 96–98
    popliteus, 98–101
    thumb, 255–256
Strengthening
    for pain management, 28
    for tendinosis, 30
Stress fracture, leg, 140–143
Stretching
    active assisted, 26–27
    client self-care, 27–28
    during therapy, 26–27
Structural integration, 4
Subacromial bursa, 194

Subacromial bursitis, 194–195
Subclavius, 165–166
Suboccipital muscles, 224–227
Subscapularis, 174–176
Subscapularis resistance test, 153
Subscapularis tendinosis, 194
Supinator, 23, 247
Supraspinatus, 182–186
Supraspinatus muscle resistance test, 154
Supraspinatus tendinosis, 193–194

T

Temporalis, 4, 5
Tendinitis
    definition of, 7
    patellar, 91
    tendinosis *vs.*, 29
Tendinosis
    Achilles, 120
    anti-inflammatory strategies in, 30
    bicipital, 194
    biomechanical deloading in, 30
    causes of, 29
    coracobrachialis, 194
    definition of, 7
    imaging of, 30
    infraspinatus, 194
    load reduction in, 30
    patellar, 91, 110
    research, 29–30
    scar tissue mobilization for, 30–31
    strengthening for, 30
    subscapularis, 194
    supraspinatus, 193–194
    surgery for, 30
    techniques, 29
    tendinitis *vs.*, 29
    teres minor, 194
Tendon, sheathed, 135
Tendon tension, 29, 32
Tenosynovitis, 7, 243–244
Tensor fasciae latae, 4, 5, 41, 42, 56, 57,
        111–112
Teres major, 4, 5
Teres minor muscle resistance test, 155
Teres minor tendinosis, 194
Test
    anterior drawer, 86
    Apley compression, 90, 104
    Apley distraction, 90, 104
    cervical compression/decompression, 206–207
    iliotibial band friction, 104

    knee flexion, 92
    Lachman, 86
    lateral collateral ligament (LCL) sprain, 88
    medial collateral ligament (MCL) sprain, 102
    muscle resistance
        ankle strain, 138, 139
        anterior compartment, 134
        biceps, 153
        coracobrachialis, 153
        deltoid, 155
        infraspinatus, 155
        pectoralis major, 154
        pectoralis minor, 153
        pronator teres, 240
        rhomboid major and minor, 155
        soleus, 123
        subscapularis, 153
        teres minor, 155
    one-legged knee flexion, 92
    patellar tendinosis, 92
    patello femoral compression, 91
    posterior drawer, 86
    SAG, 86
    transverse alar ligament, 204
    valgus stress, 88
    varus stress, 88
    vertebral artery compression, 206
Thera-Band, 28
Therapist body mechanics, 15–18
Thinning disc, 40
Thoracic outlet syndrome, 4, 190–192, 200
Thumb strain/sprain, 255–256
Tibialis anterior, 4, 5, 118
Tibialis posterior, 118
Tibialis posterior protocol, 126–128
Tibialis posterior stretch, 142
Tight muscle fiber pain, 21
Tissue, scar, 21
    eccentric alignment of, 25–26, 54
    mobilization, 30–31
Tissue compression end feel, 14
Tissue stretch end feel, 14
Toe joint play, 130–131
Traction
    knee, 96
    from leaning back, 18
    from upper body, 16
Transverse alar ligament test, 204
Trapezius, 4, 5
Triceps, 4, 5
Triceps brachii, 177–181, 247
Trigger finger, 257–259
Trigger points, forearm, 23
Twelve-steps, 5–6

cervical spine conditions, 204–210
forearm, wrist, hand, 236–239
knee and thigh conditions, 86–91
lower leg, ankle, foot conditions, 118–120
pain management, 5–29
pelvic stabilization, 40–81
shoulder conditions, 148–152

U

Ulnar adduction, 238
Ulnar deviation, 238
Upper body, traction from, 16
Upper crossed syndrome, 195
Upper trapezius, 170–175, 182–186

V

Valgus stress test, 88
Varus stress test, 88
Vascular headaches, 159

Vastus lateralis, 4, 5, 112
Vastus medialis, 4, 112
Velvet glove technique, 158–159, 214–217
Vertebral artery compression test, 206
Visualization, 18, 46

W

Whiplash, 209–210, 232
Wrist extension, 237
Wrist flexion, 237, 240
Wrist pronation, 238
Wrist supination, 238